LYING IN WEIGHT

LYING IN WEIGHT

The Hidden Epidemic
of Eating Disorders
in Adult Women

TRISHA GURA

HarperCollins*Publishers*

The names of some of the individuals discussed in this book have been changed to protect their privacy.

HarperCollins books may be purchased for educational, business, or sales promotional use. For information, please write: Special Markets Department, HarperCollins Publishers, 10 East 53rd Street, New York, NY 10022.

Grateful acknowledgment is made for permission to reprint the following: "Why You Travel" from *Zeppo's First Wife: New and Selected Poems* by Gail Mazur, courtesy of Gail Mazur; "Second Chance" from *Near Occasions of Sin* by Louis McKee, courtesy of Cynic Press © 2006; "Weathering" from *Poems: 1960–2000* by Fleur Adcock, courtesy of Bloodaxe Books © 2000.

FIRST EDITION

Designed by Lucy Albanese

Library of Congress Cataloging-in-Publication Data
Gura, Trisha
     Lying in weight : the hidden epidemic of eating
     disorders in adult women / by Trisha Gura.
         p.   cm.
     Includes bibliographical references and index.
     ISBN: 978-0-06-076148-6
     ISBN 10: 0-06-076148-2
     1. Eating disorders in women.   I. Title.

RC552.E18G87   2007
16.85'260082—dc26
                                                              2006052181

07   08   09   10   11   ID/RRD   10   9   8   7   6   5   4   3   2   1

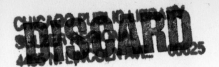
For Elizabeth

May she grow up wiser

CONTENTS

ACKNOWLEDGMENTS

My editor, Gail Winston, has supported this book beyond her call of duty. Her insights, persistence, and attention have both inspired the writing and structured it. My agent, Lisa Bankoff, at International Creative Management, is another master of her craft. She first understood the potential of the book, and then painstakingly fine-tuned the proposal, finding its "right fit."

I thank Hannah Cohen-Cline, who, while a student at Brandeis University, researched, copyedited, fact-checked, and offered insights well beyond any women of her age and experience. For editing and proofreading, I thank Joe and Mary Chadbourne, striking in their eye for detail and helpful in their suggestions. Thanks also to Jennifer Angelo, who read and commented on one of the first attempts at a chapter.

There were many people who graciously and generously offered me their time and expertise with eating disorders: special thanks to Lynn Grefe, Joanna Poppink, Katherine Zerbe, Seda Ebrahimi, Mary Boggiano, Jeannie Rust, Shan Guisinger, Lucene Wisniewski, Suja Srikameswaran, James Hudson, David Herzog, Chris Fairburn, Edward Cumella, Jim Schettler, Tacie Vergara, and the staffs at Remuda Ranch, the Renfrew Center, and Mirasol.

I wish to express my deep gratitude to my colleagues at Brandeis University. I have never experienced a group quite like them. In fact, I could not imagine having written this book without the support of our Gender, Science, and Sexuality group. Thank you, Brigette Sheridan, Mara Amster, Christine Cooper, Nick Danforth, Nurit Eini-Pindyck, Claudia Stevens, Lisa Fishbayn, Ruth Nemzoff, and Linda Andrist. And thank you, Anne Gottlieb, for your artistic direction, which ultimately inspired the last chapter.

I thank my dear friend Sharon Schnall, who supported me in so many ways: reading one of the first drafts—and also one of the last—and, in the middle, offering ideas, hand-holding, journalism war stories, and anecdotal humor. My thanks to Lauren Slater for the coffee meeting that started this whole process. And to my special friend Amy Caldwell, senior editor at Beacon Press, who walked me through the process of writing a book step-by-step, making me laugh and cry, sometimes at the same time. Tom Lavin offered me his steadfast personal and professional support; it is a gift that I deeply cherish.

My dearest appreciation goes to Steve Traina for his intimate participation in this journey—through the best moments, and the worst. And to my daughter, Elizabeth, who watched, listened, questioned, learned, and loved her mother as she embarked on one of the most exciting ventures in her life.

And finally, I cannot express enough appreciation for the women and men who offered me their stories so as to help others. I hold each in a special place in my heart, for each touched me personally. I name you all throughout the book. Though some of you are named under pseudonyms, you know who you are. And now we, the recipients of your stories, know a little more as well. Thank you for the gift of yourselves.

Confidences and Lies

One winter morning, I met my friend Lauren in a café near the campus of Massachusetts Institute of Technology in Boston. We had gotten to know each other during a yearlong science journalism fellowship at MIT and Harvard. This particular morning, we were luxuriating in the absence of deadlines and brainstorming new writing projects.

A blizzard whistled down Main Street and rattled the doors to our pasts. As we clutched our mugs, sank into upholstery, and sniffed the aroma of java, we began to confide secrets, the kind that only a storm outside and warmth within could lay bare.

Lauren told me that she had grappled with an eating disorder as a teenager. She had recovered, but it had sprung up again after her first pregnancy. She would tell her husband that she was going to the grocery store late at night. There, she would buy bags of junk food, gorge in her car, and then make herself throw up in the parking lot.

This went on for two years; she was so embarrassed that she had not gotten over bulimia by the age of 36 that she had lied to her husband and, in fact, had written a book about lying.

My mouth dropped open.

"I had an eating disorder, too," I said. "Anorexia."

I used the word "had" instead of "have" because, with years of therapy, I had recovered and gone on with life. After my pregnancy, I had done nothing like vomiting up cream-filled donuts and Bavarian coffee cake. For me at that moment, my eating disorder existed in the past tense.

And yet I wondered if it really was past, as Lauren asked me questions: How had my life evolved as I approached 40? Did I still feel the need to control my eating? Did I like my body now? And what about my 10-year-old daughter? Did I feel like a flawed mother?

At first, I answered in the detached way that I might talk about my grandmother's cataract operation. To me, battles with food belonged in the realm of adolescence, a sort of yellowed photo album that I, at 21, had set on the shelf. Since then, I had tackled marriage, infertility, pregnancy, divorce, and child rearing as a single parent. More recently, I had been watching a few gray hairs sprout, pinching the flesh around my waist, and thinking about how I would handle middle age.

Yet, as I spoke about this thing that I had overcome, I knew that I was lying to myself. I did not feel liberated—not at all. It's more like this: I have a voice in my head that whispers like a ghost. It seduces. It tells me that no one will love me if I am fat. It says that what I do is never enough. It promises that if I follow its rules, skipping meals, swimming extra laps, not eating this or that, avoiding meat and chicken and fish and dairy products, I will be safe. But most of the time I do not feel safe—just closed up and isolated.

I have tried to ignore the voice. When I scream, "Leave me alone! Let me enjoy life without these crazy rules!" it snickers and goes into hiding. Then there is silence, and for a time, even for years, I am free.

Or so I think.

But I have learned over these past twenty years, since I was diagnosed with atypical anorexia nervosa (a kind of anorexia that does not quite fit all the medical criteria), that the voice belongs to a lion with a ravenous appetite and a belly that is always rumbling. It wants to feast on my soul. And for that, the beast lies in wait as I live my life, lying about my weight and what I do to control it.

At the moments when I am most vulnerable, the beast pounces. I start slowly, skipping meals, restricting what I eat, and exercising more. I lose some weight, but never enough to crack open the fear that I felt the first time I dropped below 90 pounds at the age of 19 and could not control the urge to lose more. I can stop now. When, and at what weight, depends on all sorts of factors: therapy, supportive friends, how my work is going, my daughter, experience, and age.

If I look back and track the times when I have had a small relapse, I can see patterns. Vulnerable periods arose from stress, and emotional upheaval added more pressure. Major life transitions are the greatest danger of all: changing jobs, getting married, getting pregnant, getting divorced, and especially the postpartum period, when I experienced the terror of being a new mother. Even today as I write, I can hear the predator breathing down my neck; I know that writing this book is forcing changes, big changes, in my life.

The truth is that my eating disorder first gripped me in my teens and has not let go. Or I have not let it go. So I must admit that for my entire adult life, I have been suffering from a proclivity to relapse, a preoccupation with food and body, a residual of my atypical anorexia nervosa. In researching this book, which I did soon after that conversation with Lauren, I learned that there is a name for what is happening to me today and that there are many more women who are experiencing the same cluster of thoughts and behaviors, long after their days of obsessing over proms, pimples, and popularity issues are past.

In medical terms, we're "subclinical," or "subthreshold," which means we fall below the eating-compulsion radar. We manage—or hide—our disorders successfully. We never get to treatment centers. Some of us have never even entered a psychologist's office. The trigger for exposure is often a transitional event—the fear of hurting an unborn child during pregnancy, for example, or watching an adolescent daughter repeat the same disorder. For others, particularly women who have lived with a hidden eating problem for decades, the trigger is a medical emergency: a broken hip from osteoporosis, a pronouncement of diabetes, an electrolyte imbalance that precipitates a heart attack.

I don't know of any women who lack some sort of "food issue." I know women who count carbs relentlessly. I know women who diet on and off, yo-yoing between lost and gained pounds. I know women who are completely preoccupied with their body size, married to their StairMasters and elliptical trainers. One step further, I know mothers-to-be who wish that they could vomit more during pregnancy as they struggle to hold on to their once-slender bodies; and perhaps they do vomit, purposefully. I know one woman whose gynecologist unwittingly diagnosed her with a condition known as "hyperemesis gravidarum," which is medical-speak for serious nausea and vomiting during pregnancy. She went to the hospital dehydrated but did not vomit often enough to fit the criteria for full-blown bulimia nervosa.

Did she have an eating disorder? What does she do when she is no longer pregnant? Is there a line between "disordered eating," as the experts would label these actions, and a full-blown disease? And why does she put herself through this punishment when she is older and knows that it is not healthy? Has she grown any wiser with age?

I wanted to research the answers to these questions and more. I wanted to write this book to describe what happens to all those young girls when they grow up. We who suffer from eating disorders make headlines as kids, starving, bingeing, and purging. Society gasps at our image: the anorexics with the big eyes and protruding bones and the bulimics bent over toilets, wiping their mouths with the backs of their hands. But we grow up and society loses track of us. We get married and have our babies. Does the culture think that we all got better? Do we think that the diseases are out of our system now that we are all grown up?

I certainly thought so. When I began research for this book, I maintained a naiveté about eating disorders. This is strange, given that I had one. Still, I believed a hodgepodge of pop culture doctrine. It goes like this: Eating disorders evolve out of adolescent angst and a shaky self-image. Girls want to be popular; they see their grail in fashion magazines. They go after this image through diet, and a certain cluster of teens, because of some mysterious predisposition (maybe genetic), go overboard: undereating and overexercising in the case of anorexia, or dieting, then bingeing and vomiting, in the case of bulimia. Parents often exacerbate the problem, for example, by overtly criticizing their daughter's body. And, ultimately, most teenagers with anorexia and bulemia get better with therapy, throwing their scales into the trash bin. Granted, a small fraction do wither away in and out of hospitals until a tragic death takes them, maybe by heart attack, maybe by malnutrition. Such was the fate of pop singer Karen Carpenter, who died at 32 from heart problems traced back to her anorexia nervosa.

Now, I am finding that many of us—as well as many women who never had full-blown eating disorders but carried something of the sort with them throughout their lives—are somewhere in between. They are neither scale-less nor dead. Some have carried a residual of food compulsion throughout most of their lives. Others have flown under the radar for decades and only recently been diagnosed for the first time in their forties, fifties, even their seventies. We adult women with eating disorders represent a demographic numbering in the tens of millions, although the exact numbers are hard to tally.

Experts have long cited the figure of 8 million women with eating disorders in the United States—girls and young women ages 12 to 25. This group includes the one in one hundred girls with anorexia nervosa, defined by willful starving, and the one in four girls with bulimia nervosa, with its bingeing and purging. The number also includes the less-well-know binge eating disorder, which is similar to bulimia but without the purge step.

Anorexia, bulimia, and binge eating disorder. Eight million girls in the United States.

But this is a gross underestimate, says Lynn Grefe, CEO of the National Eating Disorders Association (NEDA). Her group estimates the number of full-blown eating disorders in children and adults to be closer to 15 to 20 million. Breaking it down, nearly 10 million have anorexia, bulimia, or binge eating disorder. These numbers don't account for the number of people who struggle with borderline conditions, which could more than double the numbers affected.

More stunning still, these numbers do not include subthreshold forms of eating disorder illnesses. We, the close-but-not-quite-there, are virtually invisible in traditional eating disorders research. And, more often than not, we are older.

"It is hard to get estimates of people who are only partially ill," says James Hudson, associate chief of the Biological Psychiatry Laboratory at McLean Hospital, near Boston, and associate professor of psychiatry at Harvard Medical School. "We just don't know."

Grefe says that she first scratched the surface when she began conducting focus groups and surveys. In her early days at NEDA in 2003, she reached out to the community to see what facets of eating disorders warranted attention.

"I need your advice," she said to a group of patients. "What can I do in my new job?"

At first, the group was silent. Then two older women spoke up.

"The first thing you have to do is tell people that it happens to us, too," one said. "And it's not because we want to be models," said the other.

What is it, then? What fuels eating disorders in older women?

In high school, I was the prim and pretty girl from the suburbs, the one who did what she was told. I packed my schedule with honors courses, earned a 4.3 grade point average on a scale of 4.0, and took calculus with all the boys. Later, I learned that brains were not an asset in the realm of teenhood and volatile hormones. I learned to hide my self. I learned to shrink from boys who flirted with me and commented about my body.

Miserable, I struggled to make sense of it all. But logic does not solve adolescence, and in the tumult of irrationality, I burrowed deeper into some mysterious haven inside me. Outside, I could not even muster the courage to look up and meet the eyes of fellow students as they passed me in the halls of Lake Catholic High near Cleveland, Ohio. At the same time, I drove harder at achieving because that was what I could do well.

But ambition is a penny with two sides. My drive to succeed won me honors and awards. But it also whittled my 5-foot, 4-inch frame down to 89 pounds. In college at a Jesuit university, I was a premed major, getting straight A's, acting in a play, singing in a traveling choral group, working with a human rights group, swimming and running daily. I was also refusing to eat anything but salad in the cafeteria. I dropped my weight in the same way I tackled a differential equation—I went at it with everything I had.

When I returned home for the first time, my parents cried and piled me into the car for a drive to a psychiatrist's office. Four years of therapy helped coax the scale back up to 110. A very kind doctor, whom I thank to this day, smoothed everything back: my brittle hair, my flaky skin, my cracked fingernails. My life.

And so I married at the age of 25. I lost 10 pounds before my wedding. People around me laughed, with the knowing laugh of the already-wed. They said that all brides lose weight. Nervous energy. But I knew better. I was dieting. I wanted to be thinner in my wedding dress. On a deeper level, I was petrified of losing myself, the self I had worked so hard to find, in a relationship with a man who had the power to overwhelm me. That is how I saw intimacy. My psyche was too fragile to allow a true relationship.

Five years later, after undergoing infertility treatment, I became pregnant. Another transition. Another place for the eating disorder to rise up. By the seventh month of my pregnancy, I had gained only 7 pounds. Stress, I told myself. I was working as a reporter at the *Chicago Tribune*, trying to hide my "condition" from my coworkers for fear of losing choice assignments. The truth is, I was almost in denial about my pregnancy because I was afraid of this baby taking over my body—and my life. Sound familiar?

But this time around, I had grown wiser about the eating disorder cycle of recovery and relapse. I knew that I needed help. I wanted this baby to be healthy—more than I wanted to be healthy myself. I quit work. I found a Jungian therapist who talked about dreams and images of plump Botticelli women. With his guidance, pregnancy became an oasis, a time-out from the eating disorder's demands, a time when I gave myself permission to be "fat."

I managed to put on 10 pounds before giving birth to a healthy 6-pound, 9-ounce girl. Then my marriage fell apart.

Two months after my daughter was born, I separated from my husband. This marked the greatest transition of my life. I had no job, no house, an infant in my care, and a custody battle that would take four years to finish. This was my postpartum. This phase, I have since learned, is one of the most difficult for nearly every woman who has had eating issues in her past.

My ex-husband worsened the situation; he used the fact that I had anorexia as a wedge to try to gain custody. As I worried that I would lose the being I had grown closest to in my life, my daughter, I almost fulfilled the prophecy my husband's attorney spelled out to the courts. I plunged to my lowest weight since that first diagnosis.

But, as I dropped below 100 pounds, I knew that if I dipped any lower, I would only feed the image that would allow the courts to take my child away. And so with that strength that age and experience afford, I managed to pull myself back together. I walked around with bags of trail mix to keep up my caloric intake while lactating. I began freelance writing. I won full custody.

At that moment, my life turned around. For some inexplicable reason, at the age of 33, I began menstruating for the first time without hormones. I gained confidence as a single mother and the rest has been a good story. I could say to Lauren in the café near MIT that, yes, for years now, I have had respite. The lion sleeps tonight.

. . .

I began this project by dusting off my scientific skills, born from my doctorate in molecular biology. I combed through medical studies in peer-reviewed journals and analyzed results as well as study design. I tapped my fifteen years of journalism experience, flying to eating disorders conferences and treatment centers, and telephoning, visiting, and checking the research of hundreds of experts in the field.

Of course, I met women. I spoke to more than three dozen women, of many different ages, in places as diverse as Brazil, France, and Twinsburg, Ohio. I read about hundreds more in case studies written up by physicians. From the anecdotes and facts that I unearthed, I have pieced together this picture of what eating disorders look like over a lifetime.

Life transitions act as chapters in this book and mile markers along the real journey that we are all taking. I begin with the transition from school to career, pass through marriage or partnership, and then go on through pregnancy, parenting, middle age, and later life. I end with a special chapter that details the healing resources available for help anywhere along the way.

Perhaps the place to begin is with the person whom I first visited: Harvard's eating disorders expert, psychiatrist David Herzog, director of the Eating Disorders Unit at Massachusetts General Hospital and president of the Harvard Eating Disorders Center in Boston. Since 1987, he has been following 240 women who sought help for anorexia, bulimia, or a combination of both. The women entered the study around the age of 25. They now average 40 years old.

"We thought that if a woman made it to 40, she would no longer have a problem," he says. "But we are seeing that this is not the case."

Most of the women in this study improved for a time, but then relapsed. In fact, more than two-thirds have not yet completely recovered, and some of them will probably remain ill with a full-blown eating disorder for the rest of their lives. Finally, it is estimated that

20 to 30 percent of women with anorexia will eventually die from the complications of their illnesses. These women have retained a preoccupation with eating—a lion like my own, lying in wait.

Different circumstances can make each woman's beast pounce. Outside of the Massachusetts General Hospital study group, there are those women who get sick later in life, women like Nilda. I met her after I learned that she had been diagnosed with anorexia nervosa for the first time at age 68. However, it is not thinness that drives Nilda, now 70. She is obsessively worried about dying. The anxiety squashes her hunger and, paradoxically, makes her hyperactive. She is afraid that if she slows down her pace, she will not get all her affairs in order and she will leave her children bereft. She feels alone, aware, and not at all ready to die.

She is quite different from Aliane, a 15-year-old girl with anorexia, who stopped eating because she wanted to be thin. That was the first reason she gave me. But when I dug a little deeper, I learned that she is disgusted by the thought of having to live with a man, take care of him, and bear his children. She is opting out of adulthood and the eating disorder gives her the out.

Nilda and Aliane are the bookends of an eating-disordered life. Their ages also mark the boundaries of this book. In between, you'll find Dana, 40, who exercises compulsively to forget possible sexual abuse; Tracy, 41, who diets and obsesses about weight while tending to two young sons; Cindy, 47, and Barbara, 54, who have had eating disorders and are now coping with teenage daughters who are suffering as well; and Rachel, 60, who hid her bulimia for nearly forty years before she could gather the courage to seek help.

These stories, on the surface, seem very different; each one of these women uses her eating disorder to serve a different purpose— Dana to quell feelings of self-loathing drummed up by violation, Tracy to vent anger at her husband for neglecting her needs, and so on.

The purpose of an eating disorder can also be different in the same woman over the course of her life. A teen might use her eating disorder as a *sculpting tool* to achieve perceived beauty; being thin means she is somebody. But, as she gets older, she might draw upon her eating issues to serve as a *weapon* against an intimate partner, an *amnesiac* against bad feelings about parenting, an *escape* from inevitable aging.

This "purpose" talk is not what we have heard in the headlines about skinny teenagers. But it is the crux of the matter. The point of an eating disorder is that women—older women, smart women, capable women, women in pain—use their eating problems to try to temper, control, massage, or unravel deep, insufferable hurt.

We used to think that eating disorders limited themselves to upper-middle-class white girls. Now reports are emerging about eating disorders breaking the bounds of African American, Native American, Latino, Asian, Indian, Fijian, Zulu, and many other communities. Poorer women are getting sick as frequently as richer ones. And researchers are now speculating that eating disorders not only mean thinness and beauty to women but also economic success and celebrity.

In writing *Lying in Weight*, I regret that I could not deal better with these developing issues of ethnicity and socioeconomic class. Because each culture has its own unique issues, trying to type all of them while at the same time defining their evolution through the lifespan would create far too voluminous a book. In addition, older women's issues have only recently been coming to light, and in the main, these first studies have dealt with predominantly white, middle-class, American-born women. Thus, I am reluctantly forced to limit *Lying in Weight* to the issues and explanations given for eating problems in this particular population of older women. While much of their struggle does apply to all women with eating disorders, I hope to explore the special issues of other groups of women in future work.

So, let's begin. When do eating problems become eating disorders, and how long do they last?

Chronicity

The Myth of Recovery

The story begins with a teenager standing naked in front of the bathroom mirror. "Who am I?" she asks, turning in profile, dissecting the reflection of her breasts, hips, and belly. As she pinches flesh and frowns, a tape in her mind begins to play. It echoes the comments of her parents, the gossip of girlfriends, and the urges of boys who might want her. The one who does not want her, the boy she has a crush on, has just blown her off. Now, facing the mirror, she hears only rejection. She blames it on what she sees, her size-6 self.

She focuses on her stomach; it is bloated. The cruelty of premenstrual syndrome, PMS. In the hopes of soothing her sorrows, she has just eaten a pint of cookie dough ice cream. Stuffed and heartsick, she looks for another way to solve her problem. She thinks, *If I were prettier, if I were a size 4, I would have gotten him. I would have gotten anyone that I had wanted. And I wouldn't be feeling so miserable right now.*

What does she do? For her, the inevitable: she bends over the toilet and thrusts her finger to the back of her throat. She tickles at first. Then she jams. She reaches that special spot and heaves up pieces of herself, the ugliness spewing out.

Then she gets up, feeling ashamed, humiliated as only others like her can imagine. She will never tell anyone. *Besides, I'll never do this again.*

But she does. Three times a day, every day.

For how long?

Media accounts do not go that far. The tale typically ends with the girl in the mirror either dropping out of the story as it goes on to sensationalize the horrors of eating disorders. Or she tells someone and gets therapy. She gets better. And the reader celebrates the happy ending with her.

But is it really the end?

Not according to medical research. Many reports track the outcomes of girls who have been diagnosed with some type of eating disorder. Anorexia nervosa, bulimia nervosa, and binge eating disorder are all clinically defined according to criteria published in the fourth edition of the Diagnostic and Statistic Manual of Mental Disorders, the bible for practitioners. (See Appendix 3 on page 315.)

The DSM-IV says that a person with *anorexia nervosa* willfully loses weight to the point of emaciation. Such an individual is terrified of becoming fat, and the fear heightens as the weight drops. Some individuals with anorexia simply restrict what they eat, while others binge and purge, either through vomiting, using laxatives, or overexercising. Since nutritional starvation usually inhibits menstruation, failure to menstruate for at least three consecutive months is one of the defining criteria of anorexia.

Individuals with *bulimia nervosa* have a very different profile. According to DSM-IV, a person with bulimia is someone who eats large amounts of food in a short period of time and feels helpless to stop. Purging follows, either by self-induced vomiting or misuse of laxatives, diuretics, enemas, or other medications, along with fasting or excessive exercise. An individual does not have to vomit to be considered bulimic. She can exercise obsessively instead. But she must cycle through the binge-purge episodes, on average, at least twice a week for three months.

Binge eating disorder is defined as bingeing, as in bulimia nervosa, but without the compensatory purging or other behaviors. Individuals with BED tend to be obese and racked by low self-esteem. They may begin to binge either after years of unsuccessful dieting (starvation prompts the urge to binge) or these individuals may use food as a means to allay their self-rejection.

Classifying patients into groups and subgroups helps researchers pin down causes and doctors decide which treatment is best. DMS-IV also gives therapists a glossary of terms to convey information to one another about their patients. And in this day and age, establishing diagnoses is necessary for insurance coverage.

But diagnoses have their limitations. Strict criteria can convey a false sense of who is well and who is not. For example, a patient in therapy can progress enough so that she no longer fits into a disease category. She no longer displays the telltale symptoms of anorexia, bulimia, or binge eating disorder. The medical community may say she is better, but deep inside she knows that something is still wrong. Perhaps she even stops treatment because she has been led to believe there is no need for it. Worse, she may find down the road that she falls right back into the eating disorder, with all its fears and rituals.

What does DSM-IV, with its pages of precise definitions, say about that? Only that she does not fit in.

THE EATING PROBLEMS THAT DON'T FIT: WOMEN WHO FALL UNDER THE MEDICAL RADAR

Dana, 40, cannot go a day without running. Every morning when the alarm goes off, she laces up. Rain, snow, or sleet, she runs outside because running inside on an indoor track or elliptical runner does not give her the same endorphin high as a forty-five-minute outdoor jaunt.

As a teenager, she suffered through both bulimia and drug abuse. Today, she has let go of both: no more bingeing and purging or smoking and snorting drugs. But she cannot let up on her exercise. She runs when she is fatigued, and even when she's injured. She has recently added a nightly twenty-minute workout on an indoor trainer. As for eating, she skips breakfast and lunch, saving her calorie quota until dinner. Even after starving all day, however, she still feels guilty about cooking herself a meal. Instead, she makes dinner for her two children—brown rice, vegetables, and tofurky (a tofu version of turkey)—and eats standing up, picking from her kids' plates.

What does Dana have? Bulimia? She does not throw up, but she does, in fact, purge through exercise. Does she binge? She says no. When asked to define the behavior, researchers can give only arbitrary answers: a "binger" is someone who eats between 2,000 and 10,000 calories in less than two hours. Because Dana does not eat that much within that time range, by definition, she does not binge. Therefore, she cannot have bulimia nervosa.

So what does she have?

How about Tracy? As a teenager, she suffered through anorexia, bulimia, and alcoholism. She sobered up and lost the binge-purge cycles, thanks to the help of Alcoholics Anonymous. But when she was pregnant at 38, and again at 40, she welcomed nausea as a gift.

"Although I felt sick, I lost weight," she says. "I was secretly glad."

Did she make herself throw up? No one but Tracy will ever know. Even if she did not force vomiting, is doing the deed "naturally" and being grateful for it considered an eating disorder?

These are the realities of eating problems for perhaps the majority of older women in Western cultures. The problems—some would call them quirks—are becoming so commonplace that experts have begun to subdivide and name them: a person who exaggerates the importance of a blemish, such as a mole, freckle, or scar, or reacts obsessively to the shape or size of a body part, such as her breasts, has body dysmorphic disorder. In contrast, a woman with orthexia abuses health foods such that when she does not have access to her special foods, say, part of a strictly macrobiotic diet, she feels extremely anxious and out of control.

Women can also have a mixed eating disorder. Called "eating disorders not otherwise specified" (EDNOS), these problems do not fit into the classic categories of anorexia or bulimia, but they are serious enough to call for therapy.

For example, Barbara, 54, dieted her 5-foot, 4-inch body down to 85 pounds in college. But she never lost her periods. In fact, after college, she even became pregnant at this low weight. Psychologists cannot classify her diagnosis as anorexia because she menstruates.

Cindy, 47, also charted in as EDNOS. She lost weight through diet and exercise but not the requisite 85 percent of normal that would position her in the DSM-IV category of anorexia. She never binged, but she purged regularly, through vomiting and overexercise. Thus, she is neither anorexic nor bulimic.

The variations go on. And they point to a very big problem. In an excellent review, published in the British medical journal *Lancet*, Christopher Fairburn, a psychiatrist and renowned eating disorder expert at Oxford, raises a startling fact: *most* eating disorders fall into the EDNOS categories. In other words, after all the hairsplitting about what defines anorexia or bulimia, most people who become ill with an eating disorder suffer from something that fails to meet the criteria for either one.

How can the majority of eating disorders not fit into given categories of disease, categories around which researchers are designing their studies and building medical understanding?

Fairburn chides the eating disorders community about the distinctions between anorexia, bulimia, and EDNOS. He writes, "The existing scheme for classifying eating disorders is unsatisfactory and anomalous. This system is a historical accident that needs to be rectified, since far more unites the three categories of eating disorder than separates them."

Indeed, researchers are trying to come up with other ways to classify eating disorders. For example, psychoanalysts have recently come up with a diagnostic manual that seeks to define mental illness by personality type rather than by symptoms. So instead of saying that someone has bulimia (she binges, then purges) or anorexia (she starves herself), psychologists would test to see whether she is one of fourteen personality types: depressive or impulsive-compulsive, for example.

In the realm of eating disorders, researchers have identified at least three personality types that describe the women who develop eating disorders. For example, some women with anorexia function very well in life. But they feel enormous pressure to conform, and they desperately need to control all aspects of their lives. Another group feels highly anxious and avoids social situations. A third cluster of women with anorexia acts compulsively and has poor coping strategies.

Yet it will be a long time before this system replaces DSM-IV. Why? The DSM-IV categorization does a great service in helping doctors define and treat the illnesses. It also helps the general public understand what an eating disorder is—and is not.

Still, the definitions need to be understood for what they are: an attempt to classify and organize. But excluding sufferers because they do not "fit in" leaves behind large, unmeasured numbers of women who could benefit from therapy. They are miserable, inching through their lives wondering, *What is wrong with me?* They believe many fallacies about eating disorders: for example, that they are diseases of young girls, and that as an older woman, they cannot have an eating disorder.

Now, because greater numbers of adult women are stepping forward, admitting that something is wrong, other myths are coming to light. One relates to who gets better and when.

>>> Mary's Magical Thinking

Mary, 36, believed in magic. She believed that when she turned 27, her bulimia would simply vanish.

The problem started when Mary was 15. She became drunk at her friend Stephanie's party.

"Just make yourself sick," Stephanie had offered as a solution.

And Mary did, even though she considered the act disgusting. A couple of months later, she did it again, this time after bingeing on food. That forged the iron loop: bingeing, purging, and starving. Between the purges Mary became so ravenous that she binged despite every attempt to stop herself.

She carried this habit with her all the way to college. At Bowling Green State University near Toledo, Ohio, her problem made her one of a growing number of co-eds with bulimia who, during the 1980s, made headlines in epidemic proportions. Mary would join her friends in the cafeteria, ostensibly lunching on salads, fruit, or yogurt. Then, on the way across campus to her dorm at Ashley Hall, she would pass by the vending machines, buy four or five Kit Kat candy bars, and eat them as she walked. The challenge was to stuff them into her mouth and swallow before she opened the dormitory doors. Then she would tiptoe with her toothbrush to the community bathroom, check to see if anyone was there, and poke the toothbrush handle down the back of her throat. She learned how to stop herself, mid-vomit, if someone else came in.

The summer after her freshman year, Mary finally admitted to her mother that she was in trouble. Her mother steered Mary to a therapist at an eating disorder center in Toledo. Mary saw him once a week, every week, until she graduated. They talked of the usual adolescent angst: relationships, self-esteem, and body image. By the end of college, she was no longer acting bulimic. Jubilant, the therapist pronounced her well.

But Mary was not convinced, even as her doctor grinned brilliantly. She smiled wanly, saying, "OK, great, good-bye."

Was she ready to strike out into the world?

For inspiration, she looked in the mirror. But despite what her therapist told her, and his impression that her symptoms seemed under control, she could only see herself as "a deer in the headlights."

Within a year, Mary was in trouble again. She took a job at a local TV station. Soon after, she began bingeing and purging at a level that surpassed anything that she had done before. She vowed to stop. She tried to run away from it by moving out to Hollywood. In the land of be-whoever-you-want-to-be, she magically thought that she could pull a geographic makeover, using distance to erase what she saw in the mirror. Perhaps she could create someone more confident, an extreme transformation, just like she'd seen so many times on TV. She boarded the plane vowing, "I will never taint the toilets of California with my vomit."

But she did. She binged and vomited as before, even as she excelled in her career as a postproduction TV producer, a demanding job that involved managing a TV show from the minute the film leaves the camera until it aired. By the time she had reached 27, her bulimia was not letting up and Mary was desperate.

Mary thought that her bulimia would dissolve at 27. Why? Nothing in her life would indicate that she was destined for recovery. But she desperately wanted to believe that it would be so. In fact, at 27, she was far more bulimic than she had ever been, despite therapy on and off over nearly a decade. But by believing the myth of recovery—that at 27 she would be ready to marry and contemplate having children, that her illness would somehow disappear—Mary did not begin the real work that would prepare her for those demanding life changes.

MEDIA CREATES THE MYTH OF QUICK RECOVERY

Perhaps Mary got her ideas from the media. It gave her stories such as the one about teen star Mary-Kate Olsen. A week after her eighteenth birthday, Olsen checked into a rehabilitation clinic in Utah to seek help for anorexia nervosa. Six weeks later, the TV star emerged, smiling, to the flash of cameras.

Six weeks. That was it. The message is that with six weeks and some hard-core therapy, a girl with an eating disorder can beat it. The story ends with Mary-Kate and her twin sister, Ashley, buying, but never living in, a 6,000-square-foot penthouse apartment in Manhattan, attending New York University, and becoming the focus of a *New York Times* fashion story with a quote from stylist Karen Berenson saying that Mary-Kate "makes skinny girls in baggy clothes look cool."

The media also presented Jamie-Lynn Sigler, a singer-actress who plays the daughter of a mob boss in the TV series *The Sopranos*. She wrote about her struggle with an eating disorder in a book called *Wise Girl*. In an article published in *USA Today*, Jamie-Lynn describes her illness, including starving, overexercising, and sliding in weight from 120 to 90 pounds. The article ends with a cheery "back to her healthy weight of about 120–125 pounds, Sigler is waiting for the new season of *The Sopranos* to debut."

Just like that. She turned 21 and got better.

These stories are informative about what eating disorders are and how they strike the prettiest, best, and brightest. But such articles are also deceiving. They leave people thinking that the disease is easily curable—that it's just a matter of finding the right pill, psychotherapy, or eating disorders center and the disease will be gone. Of course, the work of professionals at eating disorders centers and in private practice can help women make nearly miraculous progress. But the problems arise when people have unrealistic expectations about what these therapies can do, especially if the woman is not ready to begin a true healing process.

The Internet can also do great harm. To its credit, the Web offers many educational tools to help viewers cope with eating disorders. But it also posts empty promises such as Peggy Claude-Pierre's eating disorder cure based on unconditional love; and rank exploitation in the form of websites such as PumpYourAura.com, which boasts of a "Magic Cure Key" for anorexia and bulimia; or the now defunct Anorexia Q, which posted links to cabbage diet thermaboost pills, cheap weight-loss medicines, and popular fad diets.

Even reputable publications like the *New York Times* unwittingly add to misperceptions about recovery. In 1992, the *Times* ran a short piece entitled "Curing Eating Disorders," about a benefit to raise money for treatment. No reputable expert will say that eating disorders can be "cured." They can only be treated.

Semantics also cause trouble. In a 1985 *New York Times* article reporter Fred Ferretti conveyed these statistics about anorexia nervosa: "Anorexia afflicts one in 250 women, perhaps as many as one in 100, mostly from their teens to their 20's."

While the statement is accurate, it reads as if anorexia afflicts *only* women who are in their teens and twenties. No psychologist would make this claim. Yet the reader of this article walks away thinking anorexia is a disease of teenage girls.

Subtle wordplay and a plethora of false media messages left Mary believing that, like a scab on a wound, her disease would eventually just fall off as she aged, unveiling a healed self beneath. But the reality is that more older women than ever before are showing up at eating disorders treatment centers such as Remuda Ranch, in Wickenburg, Arizona.

"We are not the only treatment center seeing older patients," says Edward Cumella, director of research and education at Remuda. "So it is a pretty safe bet that this is a phenomenon."

Older women, those past their twenties, need to know that they are indeed vulnerable to eating disorders, and that their illnesses, over time, present a very different challenge than the eating disorders of adolescence.

"With eating disorders, usually, we see at least a ten-year system of waxing and waning of symptoms," says Marsha Marcus, chief of eating disorders and behavioral medicine at the Western Psychiatric Institute and Clinic in Pittsburgh, Pennsylvania. "The diagnosis is only a snapshot."

So how does one characterize a life with an eating disorder? Is it a series of climaxes and denouements, or is it a steady struggle? Do women with eating disorders recover permanently, or do they maintain a singular vulnerability, much like an alcoholic, who bears a certain "thirst" and therefore has to remain forever vigilant?

MEDICINE CREATES ITS OWN MYTHS

Society has handed these questions over to medicine. *Just tell us how long and what to do to get better.* And the medical community has answered.

Researchers have posted results from numbers of "outcome studies" that track patients with eating disorders over time. But past studies are flawed in their design and therefore give dubious results. Current studies carry their own set of problems, sometimes worsened by the patients' own reluctance to tell the truth about their eating disorders.

For example, three researchers from the University of Zurich in Switzerland tried to get a handle on the long-term picture of patients with eating disorders. Led by psychiatrist Hans Christoph Steinhausen, the team attempted to compare results from forty-five outcome studies of patients with anorexia nervosa published between 1953 and 1981 and twenty-two additional studies published in the 1980s.

While one might expect sixty-seven studies to generate much useful data, the Swiss researchers were quickly stymied. They found that they could not draw strong conclusions for two reasons: there were defects in experimental design, and researchers were tracking at different time intervals after treatment and measuring different markers of recovery. For example, the early crop of studies included only small numbers of patients and rarely went on longer than four years. A four-year study tracking teenage girls says very little about how a 40-year-old woman might fare.

Research conducted in the 1980s did a little better. These studies included more patients and lasted up to fourteen years. But the main problem (and it is still a problem) is that no one can agree on how to define the term "recovered."

The definition of this word is most crucial because it gets to the heart of magical thinking about healing. In the past, some researchers have used "normalization of eating" as a measure of recovery. This means that if a patient with anorexia does not exhibit the classic starving behaviors of the disease, she is classified as "recovered." Using this bellwether, the recovery rate varied wildly, from 30 to 70 percent.

Such a huge range in science means that the results are not accurate. But, not surprisingly, it is the most optimistic end of the spectrum that filters into public consciousness. Take the publishers of women's magazines, for example. They look for happy endings to sad stories: uplifting sagas with perky tones sell more magazines. Researchers, too, want good outcomes because those are proof that coveted therapies are working.

However, it is important for older women, intelligent women, those who believe that they might have a problem, to question the validity of these outcomes. Are these happy endings the reality?

The early studies simply cannot answer the question. They have too many design flaws. For example, Steinhausen noted that "a significant number" of the studies he analyzed did not even report weight data for the patients. "These deficits are likely to affect seriously the quality of outcome data," he concludes.

How can studies of anorexia nervosa neglect to include patients' weights?

In fact, researchers simply cannot say how many get better, let alone know the identity of the ones who recover or how the life of an older woman with an eating problem will edge along.

But good news is on the horizon. More recently, researchers have begun to crack down on such lapses in study design and ask the right questions about what happens to women with eating disorders over time.

The Rule of Thirds

Near Boston's gaslight district, at the intersection of Grove and Fruit streets, Massachusetts General Hospital buzzes like a hive. Workers clad in cotton scrubs hustle outside for a quick smoke. Meanwhile, family members scurry in past hundreds of wheelchairs, through the front entrance. Room 725 houses one of the country's most cramped clinics for eating disorders. Here, psychiatrist David Herzog, a pioneer in eating disorders research, tries to salvage lives.

Tanned from a golf outing and radiating vigor, Herzog has the aura of a rainmaker. Widely published and internationally regarded, he has amassed a team of experts and enough funds to mount a state-of-the-art eating disorders study. Between 1987 and 1991, Herzog and his team selected 246 women averaging 25 years: 110 diagnosed with anorexia, the rest with bulimia. Since then, the researchers have followed the women, wielding scales and tape measures, questionnaires, tests, and personal interviews.

The researchers check in with each participant every six months and track her current progress, rather than relying on retrospective data and self-reports of past history. The study is large by the standards of eating disorders research. It has followed the same women for more than a decade.

Meanwhile, the women, now averaging 40 years of age, have been living their lives.

How are they faring?

After seven years of follow-up, the first results have come out. Herzog's team found that most patients over time were able to reduce their symptoms, at least temporarily. Even better, a third of the patients with anorexia nervosa and three-fourths of those with bulimia had fully recovered, defined by an absence of most symptoms for at least eight consecutive weeks.

The researchers applauded the numbers; they said that most women with eating disorders are likely to recover with treatment and time. Reporters picked up the good news and wrote glorious stories of women making comebacks—women dressed in bright colors, telling their dramas on *Oprah*. Telling their stories to other women.

But what reporters glossed over, and perhaps the researchers themselves did not emphasize enough, was the rest of the findings, which were not so favorable. Recovery did not always stick. At least 40 percent of recovered patients with anorexia and 35 percent of recovered patients with bulimia relapsed within four years of getting well.

More sobering, Herzog's group found that almost 20 percent of the women with anorexia and 1 percent of those with bulimia never had periods of recovery. Eleven patients died, four from suicide. This is the highest death rate of any mental disorder; it gives eating disorders their worst face and illustrates why there is an urgent need for attention.

Another finding, this one ironic: half of the patients who had recovered from anorexia did not become eating disorder–free. They merely went on to develop bulimia, trading one eating disorder for another.

In sum, Herzog's group came up with an easy-to-remember rule of thirds: 81 patients, a third of the total, recovered and stayed well. For a second group, representing a bit more than a third, recovery seemed to rise and fall for at least ten years. And the last group, registering at just below a third, could not make any headway. Simply put, when looking at anorexia and bulimia over a decade, a third of patients will get better, a third will remain ill, and a third will vacillate between disease and recovery.

Is the Rule Really the Rule?

The Massachusetts General study is relatively strong and, because of that, practitioners in the field have generally accepted the rule of thirds. But some troublesome issues leave doubts about the accuracy of that recovery estimate.

Consider a patient in the study who reports to a researcher how she is doing. She is older now. She has been dieting or bingeing and purging for ten or twenty years. If she has not gotten better, she may feel embarrassed—enough to fudge her responses about symptoms or give false answers on questionnaires. This is easy to do, especially if she has moved away from the study site and merely has to tell her weight and symptoms over the telephone. *Oh no, I haven't binged in a year now. Really.* But she may be lying. Or she may, in fact, be telling the truth. She may have stopped her disordered behaviors at the time that researchers contacted her. But she may relapse less than six months later. Would she call back to say, *You know what, you'd better change your statistics about me?* Probably not.

Lynn Grefe, of NEDA, knows how powerful the urge to lie can be for a woman with an eating disorder. Grefe conducted her own surveys and found that the public knows a lot about eating disorders, especially in young girls. People are also aware that eating disorders represent illness. But when adults were asked the question "If you had an eating disorder, would you tell anybody?" everyone answered no.

Everyone.

Grefe explains that the disease is too loaded with shame to get an accurate counting. Yet researchers have to figure out *some* way to tally "recovery." And right now, they do so by asking each woman whether or not she has eliminated measurable signs and symptoms for a time.

"I agree, it's not a particularly fabulous definition," says Pamela Keel, clinical psychologist at the University of Iowa.

But it is the best that research can offer right now. It is also the definition that treatment facilities are using to gauge success. According to Jeanne Rust, executive director and founder of Mirasol, a treatment facility in Tucson, Arizona, eating disorders centers showcase their effectiveness by posting recovery rates of patients. These numbers come from surveys of former patients. Optimistically, top centers are posting recovery rates for adults as high as 80 to 90 percent (measured a year after treatment ends).

The rub is that they are based on the number of patients who are willing to fill out the survey or answer telephone questions, and the number is small. Most centers are getting replies from less than half of their former adult patients. In fact, Rust says response rates can be as low as 25 percent.

Such missing information poses an enormous challenge. Which former patients are most likely to lie or ignore such surveys—those who are sick or well at the time they receive the questionnaire?

Researchers do not know. Still, many generally accept the rule of thirds. For example, Seda Ebrahimi at the Cambridge Eating Disorder Center cites the rule when talking to the women she treats. But she cautions not to make too much of the number because all the women with problems throughout the world are not checking in and therefore getting counted.

"Bulimia is such a secretive disorder," she says. "I think it is underreported."

Binge eating disorder, with its stigma of obesity and unrestrained excess, shows up even less, according to James Hudson at McLean Hospital. Subclinical and EDNOS problems, as noted earlier, do not fit recognized eating disorders categories.

Yet women who are sick but not on the medical radar screen are still sick. They are simply not counted as sick. So the rule of thirds itself could be overly optimistic, and this leaves some experts wondering exactly how many young women with eating disorders get better and stay better throughout their lives.

"I have to tell you this anecdotally, because I can't get better stats," says psychologist Tacie Vergara, clinical supervisor of the Renfrew Center's Thirty-Something and Beyond Group, headquartered in Philadelphia, Pennsylvania. "The relapse rate is very high. *Very high.*"

Studies of women with anorexia and bulimia are not any more optimistic: relapse rates vary from 30 percent at six months post treatment to 63 percent within eighteen months.

This is not to say that treatment is a failure. Part of the problem is that insurance typically covers a scant twenty-one days, if at all. "The only thing that is happening for many patients is that they are not showing their symptoms for twenty-one days," Vergara says. "I want them [at the clinic] for six months, with their families, with their friends as well."

Without those circumstances, the situation becomes grimmer. Nonetheless, eating disorders experts emphasize the need for optimism. Every woman with a problem can heal, and therefore deserves a chance at recovery.

But in this push for optimism, there is also a danger: misrepresenting what recovery means. Having a history of an eating disorder, I know that promises of cures or perfect recovery can ring false. Worse, they can be a setup. I am one of a cadre of women who have eating problems because I am prone to perfectionism and overachievement. I am an intelligent woman. If someone hands me a regimen that looks like a diet and says, "Do this in eight easy steps," I react with skepticism. Worse, I may embrace the treatment and go after it with all I have. But if I slip at step 5 or slide back to step 3 or 4, then I feel like a failure. Feeling bad, I go back to the eating problem as my default. Is this recovery?

Better to give me a realistic idea of the problem that I have and what I can expect my life to become. Better to give me support and let me work my way through the mess as I try to live my life, that much more aware.

WHO ARE THESE WOMEN AND WHAT DO
THEY DO WITH THEIR LIVES?

Thus, even if the basis for the rule of thirds, including the diagnoses themselves, is shaky, the Massachusetts General study provides an obvious, perhaps more salient point: if eating disorders are amorphous, capable of different forms that play out over a lifetime, then, says Pamela Keel, "we are clearly not talking about a disorder that is limited to adolescence and young adulthood."

Indeed, roughly two-thirds of women in the study, now averaging age 40, are still sick or struggling to varying degrees. Their stories, the lives behind the numbers, open up a closet of understudied issues: What happens to job performance for these women? What kind of partners do they choose? What do such women teach their children? How do such women face aging? Do these women take their eating problems to their deathbeds?

The Massachusetts General study cannot answer these questions. It can only offer objective measures: weight, the number of times and frequency a patient vomits, the calories she consumes, scores on psychological tests.

But understanding eating disorders in older women requires stepping outside these definitions and numbers. To correct faulty myths, society must enter into the very lives of the women who have nursed an eating problem at some point in their lives. Society must ask whether these women feel as recovered as the Massachusetts General study says they are. And then, how does a woman's life unfold in the context of her own version of recovery?

RECOVERY OR REMISSION?

One group of researchers has attempted to provide a realistic picture of life with an eating disorder in recovery. Alison Field and her research colleagues at Brigham and Women's Hospital and Harvard

Medical School in Boston asked the question "What does the term 'recovered' really mean?"

"Recovery" implies that an eating disorder has gone away permanently, or at least for some period of time. On the other hand, "remission" assumes that, while symptoms are not present, the disease still exists and might reappear.

Do women recover from eating disorders or do they simply enter into remission?

To answer that, Field's team analyzed 106 women with bulimia nervosa. Each sought treatment and stopped bingeing and purging for at least four consecutive weeks. The researchers then followed the women for three more years, tracking relapse, defined by four consecutive weeks of either bingeing and purging weekly, or bingeing and purging two or more times a week.

The results were not promising: a quarter of the women relapsed within eleven weeks of stopping their bulimic patterns. By thirty-seven weeks, fewer than half the women remained symptom-free.

Because of this high rate of relapse, springing up months and years after symptoms had stopped, the authors concluded that women who are symptom-free for less than a year should not be labeled "recovered," but rather, "in remission." In other words, the disease is still present long after the symptoms have disappeared.

"Bulimia nervosa is 'an episodic disorder,'" Field writes. That statement means that recovery has good phases and bad ones, times when symptoms crop up and times when they die down.

Meanwhile, anorexia is the most recalcitrant of all the eating disorders. "If you look at the literature for effective treatments of anorexia, there are almost none," Vergara notes.

Binge eating disorder also resists standard treatment, according to Hudson.

These findings suddenly turn the whole idea of eating disorders recovery on its head. Recovery, meaning that the disease disappears forever, is a fallacy. The reality is that *time*, the length of time a person is symptom-free, becomes important in characterizing a patient's state of mind and, by extension, her health.

Chronos is the Greek god of time. The word "chronic" is defined as "lasting for a long period of time or marked by frequent recurrence." Chronic diseases in medicine, such as chronic fatigue syndrome, hypothyroidism, arthritis, and diabetes, may be treatable but not curable.

An educated diabetic never believes that her illness will go away. She never imagines that she can take a pill, have surgery, or seek out the best therapy and magically, just like that, heal her endocrine system. Diabetes is an illness that modern medicine cannot yet wipe out.

Eating disorders are like that. Field's study tells us that an eating disorder is more a chronic illness than a short-lived one.

Women with eating disorders experience something more like chronic disease: something, a demon, a voice of irrationality, endures long after the symptoms abate. Women who have had eating disorders feel this in their psyches. Dana, Tracy, Linda, Cindy, and Mary admit that something is "staying on." It might be biological, there from birth. It might be psychological, there from childhood. Either way, this predisposition clings throughout life, dragging eating disorders into the realm of chronic illness, on a par with diabetes or alcoholism.

No one would ask a recovered alcoholic to go into a bar three times a day, drink one beer, and then walk out a happy man or woman. Society for the most part understands that alcoholism lingers and a "recovered alcoholic" is a person who still has a drinking problem but who remains sober.

Yet society does not grant individuals with eating disorders the same latitude. Society expects that individuals will step into a recovery process and somehow become so comfortable with food, the monster of this illness, that for the rest of their lives they will be able to walk into their kitchens three times a day and eat just the right amount. No slipups. No relapses.

To women with eating disorders, the expectation of such resilience feels daunting—or worse. The majority choose to avoid even peering over that cliff, the chasm of recovery, for many, many years.

This is not to say that everyone who has been diagnosed with an eating disorder faces a future of hospitals and everlasting bingeing, purging, or starving. In fact, for the majority of patients, the telltale behaviors do stop or ease up, at least for a time.

But eating disorders, at their core, have an element of fallback, of chronicity.

"I look upon eating disorders as chronic, stress-related conditions," says Rust. Stress is the key, she notes. Any person will turn to her lifelong vices when faced with times of stress. In this context, stress means "big stress"—leaving school to find a career, marriage, giving birth, watching grown children move out, menopause, the death of a loved one. These are adult transitions that happen to a woman who learned to cope with life by falling back on her eating disorder, with behaviors often learned much earlier in life.

"A lot of these disorders have their roots in adolescence," Keel says, "but they tend to really have full force when these people are grown-ups."

The force is exerted because what has long ago been learned and lived with has become a vicious pattern, a nasty, an intractable habit. The teenager who solves her boyfriend problem with a diet or binge becomes the woman who does the same thing later in life, but with higher stakes. Her husband cheats on her—she diets. She loses her job—she binges and purges. Either way, she has not learned healthier alternatives. That lack of alternatives keeps the eating disorder going.

"I don't think people are finding the coping mechanisms that they need," Rust says. "And people with eating disorders use them as a coping mechanism to deal with the stresses of life."

Until a woman can learn new tools, more sophisticated strategies to getting her needs met, she will turn toward her eating disorder in times of crisis.

VIEWING EATING DISORDERS AS CHRONIC
CAN ASSIST IN HEALING

This view of an eating disorder is not entirely negative. If a woman understands the long-standing nature of her disease, she can stop trying to find cures or magic bullets—and stop feeling discouraged when immediate wellness does not materialize. Women with eating disorders do not have to beat themselves up if they are older and still struggling—or if they have relapsed after working so hard in recovery. However, individuals with histories of eating disorders who understand the nature of their disease are less likely to be blindsided by life's major stresses.

Admitting to vulnerability can bring about profound transformation. A woman can see relapse as something other than a catastrophe. A woman who has transgressed can forgive herself and move on. She can also amass support for herself when she knows she is entering a time of great vulnerability. And in treatment, recovery by a patient with an eating disorder would be seen in the same way that doctors look at other chronic illnesses, a lifelong process that ebbs and flows rather than a cure over a six-week course.

The truth is that recovery is not jumping over a line from "sick" to "well." There is only "better." And better means a spectrum of possibilities: what a woman who suffers today can expect as she looks toward her future.

There is a continuum of recovery for a person with an eating disorder. At one end there is Erin, 25. At 5 feet, 8 inches and 100 pounds, she cannot stop losing weight. She will get married next year. But today, she cannot even imagine sharing a romantic pasta dinner with her fiancé.

At the other end is Laura, 65, who had anorexia as a teen, relapsed at 48, but now no longer diets or restricts what she eats. She has gained weight and sometimes feels uncomfortable about that. But when she hears a voice in her mind that laughs and tells her, *You are fat*, she counters it with a positive one: *I am 65 and I can stand on my head in a yoga pose. I am proud of myself. And that is coming a long way.*

In between Erin and Laura are the rest: women from 25 to beyond 92 who are living with the vestiges of eating disorders. These women's stories highlight what has been neglected by the media and medical science. These women have much to say about life, as reflected through the food that they eat, their relationships, their bodily health, and their sense of who they are. They speak outside the medical arena, apart from the world of statistics and measurements.

2

Adolescence

Girls in Women's Clothing:
Eating Disorders Stunt
Psychological Development

S he sashays down the runway, and everybody is looking at her. At least that's how she sees it. A teenage girl is moving her body, not fully developed, out from the backstage of her home and into the world. She feels the spotlight shine upon her. It illuminates the awkward changes on the surface, breasts sprouting, pimples erupting.

She believes right now that life is all about appearance. But, deep within, a terrifying set of emotional and psychological changes is going on. Hormones are surging. Emotions are rushing. And new parts of her identity are swelling toward expression.

To become a whole, mature woman, she has to make a transition from childhood to adulthood. This phase may be the most demanding and difficult of her life. Her major task is to discover her identity. *Who am I as an adult?* She has to do this within the context of all the relationships in her life that have influenced her thus far.

Uncertain, she may begin by looking the part of an adult—by dressing up in a woman's clothing. The clothes are her way of saying to the world, *This is who I am*. But really, she does not know who she is yet. The development of her deeper self is much more complicated than putting on a new outfit.

And so a girl in this state of uncertainty loses her footing, at least for a time. She may express this shakiness in healthy ways: confiding her insecurities to friends, journaling her inner thoughts, painting pictures of dark emotions.

But if she feels too frightened to make the transition, if she is incapable of growing up, she will turn to unhealthy behaviors. One of these is an eating disorder. It is a tactic used to dodge a sometimes terrifying and painful transition in life.

FORCES THAT PUSH A GIRL OVER THE EDGE

Psychological Forces

There are many causes of eating disorders, and psychologists do not fully understand them all. The easiest explanation is that fashion and culture peddle the image of thinness as beauty; young girls succumb and hurt themselves in the process.

That explains part of the matter. But eating disorders are much more than the fallout of fashion opportunism. Some say eating disorders are one way to assert power in a time of seeming powerlessness. They are a voice against oppressive authority, a lifeboat in a storm of transition. Others say eating disorders are a matter of genes unleashing a drive for thinness.

Whatever the reason, all of these forces converge in adolescence. When eating disorders start here, they typically follow a pattern.

Stresses mount as new issues come up: *I have a crush on Steve, but he likes somebody else.* The old ways, the ways of a child, cannot solve the new problems: *I guess I can't throw a tantrum or complain to Mom.* A girl takes the problems out on her body: *He must not like me because my thighs are too fat.* She reduces the problem to something she can manage: *I hate my thighs. I'll go on a diet.*

And for most girls, this is where the cycle stops.

But a minority take the next step, and it is a big one. The dieting, exercise, and preoccupation with body move to center stage, taking over girls' lives, propelling them into the realm of eating disorders.

Disease usually emerges as a gradual slide: dieting evolves into perpetual starvation; or dieting forces ravenous hunger, which in turn
prompts bingeing. Or bingeing provokes extreme guilt, which leads
to vomiting, laxative abuse, or overexercise; or attempts to squelch
bad feelings with food, leading to runaway eating.

To help explain this concept in a visual way, Christopher Fairburn
came up with a simple but elegant flow chart.

In general, the progression of an eating disorder flows like this:
A woman hates herself; her low self-esteem causes extreme concern
about her shape and weight; this, in turn, prompts strict dieting.
With anorexia it stops here. With binge eating disorder, the strict
dieting leads to binge eating; with bulimia, the binge eating leads to
such guilt that it triggers the urge to vomit or purge in some other
way. In a reverse flow, vomiting, bingeing, and strict dieting all feed
back to make a woman even more preoccupied with her weight and
shape, which in turn lowers her already low self-esteem.

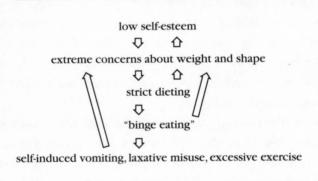

Bulimia and anorexia are but two of a wide spectrum of eating
disorders. Binge eating disorder falls into the mix as well. There
are also more minor kinds of eating and body obsessions, as noted
earlier in Chapter 1. And women can have subclinical disorders,
which include the symptoms of eating disorders but not to the serious levels that meet diagnosis.

Biological Forces

Through Fairburn's lens of eating disorders, all three are related to one another through excessive dieting, poor self-esteem, and negative feelings.

That starts it. But eating disorders take on a life of their own. They are addictions. In medical terms, this means that eating disorders involve *biology* as much as, if not more than, psychology. Eventually, a woman's eating behaviors change the circuitry in her brain.

This phenomenon is best illustrated in the Minnesota Semistarvation Experiment, conducted in 1944 by Ancel Keys and his colleagues at the University of Minnesota. The researchers wanted to observe how prisoners of war adapted to starvation and how best to rehabilitate them. Thirty-six conscientious objectors enlisted in the study and agreed to starve.

The experiment began with the participants eating normally for three months. Then the subjects' normal caloric intake was cut in half. Not surprisingly, over the next twenty-four weeks, the subjects became utterly obsessed with food, talking, fantasizing, and dreaming about it. At the same time, they became depressed, anxious, and irritable.

After the semistarvation period, the subjects were allowed to eat whatever they wanted for the next three months. They ate as if in a frenzy: they shoveled in huge meals (up to 10,000-calorie binges) but left the table complaining of hunger. They noted that their appetite ratcheted up rather than damped down right after a meal; some participants ate to the point of becoming sick—and still, they were not sated. In short, the subjects were eating as if their lives depended on it, which is understandable: they had been starving to death.

But even after they regained their lost weight, some subjects *still* indulged in strange food behaviors. In fact, the behaviors got more bizarre: the subjects, all robust men in their twenties, started to obsess about their body weight. They started complaining about fat around their buttocks, thighs, and abdomens. Some started to diet, trying to go back to their skeletal state. Losing weight and being thin somehow had caught hold of each man and, inexplicably, filled his thoughts.

This study shows the biological power of dieting. It can be addictive, and not driven only by a cultural pressure to be thin. This study was conducted in 1944–1946, and the men were in their twenties. They were not likely to care about fashion. So why should these men become obsessively concerned about fat on their buttocks and bellies?

The answer is that starvation does something to the mind. It takes hold and distorts normal thinking about food and body image. Distorted thinking describes the paradox of anorexia: women with the disease *constantly* think about food, even when they do not eat. What is going on, at the molecular level, is that a girl is splitting her body from her brain: her starving gut is trying to tell her brain's appetite centers, in loud molecular screams, "Eat!" But she forces the brain circuits that control eating to override the message. She starves in the midst of available food.

With bulimia, she starves until she can starve no longer. She gives in to the red alert, which by now is at overkill levels. She engages in a free-for-all, as demonstrated by the Minnesota men who ate frenetically when allowed to "come off their diets."

Eating disorders occur when a girl has broken her body's ability to sense hunger and fullness. For this reason, experts such as psychologist Cynthia Bulik, former president of the Academy for Eating Disorders, do not advocate diets in any form.

The majority of girls diet at some point in late adolescence but let go of the intensity after a diet or two. The most puzzling aspect of this phenomenon is why *some* girls can't stop.

To solve this mystery, psychologists have had to shine a light deeper into the psyches of girls.

There are theories of what should happen during adolescence in order for healthy development to occur. A girl is supposed to face herself in these crisis moments and learn how to deal with problems, such as unrequited love. She is supposed to shine her own light inside, take a good look at what is there, and come up with her own answers about who she is, accepting that a crush she develops may not be reciprocated. Then she might start experimenting with other ways to behave. She could even find tools other than food to deal with life's increasingly complex problems.

But by turning to an eating disorder, she is sidestepping the necessary inner work of adolescence to develop a healthy response. The great risk is that as time passes, and she reaches early adulthood and beyond, her eating disorder may wax and wane, but inevitably remain—because she has never accomplished the goals of adolescent development. Even as she ages, she remains a girl on the inside. For her, true womanhood is elusive.

>>> Jenny on the Runway

Jenny, age 32, is the niece of fashion icon Ralph Lauren. As such, she lives with an impossible legacy. She tells of it in her memoir, *Homesick*, a graphic self-portrait fashioned around anorexia and bulimia. She traces the beginning of her illness to her modeling debut at the premiere of Ralph Lauren's Little Girls fashion line.

Dolled up in gray flannel Bermudas and a purple Shetland sweater, her hair partly swept up, Jenny swaggered down the runway, 7 years old, pouty and seductive. She gave the audience an angelic vision. She was an image of opposites: in her own words, "sweet and feminine, but aloof, innocent but cultured, irresistible but unapproachable, and very, very dramatic."

Her father, head of Men's Design at Polo Ralph Lauren, was so proud. Her famous uncle was awestruck. After the show, Ralph Lauren told his brother that Jenny "was the most beautiful creature he had ever laid eyes on."

A girl goddess.

She never forgot that moment, or the urge to re-create it. She tried to, many times, first through lessons three times a week at the Harkness Ballet School in New York City. Then she attended ballet camp in the Berkshires, in western Massachusetts—a jungle of competing dancers. Finally, the pressure to have the perfect body became so great so early in her life that she fought back with what amounted to a vow to starve herself.

By 10, she developed anorexia; by 15, bulimia. She entered a catastrophic cycle of bingeing and purging through vomiting, laxatives, running, gym workouts, and exercise classes. By 24, she had so abused her body that her upper bowel broke loose and wedged in the space between her vagina and her anus.

Through her twenties and into her thirties, her obsession with her body took her from doctor to doctor, through surgeries and chronic pain, hospitals and eating disorders clinics, alternative therapies and psychic healers. Underneath all these efforts lay an enduring homesickness—a longing for the sense of safety that she felt as a girl but could not re-create for herself as a young woman.

While raised under extraordinary circumstances, Jenny typifies the ordinary progression from a young healthy girl to one with a full-blown eating disorder. Hers began with a problem: how to handle the pressures of an environment highly focused on physical image. She chose a body-based solution in part because her stresses were already body-focused. She turned to dieting and exercise, an obvious answer for her. Over time, Jenny's behaviors grew so out of control that they stifled any possibility of normal adolescent development.

"When I was sick, I was very checked out," she says. "I was on vacation, let's put it that way."

Until recently, she had no energy left to put into the hard work of finding new ways to handle adult situations, such as who she was underneath the image of "girl goddess." In a dark way, her eating disorder served a purpose: by getting sick, Jenny found a way to flee the pressure and hide backstage.

But a vacation from life, however necessary for survival, does not solve the larger issue of identity development during adolescence. This takes place through a series of tasks. If completed, they will allow a girl to find out who she is and how that persona will manifest itself in the world.

To understand what is going wrong when an eating disorder disrupts psychological development—and why some teenagers get them and others do not—it is helpful to explore what normal development looks like.

DISCOVERING WHO I AM:
THE MAJOR TASK OF ADOLESCENCE

Developmental psychologist Erik Erikson described adolescence as a singular and intense phase in the overall development of a child. By this time, the healthy child has developed trust, autonomy, initiative, and the ability to be productive. Adolescence is the next step. But it is by no means a simple one. It is a battle, the last stand of childhood.

A teenager senses that new responsibilities are arriving. This is nothing new. When she was younger, she first developed by experiencing new demands: for example, her parents wanted her to crawl, walk, then ride a bike; her teachers encouraged her to read. The girl experienced her parents' and teachers' wishes as subtle imperatives. She reacted to these and her own internal drive by trying out new behaviors. The ones that worked, she kept. Others, she discarded. In this way, she developed.

And then she hits adolescence. It is as if someone has come along and raised her developmental bar by an order of magnitude. Everything begins changing at once, and the changes do not always move in sync. Her body grows in spurts. Sexual maturation begins. Her mind develops rationality and abstraction. Because of this, the world beyond her family opens up. She begins to recognize the vast culture out there and its often conflicting values. She is measuring herself against these observations and getting frustrated when they contradict what she senses inside herself.

To become a healthy woman, this girl has to complete a mission: she has to develop an identity, a self that abides no matter what form the outer body takes or what circumstances shape its world.

There are girls who really struggle with this task. They become extremely vulnerable. A fragile teen can take her struggle with identity out on her body. She is the girl who turns to dieting, exercise, or more extreme behaviors as a stopgap for her developmental shortcomings. Her body dissatisfaction, a common component of adolescence, is evolving into disease.

Why does it happen to her?

NATURE VERSUS NURTURE:
WHO IS PREDISPOSED?

Some girls can master the daunting tasks of development. They are "sturdy souls," says Joanna Poppink, a private therapist in Los Angeles who specializes in eating disorders. "But somebody else might not be quite as sturdy and needs another way to take care of herself."

Psychologists describe her as "anxious," a "perfectionist." (With bulimia, those who are predisposed are also "impulsive.") She is a worrywart, thin-skinned. Things get to her. In a positive light, she is intelligent and driven. In a negative one, she is extraordinarily hard on herself; she does not feel worthwhile unless she accomplishes the ultimate.

To understand the mind-set, try this: imagine that a girl is eyeing a billboard showcasing the image of one of those trim, breathtakingly beautiful young women. What does she see? Is she amazed, awed by the perfection of that body? Or does she feel defeated, knowing that she will never look that way? What does she do? Go on with her life, unphased? Or does she feel a tinge of inadequacy? Maybe she skips the cream cheese on her bagel that morning.

Girls with a predisposition for an eating disorder do not get off that simply. Their nature forces them to measure up. They experience a profound internal compulsion. It is the voice of an authoritarian parent; some call it the beast within. It forces them to aim for impossible standards and, at the same time, forbids them from experimenting with other ways of being.

This combination of traits makes *her* the one who gets the eating disorder, while others, faced with the same gauntlet of adolescent challenges, simply remain unhappy with their bodies or turn to some other vice such as drinking, drug-taking, or outward-directed violence.

When psychologists talk about "predisposition," they include both genetic and psychological factors. Individuals have particular brain chemistries and innate personality styles, thought to predispose a person to an eating disorder. There are also environmental factors—how one is raised. Cynthia Bulik explains the fateful combination of genes and environment this way: "Genes load the gun; environment pulls the trigger."

So a girl is born with the genes that form her brain connections. Those create the idiosyncrasies of her personality. Her family and culture fertilize her developing mind and body. She learns to absorb all the emotional undercurrents among people in the room. Perhaps her family has reinforced the duty to please. Perhaps she is a protected child; she has not been given the chance to try things on her own; or when she has, she has been shot down with criticism. She was born, or has learned, to be terrified of making mistakes, frightened of doing so beyond the norm. She is, developmentally, a child lost in the big city, searching for her mother to take her home.

Those without an eating disorder ask, "How can someone override hunger, a drive as vital as life itself?" Fear, another biological drive, can do it. A person who faces danger will feel the urge to fight or flee before the urge to eat. It is Biology 101. A Neanderthal does not feast while it is battling a tiger.

A girl who moves from body dissatisfaction to genuine eating disorders reaches puberty at a fearful disadvantage. She already carries high anxiety. Then, when she faces the stresses of adolescent transition, boom! They pull the trigger of her genetically loaded gun. She is in the realm of fight-or-flight. She uses food to fight: *Fine, just try to make me eat.* Or she flees: *No one will expect anything of me if I am sick.*

"The eating disorder is a very creative act developed by a desperate and strong person who is fighting as hard as she can for her life," says Poppink.

When Poppink used the words "her life," she means that the girl feels like she is either "going to die or go crazy." Her sentiment bears truth. If she were to develop properly, she would lose the identity of "girl." But she does not realize that she would replace it with the positive identity of a woman.

THE EATING DISORDER, USED AS A CRUTCH

It is at this psychological crossroads that the eating disorder enters the scene. It offers to rescue this kind of girl by promising to make development easier.

But eating disorders function like a crutch for a severely broken leg, one that does not heal. The crutches support for a while, but the leg weakens. When the crutch has to go, the girl is in trouble. She cannot walk unassisted with an atrophied leg. Worse, her whole body has weakened while her leg was casted.

Just as neonatal researchers try to trace the cause of an infant's physical abnormalities back to what might have happened in the womb, so psychologists try to understand the symptoms of a patient with an eating disorder in terms of thwarted tasks in psychological development. But recovery is a painful process because it means, first of all, removing the eating disorder "crutch" to examine the underdeveloped self. Recovery also requires going back and identifying where and when the initial harm was done and then undergoing psychosurgery to repair the injuries incurred, for example, through childhood trauma, incest, or dysfunctional family dynamics.

But the focal points are quite different for every girl with an eating disorder. The behaviors she shows may appear similar enough for categorization: she starves—anorexia; she binges—binge eating disorder; she purges—bulimia. But this is simply the surface. Underneath, every girl is unique in why she chooses her eating disorder. And the places in her development that are stunted, allowing the eating disorder to develop, will also vary.

In his book *Identity and the Life Cycle,* Erikson described development of identity with words that scientists often use to talk about the physical development of an embryo in the womb.

"Anything that grows has a ground plan," he writes, and "out of this ground plan, the parts arise, each part having its special ascendancy, until all parts have arisen to form a functioning whole."

With an embryo, parts mean physical limbs and organs, the stringy spinal cord, for example, or a muscular heart. Each has a proper time when it should develop and begin to function. Each develops on its own and, if all goes according to plan, a whole, healthy baby pushes out into the world, ready to take on life.

Psychological development unfolds in the same way, albeit more invisibly. The parts of identity are more abstract. In her book *Reviving Ophelia: Saving the Selves of Adolescent Girls,* Mary Pipher describes these parts of the self as a group of interacting mini-selves. There is a physical self, made up of skin, bones, and biochemicals; an emotional self that laughs and cries; and a thinking self that analyzes and keeps it all together. There is an ambitious academic self that sometimes becomes a career self. There is a desirous sexual self, as well as a questing spiritual self. Finally, there is a social self, nurtured by family and, later, by the surrounding culture.

Each mini-self has a job that must be completed in order to propel a girl into womanhood. And the selves, while developing on their own, also have to interact in harmony to create a viable, whole self. In fact, it may be helpful to view the self-consciousness that adolescent girls often experience as girls "taking themselves apart," trying, as a puzzle, to reshape the individual pieces. Maturity, then, comes when a girl, in the context of her relationships, can reassemble the pieces into a new self-portrait, herself as a woman. But if a girl allows an eating disorder to enter, it distorts her picture and prevents it from evolving into what it could become.

An eating disorder can fit into any part of development and slowly but powerfully disrupt proper development of the whole.

HOW EATING DISORDERS DISRUPT THE TASKS OF ADOLESCENCE

Coming to Terms with the Physical Self

Normally, a teen's body changes in size, shape, structure, and chemistry. A girl shoots up. She rounds out, spreads, and softens. These physical changes do not occur all at once: her legs lengthen faster than her torso, her feet sooner than her arms, and she looks gangly, awkward. Her body begins to behave erratically.

Hormones are surging in her system. She is experiencing streams of estrogen, adding fat cells to hips, thighs, and breasts. Spurts of progesterone cramp her abdomen and blotch her face with pimples. She feels batted about by these currents of biochemistry and can't help but become preoccupied with all the ways her body is changing.

Preoccupation is normal. In fact, an adolescent girl can use it to her advantage. If she can accept her physical self as a gift and create her own ideal for herself, she will reach adulthood having redefined physical beauty on her own terms.

But some girls—in fact, most—tilt preoccupation to the negative.

"With early adolescence, girls surrender their relaxed attitudes about their bodies and take up the burden of self-criticism," writes Pipher.

Girls of this age hear external criticism and make it internal. They own it and become it and, feeling bad, try to unload it. They live in a world where accepting their physical selves is nearly impossible. Fashion magazines and music videos often dismember women's bodies with close-ups of a specific part. A $40 billion diet industry and an exploding $9.4 billion plastic surgery business send out the message: *Your body is flawed as it is. But you can achieve perfection. In fact, you must.*

"The increasing pressure to be thin and the unrealistic images portrayed in the mass media may have a devastating effect on women's self-perceptions, self-esteem, and identity development," writes researcher Sherry Turner in a paper demonstrating that viewing the covers of fashion magazines for a mere thirteen minutes can significantly lower a girl's self-esteem.

Indeed, eating disorders experts are quick to cite how culture has slimmed down the beauty ideal. From the 1960s on, for example, the average weight of a *Playboy* centerfold and a Miss America Pageant contestant has dropped steadily, compared to the weight of average American women, who are getting heavier. By 1988, nearly three-fourths of *Playboy* models and two-thirds of Miss America contestants weighed 15 percent below their expected weight for age and height.

Fifteen percent. That is the boundary between subthreshold and true anorexia nervosa. What this means is that women in their twenties and thirties today came of age with anorexic models as their ideal of beauty. The impact cannot be overstated.

Just as impressionable girls are becoming rounder, the culture is telling them that their budding physical selves are all wrong. Girls learn that they are supposed to be flatter, skinnier. They react, not surprisingly, through their physical selves.

Recent news stories now decry the emaciated state of today's top fashion runway models. Still, an estimated 42 percent of elementary school students between first and third grades want to be thinner. And 81 percent of 10-year-olds are afraid of being fat. Girls feel the effects more than boys. Even underweight girls think they are overweight, and thus hate their bodies. And body dissatisfaction has gone global, plaguing girls in Great Britain, Australia, New Zealand, Brazil, Israel, Japan, Sweden, Croatia, Mexico, Fiji, China—even in the most rural and deprived parts of South Africa.

Feeling bad about one's body leads to attempts to change it. Dieting usually comes first. Girls younger than 9 are now dieting. *Teen Magazine* reported that 35 percent of girls ages 6 to 12 have been on at least one diet.

The promotion of dieting gets a helping hand from corporate opportunists who profit handsomely from girls' insecurity. Some analysts claim that the thinning out of models over time is not accidental. By marketing ideals that are impossible to achieve and maintain, the cosmetic and diet product industries have drilled an infinite well to plumb for profits. Why not cash in on women's self-castigation? Why not instigate it?

And here, in the realm of the physical self, the eating disorder fits in snugly. It typically starts with unhealthy dieting or exercise. One diet leads to two and two leads to more. More leads to compulsion. According to the research group Anorexia Nervosa and Related Eating Disorders (ANRED), more than a third of "normal dieters" will eventually progress to unhealthy, compulsive dieting. This includes fasting, skipping meals, excessive exercise, laxative abuse, and self-induced vomiting.

Today, one of every four college-aged women uses such unhealthy methods of weight control. And so an eating disorder begins.

This is how Jenny Lauren fell into trouble. She began with an excessive preoccupation with her body that was fueled by a cultural prerogative. "I wasn't the only one taking two of Gilda's aerobics classes a day," she says. "Even today, there are women walking all over the streets of New York in their tights and leotards with nothing covering up."

But instead of looking to the models for inspiration, Jenny would do better to look at real people: photos of friends, goddess images from antiquity, women depicted in works of art, film stars of the past, and the varying naked bodies in girls' locker rooms. She could look to other aspects of herself that have nothing to do with appearance.

Jenny did look elsewhere. She made several pilgrimages to Abadiânia, Brazil, where a healer named João de Deus (John of God) sees people with ailments from all over the world. Jenny saw him, too. She also witnessed humanity, many people with broken or ailing bodies. They changed her outlook. "Barely anybody there cares what anybody else looks like," she says. "When you look in someone's eyes, there is only a warm smile. That's what enhanced my life."

Taming the Emotional Self

Parents of teenagers say, "Hormones," and other parents nod knowingly. Hormones whip a girl from calm to anxiety, from euphoria to hysteria. She is trying to deal with an emotional self so immature that minor events trigger big reactions and major events trigger a bored "Whatever."

Emotions often cause her to lose perspective.

Vassar College psychologist and neuroscientist Abigail Baird knows why. To explain it, she came up with what she calls "the ugly-sweater theory." Basically, if a seventh grader walks over to another seventh-grade girl and says, "Your sweater is, like, hideous," the day is over for the girl in the sweater. Game. Set. Match.

Baird is studying what happens in the brain during these moments when emotions swamp logic. She is creating a brain map of the teenage emotional self.

While formerly at Dartmouth, she and her assistant, graduate student Jane Viner, ran a study in which they put seventh-grade girls in magnetic resonance imaging (MRI) scanners, which measure those parts of the brain that become active under different stimuli. One group of girls looked at pictures of other girls who showed hostile facial expressions. A control group saw photos of similarly aged girls showing nonhostile facial expressions. The facial expressions pictured were meant to simulate the cattiness found in the hallways of middle school and high school hallways. After the girls saw the photos, they completed surveys about how they were feeling about themselves.

As expected, Baird found that girls who viewed the negative photos scored lower on surveys of self-esteem than the control group. More enlightening, Baird could actually see what this self-loathing looked like in MRI images of the girls' brains. The amygdalan areas of the brain, which govern emotions, were stimulated in girls who viewed the negative photos. Meanwhile, the prefrontal cortex, which controls higher-order thinking, did not light up as intensely. Girls who viewed the photos of nonhostile girls did not show these same brain patterns.

This suggests that girls confronted by "mean girls" are swamped by their emotional selves. They lose the rational pieces of their mind, literally, and thus, struggle with feeling bad about themselves.

Emotions buffet and mislead a young mind, but some girls manage to hang on. They ride the turbulence and land on the opposite shore of adulthood, worn and torn, but pulsing and breathing. Others do not.

As psychologist Charlotte Kasl explains in her book *If the Buddha Got Stuck*, a girl has to learn how to sit with painful feelings and ride them like rapids. As her emotions are flooding in, she has to hold fast to herself and say, again and again, this, too, will pass. She has to engage other parts of herself to help tame her emotions. For example, by developing her thinking self, a woman can work toward balancing her emotional self.

But if she cannot achieve that balance, an eating disorder offers a seductive but false solution. Again and again, experts say that women use their eating behaviors to temper or soothe powerful emotions: Binges squelch feelings of depression, anxiety, stress, and boredom. Anorexia numbs all feeling. Bulimia gives a high through bingeing and a catharsis through purging. A girl with an eating disorder uses these behaviors to manage her emotions, but in doing so, she never develops healthier management skills. She will go through life with the deficit, often returning to her eating behaviors as a default, unless she is willing to develop other coping tools.

Discriminating and Reining in the Thinking Self

Teens often do not reason, and often, one cannot reason with them. In developmental terms, only the brightest adolescents are moving forward into "formal operational thought." This is a style of thinking that emphasizes logic, problem solving, and the idea that there are many solutions to any one problem. For example, an adolescent gets a D on her essay about Shakespeare's *Hamlet*. Her reaction is, *My teacher hates my guts,* as opposed to *I should go ask my teacher why she gave me the low grade.*

In addition to such unreasoned responses, most adolescents have not yet developed the capacity for balanced assessment; they tend to think in extremes. *Everyone hates me.* Or, *Everyone loves me.*

Adolescents also tend to overgeneralize. One event, one offhand comment, becomes a prognosis, good or bad. If she fails one test, then from now on she will fail *every* test. In fact, she now deems herself a *total failure* after one bad test score. As the irrational thinking picks up steam, she thinks, *Why should I study? I am just going to fail anyway.*

This is extrapolating an entire future from one negative moment. Most teenagers will do it. Then, as the moment changes, their entire reality also changes. It looks psychotic—and doctors would consider the behavior to be so if it were happening to an adult. But it is normal in adolescence; in fact, there is evidence for this unwieldy thought process in studies of the brain.

In their work with girls' brains and emotions, researchers Baird and Viner wanted to find out whether a thinking self could be used to temper an emotional self. The researchers came up with a ten-week course that taught girls how to cope with aggression in relationships. The course consisted of worksheets, role-playing, and other exercises to help seventh-grade girls understand their emotions better.

After giving half the girls the course—the other half had a study period for a comparable amount of time—Viner brought the two groups of girls back to the MRI scanners. In a repeat of the original studies that mapped out the brain on emotional overload, girls who had not taken the ten-week course and saw photos of "mean girls" again showed robust brain activity in the amygdala and other brain regions known to elicit emotions.

But girls who had taken the course showed a different response. In addition to the emotional centers of the brain, these girls activated thinking regions of the brain, areas known to rein in impulsiveness. According to Baird, the girls had "acquired some new cognitive strategies."

And they felt better about themselves, as measured by surveys of self-esteem.

Thus, one task of the thinking self is to temper the emotional self. A girl has to find the real message in what is happening to her in the moment. She has to apply logic: *There will be other tests that can help me boost my grade back up.* Or she can brainstorm alternate explanations: *My D could be the result of the all-nighter that I pulled to write the paper.* Or she might come up with alternate solutions, such as, *I'll ask my teacher for tutoring.*

But a certain girl, the one who develops an eating disorder, never gets to this level of thinking. She stays at the all-or-nothing phase of extremes. In fact, her eating disorder is an expression of her immature thinking patterns: she is either starving—eating nothing— or bingeing—eating all. She cannot find the middle ground, a skill of a more mature woman.

Venturing Out with the Academic and Career Self

As girls reach adolescence, many of them bury their academic selves. Boys tease or ignore girls for many reasons: competition, insecurity, or lack of understanding, to name a few. She boils this down to *If I'm too smart, he won't like me.* And being liked means everything at this age. Added to this, popular girls will label a smart girl as a "brainiac" and shut her out of social circles. Fearing this kind of shunning, many girls going into high school willfully dumb down their academic selves.

Researchers are still trying to piece together exactly why. Pipher points out that girls tend to thrive in smaller cooperative environments. Girls would rather maintain their friends than compete for a deserved award.

Enter math, science, and problem solving—skills that are becoming more important in an increasingly tech-savvy world. Studies show that teachers teach these subjects and skills differently to boys and girls. For example, when students hit a snag in problem solving, teachers tend to rescue girls, while they encourage boys to figure their way out. Teachers may think they are helping girls in this way, but by providing the extra help, a teacher may actually be doing harm. Research shows that giving too much help fosters dependency and undermines mathematical confidence. Girls who experience extra attention often walk out of their math and science classes unsure of themselves.

This practice has repercussions as girls move into their twenties and venture into the workplace. They experience stark gender gaps in pay and opportunity. In 2004, for example, female executives and managers, including chief executive officers and chief financial officers, earned only 70 percent as much as their male counterparts. Female attorneys made less then three-fourths of male lawyers' incomes. Female doctors and judges earned only half as much as their male counterparts. The disparities go on, from architects to biochemists to entertainers. This sends a sobering message to teenage girls, who are trying to stitch together their new academic selves. They hear "Just Do It" from Nike, but when they take a job, they soon realize that they cannot "just do it," at least not at a pay scale on a par with men.

Some women react in anger. Others pull back, choosing to fight what they see as failure by *not* trying. Erikson notes that entering a world of limited opportunity can damage the formation of healthy self-esteem. In order to develop a healthy academic self, and perhaps a vital career self, a teenager will have to let her intelligence and ambition shine. She will have to balance the desire to fit in with the desire to succeed. She will have to identify what success means to her and start drawing from her other selves to achieve that. Tapping her thinking self, for example, she maps a strategy for a career plan. Her emotional self can guide her by genuinely responding to internal cues about her likes and dislikes. She will have to find teachers and mentors to help her overcome the obstacles hindering her success. She will have to find her own voice to speak out about what she wants to achieve.

Some girls, like Christine, never seem to make it.

>>> Christine's Disillusionment and Her Eating-Disordered Solution

As far back as she could remember, Christine, age 34, had wanted to be president of the United States. In fact, her high school classmates introduced her as the future president when she gave her graduation speech as valedictorian.

She had a plan: She would go to college, double-major in English and political science, go on to law school, then practice law for a year. After that, she would run for the House of Representatives and the Senate. She would get appointed chief of staff to the current president of the United States, and wrap it all up with a rousing presidential campaign of her own.

She got as far as college in Arizona, where she worked on Dan Quayle's presidential campaign in Scottsdale.

"Then I woke up," she says.

She witnessed the disingenuousness, backstabbing, and economics of real politics. They disgusted her. "It's all about who can raise the most money," she says.

Having lost her young girl's dream, she floundered. She took on a series of minimum-wage jobs, including one at a gym. One of the patrons told her about a part-time job writing for the San Francisco Giants' new website. Bright and eager, Christine got the job. But as she began working, she experienced discrimination from players, scouts, and managers, who badgered her with questions that showed doubt about her abilities.

Meanwhile, Christine earned a spot on the show *Who Wants to Be a Millionaire?* She became the only female contestant in her group and, at 28, by far the youngest. Confident, she flew out to New York and envisioned herself a winner. But as she played the game, being filmed for millions of viewers, she choked; she hit her buzzer less than a second after another contestant hit his. She came home humiliated, suffering her loss in a deeply personal way.

"I saw myself on TV and thought, 'You are a big fat loser,'" she recalls.

So she joined Weight Watchers and, after officially quitting at 5 feet, 4 inches and 117 pounds, she began a steady slide into anorexia for the first time ever in her life. Spring training season rolled around and Christine returned to the Giants weighing 87 pounds.

"Everyone looked at me, especially the scouts, and their jaws dropped," she recalls.

One man even asked her if she had cancer. When she said no, he replied, "But you lost a whole person."

She had. And she kept losing more, right up until she entered treatment at Remuda Ranch in Wickenburg, Arizona. "I was definitely gone," she says of that time. "None of me was left."

Christine, with large ambitions for herself, might have overreached. Entering the real world, she was quickly disillusioned. Perhaps, as Dartmouth researchers Baird and Viner discovered, she needed to develop the rational skills to help her come up with a game plan to achieve her career goals. She needed to develop her thinking self to give her

career self its context. But it appears that she missed this developmental milestone. Instead, Christine transformed her perceived failure
to succeed at a wildly optimistic career goal into a failure of her body.
In a typical pattern, she began to diet and exercise. She seized on this
new identity as an über fit woman as a substitute for a career self. She
was good at losing weight, better than anything that she had tried
thus far. The actions rewarded and reinforced the eating disorder in
her life.

The irony of an eating disorder is that the girl who can drive herself past hunger is the same girl who can drive herself up the corporate
ladder. It's a matter of where she channels the energy.

Owning the Sexual Self

Sexuality during adolescence looks like an accident waiting to
happen. The biological self skids into other selves as teens develop
the physical but not the emotional capacity to deal with a full-
blown sexual relationship. Nature has played a dirty trick, priming
girls' bodies to bear children while they are still children themselves. In another time, and still in some cultures today, girls menstruate at a later age and have their babies shortly after the onset of
menstruation.

But in the United States, the biological self speeds far ahead of
emotional maturity, with girls menstruating far earlier than their
recent ancestors. Such physical precociousness is linked to sexual
awareness and activity at ever younger ages. Yet, according to Pipher,
girls have not yet developed their emotional and thinking capacities
to be able to negotiate a healthy relationship.

The contemporary sexual landscape is a wild place. Today, boys
and girls freely mock each other's physical characteristics, from
tongues to pubic hair to periods to prowess in oral sex. Adolescent

teasing today has reached the level of sexual harassment. It is often graphic and mean-spirited.

In a survey of 2,036 college students, aged 18 to 21, the American Association of University Women found that more than 60 percent of women had been sexually harassed. Such harassment is defined as any unwanted and unwelcome sexual behavior that interferes with one's life. Ninety percent of the students never reported these behaviors to campus authorities, even though more than half the women said that they felt self-conscious or embarrassed because of the incidents.

However, harassment may be just the first in a series of violations to the sexual self. Jay G. Silverman, director of violence prevention programs at Harvard School of Public Health, found that nearly one in five sexually experienced adolescent girls in the United States reported being physically hurt by a date in the previous year. By comparison, only one in twenty-five girls who were not sexually active reported being hurt. Dating violence is abhorrent and unacceptable. But Silverman's data show that girls experimenting with their sexuality are getting slammed harder.

In an ideal world, an adolescent girl would emerge from her parents' home to encounter an environment that nurtures her budding sexuality—defined not only as sexual behaviors like touching and intercourse, but also as attitudes and behaviors that empower her to become the lead actor in her own sexual drama. Unfortunately, such a protective sexual haven does not exist today. Girls are strutting their sexual selves in a world of insanely contradictory signals.

On one hand, religious and morality-oriented organizations flash the red light at sexuality; sex is sinful and girls must say no to preserve the sanctity of their bodies for marriage. On the other hand, the media beams the green light on sexuality, bombarding young girls with images of navels and nipples and women dressed up in gauzy frippery.

There is a word for this: objectification. It means that women become sexual objects, their bodies and sexuality linked to products that are bought and sold. Objectification steals a girl's dignity, turning her into an object for others to steal or buy. Objectification also convinces women that sexuality is tied to body appearance. The logical extension of that is not hard to imagine: sexual power translates into weight issues.

Magazines have capitalized on the connection. Looking at the covers of women-targeted magazines, one sees that messages about men and relationships are placed next to headlines about weight loss. Girls read, "50 Guys Who Want to Marry You," next to "The New Diet Drug" and "The Best Sex He Ever Had: Steal These Secrets," paired with "Remake Your Shape."

These ads are encouraging girls, and eventually young women, to find out what "men really want" rather than what their sexual selves really want. But if a girl succumbs to the messages in their contemporary context, she may lose not only her virginity but also her sexual self in the bargain.

A girl who experiences objectification has trouble shining light on her developing sexual self because she has learned that something about it is dirty. The message she has internalized is that if she shows her sexuality, then she deserves to be objectified, even abused.

In order to develop sexually in a climate of sexual danger, a teenage girl has to hang on to her sexuality, or try to recover it. To do so, she must find ways to honor her inner ripening and avoid its exploitation. She has to understand that sexuality is more than her body; it is her way of being intimate in relationships. She has to search for what her sexual self wants—perhaps relationships that are close emotionally and spiritually, as well as physically—rather than what "men really want." She has to learn how to say no when circumstances are wrong and yes when they are right.

But some girls walk into adolescence after suffering a huge blow. Sexual abuse makes girls extremely vulnerable to an eating disorder. A girl turns to eating for body reshaping to express, metaphorically, what has been done to violate her.

If a girl cannot find room to experiment with her sexual self in a safe context, she is at risk for an eating disorder. If her body has been physically or sexually violated, she is also susceptible. In a study published in the *Journal of the American Medical Association*, Silverman and colleagues found that high school girls who had been abused were three to four times more likely to take up eating-disordered behaviors such as the use of laxatives and vomiting. The same group also was more likely to use drugs or alcohol, get pregnant, or attempt suicide.

Other researchers have suggested that eating disorders work to numb the rage and other intense feelings stemming from abuse. If a girl has no means to process what has happened to her and to reclaim her stolen sexual self, she will bury her feelings. However, they will not disappear. They will percolate below the surface, rising up unbidden. And when they do, the eating disorder will flare up. An eating disorder can serve as an escape, a pacifier, a distraction— even a narcotic. Bingeing on food and overdoing athletic workouts produces a high that takes a girl out of her emotional self.

>>> Jody's Story of Abuse

Jody was molested from age 3 to age 16 by her older brother. In one of the more graphic and heartbreaking cases of eating disorders, she became both promiscuous and bulimic.

While her brother crept into her bed night after night, she felt both invaded and aroused. Her sexual self had been awakened, but too early and in the wrong way. The result was an unhealthy split in her sexual self. Jody felt conflicted: she wanted to "turn on" sexually and to repress her sexual feelings. At 8, she did the latter by bingeing and purging. Boxes of donuts, slabs of cake, and then trips to the bathroom to vomit it all up.

Her mother knew about the bulimia. She saw it happening. But she did nothing, except to tell Jody that if she continued, she would get fat. Jody's mother also denied the sexual abuse when Jody, at 16, finally spilled her secret. Instead, Jody's mother accused her of lying, and from that Jody learned that her sexual self was shameful, to be put away and never talked about.

But "dirty" emotions remained, rooted in her psyche. She turned her anger at her family into an eating disorder.

Jody's words to describe her feelings are graphic, fierce, and tortured. They are not pleasant. Nonetheless, they poignantly express the distortion of thinking and the destruction to the self that is possible when a girl is sexually molested.

Every time her brother touched her, she says, "I wanted to spit puke out of my vagina into his face. But my vagina would not do that. It was turned on instead of turning off. My body was violating me. So I spit puke out of my throat instead."

Eventually, Jody discovered cocaine. It worked even better as a mind-numbing strategy. And she lost weight as a bonus. It was only at age 42, when she entered a rehabilitation facility, that she was able to get "clean" from her drug and eating habits.

To work through her issues, she first had to set aside her crutch. Then she had to face her emotional self. She did this during rehabilitation, where therapists gave her a safe place to express her feelings. Counselors also helped Jody to develop a thinking self, with tools to discriminate between destructive and fulfilling intimate relationships. Jody has learned how to determine who is a kind and gentle partner and who is not. She has learned to assess the difference between danger and excitement in sexual situations. And she has grown more comfortable within her physical body, a body whose natural sexual sensations no longer fill her with guilt.

Finding Meaning Within the Spiritual Self

The character of Harry Potter touches a cultural nerve. His story and all such fiction built around knights and wizards and magic fill a void, a longing that first opens up in adolescence. This longing is a quest for deeper meaning in life. Teens start looking for answers to the big questions: *Why am I here? Why does suffering happen in the world?* This is the realm of the spiritual self. A teenage girl wants to understand, at the deepest level, that she is part of something much larger than her self. And sometimes when she gains that understanding, it is at a gut level.

She may love the exuberant sensation of being absorbed into something larger: rock concerts with other people gyrating around her; iPods drowning out sounds of the real world in favor of throbbing rhythms and shocking lyrics. She may build an alternate reality through instant messaging and chat rooms. Or she may embrace ideologies, embracing causes and "isms"—environmentalism, human rights activism, feminism, vegetarianism. She may even try religious exploration, embracing the practices of her family; or she may rebel and seek belonging in an alternative cultlike group.

But problems can emerge if an individual overidentifies with any particular group. A vulnerable teen, one prone to an eating disorder, tends to conform at the expense of her own internal self. Or she will let the group tell her who she is without doing the hard work of her own discovery.

How this relates to eating disorders can be seen in the Internet-driven subculture of those who have anorexia or bulimia. There the disease takes on the force of a religious doctrine. "Pro-ana" (for anorexia) and "pro-mia" (for bulimia) websites have cropped up to establish solidarity around having an eating disorder. In fact, the trend is spreading, according to researcher Anna Bardone-Cone. In preliminary work, she has counted more than four hundred pro–eating disorder websites.

Girls who identify with and participate in these sites attempt to "transcend" their culture, setting themselves above all others as the starving, self-abusing saints of old once did. The saints had God as their pinnacle. Girls with eating disorders today have no such higher ideal guiding their actions. So identification with the group, a natural sentiment in adolescence, goes horribly awry.

Instead, girls have to do their own soul-searching. They have to find the behaviors that make larger statements to the world—for example, eating no meat, an action that may say, *I don't agree with exploiting animals.* They have to find teachers, spiritual directors, or groups that help them make sense of injustices. They have to understand that the world can be a safe, meaningful place.

Authenticating the Social Self in the Family

Just as parents hold up a toddler when she takes her first steps, a family can support a young girl taking her first steps into the world. There is a push-pull to this. Too much help from parents, and the child fails for lack of opportunity. Too little help, and she falters for lack of resources.

Given either too much or too little attention from parents, a teenager will lose confidence as she strikes out to develop her social self. She is at the place in her life where friends' opinions often hold more sway than those of family. At the same time, peers can alienate, frustrate, or torment her. Other relationships may not work like the familiar family dynamics she is used to. Teachers can play favorites, for example. Bosses can fire her on the spot.

She is confused about how to behave in all these new relationships. But wanting to be independent, she stubbornly hides the truth: she is afraid to be out in the world, so she picks fights with her parents or siblings. These confrontations can signal that she is hanging on to her parents while appearing not to. These fights may even help her save face, particularly if conducted in front of her friends.

Constant fighting can also mean that her parents are hanging on too tightly. If she feels that her parents are limiting her options, if she realizes that she is being asked to repeat what her parents have done or to enact their dreams without being allowed to find her own, she will rebel. Conflict can also be a means of asking her parents to let her go.

According to Pipher, girls today are pressured to abandon their families and join their peers at a time when they may need their parents' guidance the most. When girls venture out into the world, often it really is too much for their adolescent psyches to handle. Culture bombards adolescents with junk images and mixed messages about body and sexuality. Gender rules are ambiguous and changing. The social self wobbles more often today than in decades past, in part because of the whims and pressures of mass media. Parents are caught, sensing that their teenagers need help but also feeling uncertain about how much or what kind of help to give.

To develop her social self, a girl has to learn balance. She has to move from *dependence* to *interdependence* with her parents. As she learns this skill at home, she can apply it to her peers and other relationships outside her family.

This does not mean completely cutting off her family. If she detaches before she is truly ready, she will either re-create immature attachments to others she meets or remain attached to her parents in darker ways, through fighting or rebellion. The goal is to take little steps toward interdependence, just as a near-toddler lets go of her mother and walks three steps toward a new support at the coffee table. As her social self strengthens, a girl will be able to take more steps until she has developed a mature social self.

>>> Molly's Food Fight Against Her Parents' Prohibitions

Molly, 40, grew up in a Montana household in which her parents forbade almost everything except crunchy organic fare. In her parents' view, eating Oreos was the equivalent of "masturbating on the kitchen table." The minute sugar entered the house, Molly's parents tightened their lips and pitched the offending granules into the trash.

But even the strictest prohibitions could not keep out a culture flooded by junk food. Molly's girlfriends happily fed her Lays potato chips and sugar-laden Pixie Stix. She ate like a prisoner just released from a concentration camp.

She ate and gained weight. Her parents noticed and cut back further on her diet at home. Molly, in turn, began sneaking forbidden foods. This evolved into bingeing, and as she grew heavier and her parents criticized her weight more, she turned to routine vomiting. She binged and purged so rabidly that, at times, she became hoarse from the rawness in her throat.

Molly used food to fight in the most literal sense. But the deeper battle was a struggle to assert a social self in need of independence.

Molly was not independent. Because of her parents' food-choice encroachments, she had not developed her own skills at balancing food cravings and satiation. Her immaturity followed her to college, where her eating got so out of control that she gained 30 pounds in six months and had to quit school after one semester.

After that 1982 fall semester, Molly moved back with her parents and worked at a series of low-paying jobs—from fast-food service to shelving books at the public library. She drifted that way until 1989, when she boarded a plane for France. At 24, she landed at Charles de Gaulle International Airport in Paris—no job, a little money, and no knowledge of French. She was convinced that a place as "magical as Paris" would sweep away her eating disorder and give her a place in the world.

The strategy backfired. Molly ate and threw up on the steps of the Opéra just as easily as she did in the bathroom at the Missoula Public Library. In fact, her bulimia erupted with far more extreme modes in France; the food was enticing. Yet, on a subconscious level, Molly was using her bulimia as a way to avoid social maturity.

"Without bulimia, I don't think I could have done it," she says, referring to her two years in France. "Because at the end of the day, after figuring out how to get home on the right bus, the only thing on my mind was, *Where can I get some food and where can I throw up?"*

Bulimia promised to coddle her social self, out there in the world without her parents. But the eating disorder eventually became her parent: harsh and unforgiving.

As a testament to the impact of an overprotective family on an identity, young women with eating disorders often get angry or "divorce" themselves from their families as they recover. This is one way of working out the separation that should have occurred much earlier in adolescence. The eating disorder has served as parent, and must fall away, just as the parents' roles as protector and nurturer should fall away as a young woman learns how to take care of herself.

This shedding of a worn-out paradigm happened to Molly, at age 31, after she checked into Ballard Medical Center in Seattle, Washington. Although her parents were initially supportive and helped her pay for treatment, they did not come to the hospital to attend a program for families. In fact, after Molly told them that she was entering therapy, they never spoke to her again. Now, almost ten years later, her mother and father still refuse even to answer her letters. Her parents live a mere 60 miles away.

Molly's parents controlled too much, just as Jody's parents provided too little. Yet Molly sees a silver lining to her parents' exit from her life. She found that she could do the work of recovery unimpeded by their criticism. She also engaged the help of a therapist, who advised with a kinder maternal voice. In this way, the therapist was like a temporary mother to Molly's redeveloping social self.

For example, the therapist taught Molly about the link between dieting and bingeing. Molly listened and was able to begin her recovery by stopping the dieting. Next, the therapist taught Molly how to use her mind to moderate her emotional self. She had to fill her kitchen with her favorite binge foods—$200 worth of Häagen Dazs ice cream, M&M's, and, of course, Oreo cookies—and had to live with them in her home, eating only a few at a time, no bingeing, no purging. Before long, her real self had started making the rules.

"To this day, when I open my fridge and see chocolate in there and ice cream, I just grin," she says, "because I can't believe it can live in there and not yank me in."

But it does live there, and she lives with it, in balance.

Authenticating the Social Self in the World

Finally, the girl goes out into the world. Erikson says that in order for a girl to reach her potential, her developing self must know that it can master its environment outside the family. She has to feel that her options are wide open. She has to believe she has an equal shot at achieving what she wants. If there are cultural messages that limit her potential, a girl—particularly one astute enough to know she is limited—will flounder, no matter how resilient her other developing selves.

The environment in the United States does not support this social development. In fact, U.S. culture discourages girls from becoming their authentic selves. For example, the culture does not encourage the emotional self to express anger. A girl may cry but not lash out. And the culture frowns upon her sexual self. She may bleach her hair blonde and sway her hips cutely, but what would happen if she wanted to discuss a subject such as masturbation, which is taboo in the cultural mainstream? Our culture limits her academic self. She may get a doctorate in computer science, but not earn a salary equal to that of her male counterpart.

In other cultures, the prohibitions on women are even greater. The news is full of stories about women being silenced, having their faces covered, being married off as children, being raped by husbands, being stoned and slain for reasons having to do with gender.

In short, much of culture obliterates parts of girls' selves. A girl without a strong social self responds to the imperatives by boxing up those offending pieces and stowing them away in a psychological attic. The situation is worsened when a culture is too restrictive or at odds with a girl's developing sense of self; the girl may rebel as if she has an authoritarian parent. Girls growing up in cultures in transition or as the daughters of immigrants often experience clashes in values: their mothers adhere to traditional values while they try to embrace new ones.

Perhaps the most striking global illustration of this dynamic has come from anthropologist and psychiatrist Anne Becker's work with teenage girls in Nadroga, Fiji. In 1995, the village chief introduced television into the village. Within three years, almost a third of the girls had developed eating disorders, wanting to diet, vomit, or exercise excessively. More than 11 percent of those surveyed became fully bulimic. The majority, 83 percent of the girls surveyed, blamed their change in attitude on the media.

While it would be easy to blame this startling change on "culture," Becker, who is now director of the Adult Eating and Weight Disorders Program at Massachusetts General Hospital in Boston, investigated the problem further. She noted that the country is undergoing a dramatic shift from an agrarian to a Westernized economy. Fijian girls want to go to work. Employment as a flight attendant on Air Pacific is a dream job. These girls cannot rely on their mothers to help them navigate the new cultural terrain, so they are turning to TV characters for a blueprint of how to make it, equating her body shape with her power as a woman of the world.

"I want to be like Xena so that I can protect myself by getting all those manly skills," says one Fijian girl. "When I come across some kind of different, difficult situations, I can just use them in order to defend myself."

This situation echoes that of young women in the United States in the early 1970s. American girls at the time were faced with new opportunities in the world but had few skills or female mentors to guide them, including their mothers. Kim Chernin, in her book

The Hungry Self, writes that this generation of mothers had been schooled in "femininity," using appearances to please others. Girls who experienced this collectively had more trouble developing their social selves and therefore their whole selves.

"The present epidemic of eating disorders must be understood as a profound developmental crisis in a generation of women still deeply confused . . . about what it means to be a woman in the modern world," Chernin writes.

Thus, developing a cultural self, in this context, means not only developing a physical self apart from fashion images of models, actresses, and ballerinas, but also realizing a desire to succeed. Girls want to have a voice in their societies. If society will not let them, the result can be an eating disorder, a weapon against oppression.

>>> *Paola Straddles Two Opposing Cultures*

Paola, age 35, is a smart girl, bright enough to become a lawyer in Brazil, where doors were once closed to female attorneys. While cities like São Paulo, where Paola lives, are experiencing a boon in job opportunities and Western-style development, rural areas are still largely traditional. This transition has been creating social tension, and Paola is trying to resolve it with purging-style anorexia.

Paola was raised during the 1980s by a stay-at-home mother who believed all women should do the same. Paola's mother was terrified by recent social changes, and she fought for her daughter's destiny like a tigress whose cub might be stolen away.

Paola brought home schoolwork marked with A's, and her mother punished her—to keep her from taking the accomplishment too far. "Too far" meant Paola would be lost to change. When Paola won awards in school, her mother beat her. When people commented that Paola was beautiful or smart, her mother called her daughter "fat" and mocked the girl's breasts.

This began the push-pull of independence and dependence. Paola dreamt of earning enough money to move out on her own—she seemed to succeed. At 11, Paola worked in a store; at 12, a preschool; at 15, a bank; and, at 17, she moved out. She went to junior college and paid her way by working at an insurance company. Later, she attended law school and apprenticed all the way into a private practice.

But dependence asserted itself in tandem: Paola developed an eating disorder. At 11, she was dieting and taking laxatives as well as her mother's diuretics, prescribed for a heart condition. By 12, she was vomiting as well. At 15, she had dropped from 117 pounds to 93. The doctors initially missed the diagnosis because Paola also had a kidney problem. This masked the fact that purging, laxatives, and diuretics were throwing off electrolyte levels in her body.

At 24, Paola experienced a potassium deficiency so severe that she fell into a coma. But she recovered and, at age 26, she was back at work. In fact, she was invited to run the São Paola branch of her firm's law office, a job she enjoys and the only pleasure she claims she has today.

But Paola keeps mainly to herself. She does not date and continues with symptoms of anorexia and bulimia, even after her hospitalization for coma. She is currently going for therapy as an outpatient at PROATA, one of two public eating disorders clinics in São Paulo.

Her parents have talked with counselors in the program, and while her mother seems more reasonable, Paola feels guilty about her success and remains a product of the culture in which she was raised.

"When I am accomplishing, I feel like I am being bad or hurting someone," she says. "Purging feels like penance for accomplishing things."

In her book *The Drama of the Gifted Child*, Alice Miller writes that girls are often forced to choose between being authentic and being loved. By being punished as a child for achieving her goals, Paola was forced to make that choice. The eating disorder emerged as a solution, a means of atonement by which Paula could realize her social self. At the same time, her eating disorder numbed her emotional self and, therefore, would not let her achieve her dreams.

To heal, Paola will need to accept the idea that she can be both successful in the workplace and loved. She is just beginning that task with the help of her therapists at PROATA. This culture, with a different set of values, is helping Paola grow a new self. She is beginning to balance her professional and emotional selves rather than having one fight against the other.

The runway from adolescence to the adult world is clearly perilous. A girl with a certain predisposition tends to hit a bump and trip. But even if she does stumble or fall, she is not doomed. As an adult woman in recovery, she can climb back up, brush herself off, and resume her task of growing up. Then she can look back at the impediments that tripped her up; she can better understand the various problems that caused her disease.

This chapter has taken those pieces apart, using real-life cases of girls with eating disorders as illustrations. A young woman can undertake this forensic examination of her own life. In discovering the deficits, she can start to develop personal understanding, as Jody, Molly, and Paola have done while in therapy. While that development is progressing, a girl can draw from parts of herself that are stronger to balance out those that are weaker. Jody turned to her social self in a therapeutic community to heal her abused sexual self. Molly employed her thinking self to help repair wounds in her family social self. Paola focused on her accomplishments, her career self, to help her deal with cultural conflicts. If a girl is willing to work at these tasks, she can take a second walk down the runway. But being older, she can do it as a woman, all dressed up as her real self.

3

Young Adulthood

She, He, and It:
A Lover's Triangle

A woman with an eating disorder meets a man and falls in love. The couple decides to live together. As she packs up her things for the movers, she dwells upon her prized possession: a silver tea set given to her by her late grandmother. She wants to keep it close because it reminds her of sharing scones and secrets on those special late afternoons so long ago. So she wraps the precious tea set in soft clothes and carries it around in a backpack.

She cannot let it go.

Then the woman's partner arrives with his belongings and asks what's inside the backpack. She says, "Something personal." And he waits for her to say more. But she does not. He does not press her; after all, partners want their space. But over time he becomes jealous of this thing that she holds so close but will not tell him about. He never dares to open the backpack because he is afraid of what he might find and what the finding might do to change their relationship. The backpack sits between them unopened.

. . .

The transition from individual identity to intimacy is all about shedding baggage—even deeply held attitudes. It's about a woman adapting the norms of her childhood to the home she is trying to create with her partner. It is also about learning new ways to adjust to this new reality of togetherness.

Yet letting go of the past can be painful. This is why an adolescent shies away from intimacy. She is not ready for it. Insecure and not yet sure of her identity, she wants to hang on to some semblance of her childhood. In such cases, an adolescent self will be able to go only so far in a relationship with a potential partner. The relationship cannot be one of equals.

However, as a healthy teen completes the tasks of adolescence, she becomes more confident. She begins to reach out toward friendship, teamwork, leadership, love, and inspiration. She desires this closeness. In fact, the desire begins long before sexual relations do. Intimacy starts with substitutes for love—endless talk at slumber parties, emoting in chat rooms, discussing plans, wishes, and expectations in long phone conversations. The goal is to define oneself in words and ideas. In this way, she makes her new concept of herself tangible and unveils it to the world.

"It is only after a reasonable sense of identity has been established that real intimacy with the other sex is possible," writes Erik Erikson.

And then a woman meets a man.* They believe in their match. They agree on certain things, especially that life is better together than apart. Maybe they decide to enter into a committed partnership; they achieve what Erikson refers to as "genitality," defined as "the capacity to develop climactic mutuality." Perhaps they move in together, or marry.

---

* For the purposes of simplicity and due to the paucity of information about homosexual couples, "partner" in this chapter will be referred to as male.

With these changes, the woman's identity has to shift. She quickly realizes that the rules of a single woman do not always apply, and that she will have to discard the ones that no longer work. At the same time, she will have to master a whole new set of skills, negotiating, compromising, and realizing her needs in the context of her partner's needs. Overall, she will take on a new identity of "significant other" or "wife" and integrate this into her previous sense of self.

THE EATING DISORDER AS PRIMARY LOVER

A woman with an eating disorder cannot do this. First, she did not define her identity in late adolescence. Insecure and perhaps even ashamed of her arrested development, she may hide her underdeveloped self, seeking out only superficial interpersonal relations. She may try relationships with various partners, and fail at true intimacy again and again. Or she may pursue a relationship, hoping that her partner will do her "inner work" for her.

"Tell me who I am," she begs her partner. "Am I pretty? Am I smart? What do you like about me? Will you love me forever?"

Her partner may try to do her bidding, answering the questions, hoping not to make a mistake. But he will undoubtedly fail because he cannot tell her who she is. At the same time, her constant demands make him feel burdened and overwhelmed.

So this becomes a love story about a woman who is already stalled or stuck in development and a man who is grappling with his own dreams and developmental issues. They bring themselves to the table, as all couples do, and ask, "Your needs or mine? Whose take precedence? How do we decide?"

But there is something else that makes this negotiation impossible: her eating disorder. It has helped her in the past by giving her a purpose. Getting and staying thin is her goal. In focusing on that, she feels in control, full, and safe. Still, the eating disorder has shut a door on explorations of who she *can be*. If she cannot grow, she cannot evolve *with* her new partner. She is stuck. And he is forced to fit into the narrow confines of her life.

What kind of relationship do they create?

That depends on the nature of the eating disorder and the couple living with it. Some women bring to the relationship an eating disorder that they acquired as teenagers. Others may simply bring an unformed self—and an eating disorder yet to be realized. Or a woman may come to the partnership partially recovered. *I no longer have my symptoms; I am not throwing up. I weigh enough. So what's the problem?*

The issue is that the eating disorder is kicking in or gaining momentum, and because of its power, it is likely to win out as her primary lover. Her relationship with food starts competing with her relationship with him. And if she feels that she can depend on it more than on him, as is often the case, they move into a perverted triangle: she, he, and it. The eating disorder stands between them, blocking intimacy.

As with any love triangle, she may try to juggle a commitment to her disorder along with a professed commitment to her partner. She may do that for the duration of the relationship, bringing on jealousy, shouting, fights, and silent passive-aggressive warfare.

In the end, she must choose. If she opts for the eating disorder, the relationship will fall apart or subsist for years on a superficial level. But if she opts for him, she has a daunting task: she must let go of the eating disorder. This is the only act that will allow the relationship to breathe, to animate.

THE PARTNERSHIP CAN TRIP THE EATING DISORDER

Researchers are now looking more closely at the dynamics of couples in which one partner has an eating disorder, and this scrutiny has revealed an entirely new dynamic. When an eating disorder sits in the middle of a marriage, it may not be because the woman is bringing it to the relationship; rather, the relationship is bringing the eating disorder to her. Bad relationships or even the external stresses of partnership—who moves where for whose job, for example—can tip a fragile woman toward eating issues that help her cope.

As more and more married women with eating disorders are showing up in therapists' offices, marriage counselors are contemplating not only how the eating disorder is affecting the relationship, but also how the relationship is affecting, and sometimes triggering, an eating disorder.

Not surprisingly, researchers are now looking to couples counseling as an avenue of treatment, along with individual therapy. The idea is to help women sort through their unresolved issues, and to allow men to sort through their baggage as well. If together they can find and use therapy and communication tools to build their relationship, they can salvage what is necessary and leave behind what is not.

The dynamics are complex and best understood by looking at them from three different perspectives: hers, his, and theirs. The goal is to understand what each partner is bringing to the relationship, what each had hoped to get from the other, and, ultimately, how the eating disorder can be taken out of the partnership. If together they can do this, the couple has a chance not only to survive but also to thrive in a new relationship built on true intimacy.

FROM HER PERSPECTIVE

A woman with an eating disorder, one who is partially recovered or perhaps on the brink of healing, comes to a relationship in an adolescent phase of her psychological development. She is weighing the prospect of a partner, not yet having realized her true self. As a result, she acts in one of several ways: She may choose someone whom she hopes will correct or compensate for her adolescent deficits. Or she may subconsciously select a partner who re-creates negative patterns from her youth. In another scenario, she may deify a lover, making him into some fantasy figure who will save her. If she has not yet individuated in a healthy way from her parents, chances are that she will try to re-create a parent in her partner.

This troubled woman, no matter how severe her eating disorder, falls into one of a handful of categories. What follows are descriptions of the potential patterns that weave through her primary relationship. These are by no means clear-cut: a woman may find parts of herself in each category. But overall, the descriptions will help illuminate why a woman with an eating problem is behaving as she is with her partner, and why she chose him in the first place.

The Loner, Harboring Her Secret

With eating disorders, "the whole thing is based on secrets and denial," says Lucene Wisniewski, clinical director of the Cleveland Center for Eating Disorders in Ohio.

Hide your food in the napkin. Brush your teeth when you are done vomiting. Put him off the scent.

And the deepest secret: *If he gets to know me, he will stop liking me because I am never going to be enough.*

For one category of woman, the loner, entering into a relationship means exposing this and all of her secrets. She figures that it is better to keep to the surface, which, if she works hard enough, can at least make her *appear* perfect. This type of woman may be willing to date but usually forgoes a partnership, assuming that it is better to be alone than to be exposed as struggling with intimacy.

Studies show that the kind of girl with an eating disorder who makes this choice tends to have restricting anorexia, that is, anorexia in which a person starves but does not purge. For example, Finnish researchers found that girls with anorexia dated less and had less interest in doing so than those who had bulimia. In another study of 193 patients, twice as many married women with eating disorders had bulimia as opposed to restricting anorexia. The message here is that fewer women with anorexia tend to marry as compared to those with bulimia.

Why? Perhaps restricting food is merely a metaphor for how she inhibits herself in many other areas of her life, sensuality included. Studies show that girls who have anorexia have more negative attitudes toward sexuality than girls with bulimia. Indeed, women with eating disorders, anorexia in particular, hate the sensation of being touched.

"She does not want anyone to touch her 'fat,'" says David Herzog. For her, fat is a metaphor for self. She is afraid that he will come close and palpate, *feel* disgust, loathing her in the same way that she already loathes herself.

Another reason for the inhibition: the act of starving changes the body, blunting the neurochemicals that control sexual mood.

"If you lose weight, your libido goes in the toilet," Wisniewski says. "These women are either not having sex or faking their way through it."

And yet this woman yearns for connection. Deep down she *does* want to feel a partner stroking her body, stimulating her mind. She wants to touch him in return. Tragically, she cannot engage this way. The fear of exposure is too powerful.

Mary Pat is one of these women. At 34, she has never been on a date in her life. Abetting her problem is this reality: Mary Pat has not lived in any one place long enough to start an intimate relationship. She has moved twenty times in the last seven years. Every three months she uproots—from Ohio to Alaska, Rhode Island to North Carolina, and many places in between.

Why?

"I figure I might as well leave first before they leave me," she says.

Afraid of having people really know her, Mary Pat is avoiding intimacy. At the same time, her strategy of moving has made things worse. She is lonely—deeply, achingly isolated. To deal with that, she has developed an eating disorder, diagnosed as eating disorder not otherwise specified (EDNOS). It has starving behaviors that qualify as symptoms of anorexia. But she also purges with laxatives and obsessively exercises. The behaviors work, more or less. For a short time, they dampen the sting of loneliness. But by engaging with her disorder, Mary Pat, who was recently hospitalized for depression in conjunction with an eating disorder, is starving her social self, which, if given a chance to develop, would help her to connect to true friends and lovers.

The Ambivalent Partner: Together But Separate

Some women, like Mary Pat, avoid any intimacy. Others venture forth but only partway. They pick a partner who will keep his distance: a person with a low sex drive, a narcissist, a loner, a man who travels frequently. He does not ask her many questions and is content to live with a superficial self, which is all that she can give him.

The strategy is to be with him but also to keep her eating disorder. It is like being married and having an affair. She juggles two lovers. Or she builds a wall around herself, hides behind it when she engages in her food rituals, and then, once in a while, steps out of her fortress to meet her partner.

Stephan Van den Broucke, a social psychologist at Katholieke Universiteit Leuven in Leuven, Belgium, conducted a study that illuminates this kind of woman. He compared three groups of couples: those in which one partner has an eating disorder, those seeking counseling for marital troubles but no eating disorder, and a control group with no reported marital problems and no eating disorder.

After observing the partners' interactions, Van den Broucke found, not surprisingly, that the three groups form a spectrum of happiness: couples without an eating disorder or marital woes showed the greatest satisfaction in their partnership; couples with marital problems and no eating disorder fared the worst; and eating-disordered couples fell in the middle.

This seems like good news for a couple with an eating disorder between them. But there was a glitch in the study results. Couples in which one person had an eating disorder fought less because they interacted less.

"They are avoiding dealing with conflict-ridden issues altogether," Van den Broucke says. "There is no discussion at all. Not even in an escalating way."

The couples with eating disorder issues are avoiding conflict not because they are working in harmony, but because they are orbiting in two separate spheres.

"Eating disorder couples have the propensity to censor their negative communication, but they also fail to provide each other with positive messages," says Jan Lackstrom, an eating disorders therapist at the University of Toronto. "Their communication is not hostilely destructive, but somewhat bland and unrewarding."

This is how Erin, 25, manages to keep her relationship going. She is a biologist who was diagnosed with anorexia nervosa. After she left an outpatient clinic four years ago, she took off the weight that she had gained and fell back into her old patterns.

She met her partner—a manager at a restaurant where they had both worked. They dated and, a year ago, they became engaged. This should make her happy, but instead Erin senses that something is wrong. She avoids thinking about the wedding and has not yet set a date. Instead, she fixates on her 5-foot, 8-inch, 100-pound body, her size 0 jeans bagging out on her. She has taken up an extreme regimen of dieting, running, and weight loss. It has taken over her life, coming ahead of everything, including her relationship with her fiancé.

In the mornings, when she sleeps at his place, she feels so compelled to run, she cannot stay in bed with him. The couple rarely eats meals together, in part because they work different shifts. Erin admits that scheduling is probably an excuse; if her fiancé were to pop into her work one afternoon and say, "Let's go for lunch," she would "freak out," obsessing about the calories and fat that she inevitably would have to eat. She probably would not go. And she feels horribly guilty about that.

"I should be able to go home, have a lovely dinner with my fiancé, and get it on," she says. "But I feel so disgusting and concerned about my weight, I just want to curl up in a fetal position and watch Must See TV."

Erin and other women like her have pseudorelationships, picking men who will accept distance and sexual frigidity as the norm. The men, in turn, have their own reasons for attraction, ranging from insecurity about their own masculinity to simple acceptance of what becomes the status quo in a relationship.

Erin's anorexia has caused her hormones to act as if she is in perimenopause. She has lost her sex drive and bemoans that. But she is not about to give up her disorder. So as long as he lets her keep her behaviors, which she tells him are mere eccentricities, she will stay in the relationship. And unless recovery happens, both will stay, more or less, in their separate worlds.

Forever a Child: Partner as Pseudoparent

If a woman is entering a relationship with a girl's sense of self, she is going to act like a girl in that relationship. For example, she may fixate on her appearance, a leftover of teenage preoccupation. She may make snap judgments or be afraid to decide anything for herself. She may even throw tantrums. These alone are red flags for any adult relationship.

"How do you have emotional intimacy if you cannot respond to someone without freaking out?" says Wisniewski. "Even in physical intimacy, she has to be able to say, 'This is what I want.'"

Many of these women have problems detaching from their families of origin. Psychologists have a theory of attachment. It asserts that in times of threat, infants will want to be close to their parents, physically and psychologically. If the parents respond adequately, the infant carries a sense of security into her adolescence and adulthood. That sense of safety will guide her future relationships.

If the parents fail to respond, however, she will experience later problems, eating disorders among them. In a study of 306 undergraduate women, researchers found that those who reported the highest level of alienation from their fathers also showed the greatest symptoms of depression and eating disorders.

In terms of intimacy, a girl will assume responsibility for her father's absence, physical or emotional. She will then go on to re-create the dynamic, looking for a man who will treat her as his child or, at the other extreme, ignore her as her father did, giving her only a shadow of himself as he lives in emotional retreat.

Tracy, 41, exemplifies one variation on the theme. She grew up in Horsham, Pennsylvania, the daughter of an architect who was a project manager in the U.S. Air Force. She characterizes her father as an emotionally unavailable workaholic who "could not relate to his three daughters."

Tracy tried to fill the void. Starting at 12, she experimented with alcohol and dieting and purging. Later, a full-blown alcoholic and bulimic, she went away to Virginia Tech, in Blacksburg, and majored in architecture. "I wanted to follow in my daddy's foot-steps," she says.

In an act of rebellion, however, Tracy changed her major to fash-ion design. The move was meant to thumb her nose at her father—and she regrets it to this day. It did nothing to resolve her anger at him, as she had hoped.

"I had no self," she says.

Instead of going through the painful task of self-discovery, Tracy "fell in love every other week," hoping to borrow the identity of somebody else.

She spent the next decade in a quagmire of bad relationships in-volving men who cheated on her. She relied on food and alcohol to soothe her humiliation. After she got sober through Alcoholics Anon-ymous, she gravitated toward an easy substitute: dieting, purging, and exercise.

She eventually met her future husband, Tim, while vacationing at a beach house in Bay Head, New Jersey. In a conversation on the beach at three o'clock in the morning, he told her that both his father and grandfather were alcoholics; later he proceeded to get drunk and pass out on the floor of her bathroom. Tracy says she "knew that it was a bad idea to get into this relationship," yet she went ahead. She was attracted to Tim's ambition and the financial security he offered.

"I married the potential," she says. "I married my father."

Now, having been with him for the last seven years, Tracy battles the same sort of emotional withdrawal from her husband that she experienced from her father. Tim travels constantly for work and for his passion, go-cart racing.

Over the years, Tracy has recovered from bulimia and now has a less serious preoccupation with food and appearance. She has a subclinical problem. But the disorder has its remnants in the dynamic of how the spouses relate to each other.

When Tracy gets angry and voices her unhappiness, her husband blames her. And she blames herself, an old childhood habit. Then she works harder on changing herself. She focuses on her spirituality through participation in a church group; her weight, through dieting; and her appearance, through fancy clothing.

It is a set of compulsions that she cannot seem to leave behind.

"I regret that I have not done enough work on myself to be with someone other than a guy with this background," she says. "But I accepted that night, 'This is the guy who I am going to be attracted to.' 'This is somehow my path.'"

The Goddess: Preoccupation with Perfection

A fourth type of woman is one who strives to be perfect, to the point of seeming ethereal. She cultivates her image, her appearance, and her competence. Through these expressions and her body language, she promises any potential partner that she is going to be kind, nurturing, undemanding, and affirming. She promises to be her man's earth mother or angel.

Joanna Poppink, a therapist in southern California who works with eating-disordered couples, says that many women with eating disorders need to get to a state of perfection because their self-esteem is so low that they cannot tolerate any criticism.

"If you are perfect, then you are beyond criticism," Poppink explains.

In Hollywood, where many of the therapist's patients live, such women abound—goddesses with eating disorders.

The goddess attracts many partners. Men are positively bewitched by her image. Her goal is to maintain her place on the pedestal. When choosing a partner—and she has many to choose from—she may pick a god. Now they are two divinities, each one perfectly enhancing the image of the other. She throws him great parties and plays the trophy wife that he thinks she is. He, in turn, performs for her, affirming her image of perfection.

In another scenario, the goddess may choose a worshipper. This man is obedient and compliant. He will treat her as she thinks she should be treated. He initially falls in love with her beauty and, through his unquestioning devotion, reinforces her fantasy that she is perfect. They think they are entering paradise, but instead, they are falling into a sinkhole of impossible expectations.

What she may not understand is that she is becoming dependent on him because she needs his constant reinforcement. And he, by adoring her, is pressuring her to continue to be perfect.

The eating disorder slips in easily because it is part of her strategy to achieve perfection—through a thin, wispy physique. At the same time, it also siphons off some of the pressure: if she focuses on only her weight and appearance, she simplifies her deeper issues with self-esteem and avoids having to confront them head-on.

But if she wants to recover, she may be setting herself up for a much harder journey. To recover, both she and her partner are going to have to ease her off the pedestal.

Can they?

Carrie's story illustrates how it might work. She met Eric while she was a contestant at a beauty pageant, dressed as the Statue of Liberty

"She had this air about her," Eric recalls. "Like, 'I'm all that. My stuff doesn't stink.'"

The truth was that Carrie felt as insecure as ever. At 19, she had just been through therapy for anorexia nervosa. She had dieted and exercised her 5-foot, 5-inch frame of 150 pounds down to 93. In time for the pageant, she had gained back 10 pounds. But through all these efforts, she had not yet gained a sense of self.

That was where she was in her psychological development when she met Eric. The couple hit it off. He fell in love with a beauty queen. She liked how readily he listened to her.

On their first date, Carrie was forthright. She told Eric about her troubles with anorexia nervosa. She explained what weight and food meant to her and the many fad diets she had been on. She talked about her dream: winning a state title in a pageant. Thinness was key to that goal. It was her quest for identity.

Eric understood his role: "Basically all I could do was be there for her if she needed something," he says.

And he has. Throughout the years of their marriage, Eric rallied around Carrie as she continued her efforts at recovery and fought hard for her goal: eleven years of competing on and off in pageants. In the end, he held her hand as she won the title of Mrs. Ohio, the married woman's counterpart to Miss America.

Ironically, Carrie used eating disorders as her "platform," a description that a contestant uses to define herself. Carrie told the judges that if she won, she would become a spokeswoman for eating disorders awareness. Wearing the crown, she would give talks about her past and bring the issue to public attention.

That is what she is doing even now, at 32, as she still struggles with her subclinical issues. Her weight is in the normal range, but she still has compulsions about food. She has to control her portion sizes, counting out twenty-four Frosted Mini Wheats in her cereal bowl every morning, for example. She will not eat foods that touch each other on her plate.

Eric takes it all in stride, saying he feels lucky to be married to her.

"If you've seen her," he says, "she is gorgeous. And I am just a schmo."

Carrie has come a long way. But for her to feel even more comfortable about herself, she will have to hand in her crown and trust that she is lovable, even if she were to grow old and fat. And Eric will have to be able to support her, even then.

FROM HIS PERSPECTIVE

Layered on top of the myth that only adolescent girls get eating disorders is the fallacy that married women with eating disorders must have gotten them as young girls. One step further, and a myth forms about the partners of these women: they must be attracted to women who are ill, many of whom have been so since they were teenagers. Therefore, the partners, in choosing such a woman, must be ill themselves.

What kind of man would partner up with a woman who might put him second to her relationship with food? What kind of man would marry a woman who barely eats and weighs 85 pounds?

Most likely an "immature" one, according to British psychiatrist Peter Dally, who championed novel approaches to treating eating disorders until his death in 2005. Dally was one of the first researchers to look more closely at men who married women with eating disorders. As senior consultant psychiatrist at the Westminster Hospital in London, he observed forty-five husbands of his female patients and fit the men into three categories.

Overall, Dally believed that a husband picked this kind of wife because she, being sick, did not threaten his fragile sense of masculinity and self-esteem. Thus, both partners were suffering developmental flaws. As such, the couples could build only poor foundations of intimacy.

What follows is a distilled version of Dally's observations combined with more recent clinical observations that reveal the kind of men who partner up with women who have eating disorders or simply disordered eating.

While developmentally mature men do sometimes partner with

developmentally immature women with eating disorders, as Dally suggested, this is not always the scenario.

The Nice Guy: Passive and Compliant

The most common profile Dally observed was men who are passive. These men, more than half of the study participants, avoided conflict. They compromised, conceded, cowered, and sacrificed their own needs, appearing to want only to be accepted and loved.

"He is genuinely bent on doing good," says Blake Woodside, who specializes in eating disorders and marriage at the Toronto General Hospital Ambulatory Care for Eating Disorders. "But sometimes, taking care of her is a distraction from a problem that he himself has."

This scenario may have happened with Eric and Carrie. Eric had been raised by an alcoholic father and a passive mother. He had buried his issues with his dad in his exuberance over being with Carrie and his worry over her welfare.

But Carrie had been working hard to recover and was well on her way to learning how to identify her needs and assert them in her marriage. This became evident after Carrie gave birth to their son. She had a dream that Eric's father, who kept guns in his house, had killed their son in a bout of drinking. Carrie told Eric that she would not tolerate her father-in-law drinking around the infant. And, at that moment, Eric realized that he had to confront his lifelong problem.

He did, drawing a line in the sand. He told his father not to drink around the boy. But when Eric's father defied the ultimatum, Eric cut off all relations with his parents. "I told them, 'I'm done,'" he says.

But the issue is far from resolved. Eric has more work to do, and he will be able to do it only if Carrie's issues stay on the back burner for a time.

Dally says that, in a very unconscious way, a husband may actually welcome his wife's crises: it means that she needs him and he can rescue her. He feels stronger. She, in turn, feels good about being rescued, and so she continues to need him and the relationship. This can feel reparative to the partners.

The same theme holds in the area of sexual relations. A man may actually want a woman with a limp sex drive; if his partner is struggling with issues of libido, like Erin, there is no pressure on him to perform sexually.

However brilliant a solution this seems, the outcome can be dangerous. He is connecting to her in her illness, consciously or unconsciously. Thus, she will sense, *This is why he is with me*. She will think, *If I give up my eating disorder, where is that going to leave our relationship?*

Indeed, lifting the eating disorder would mean ending the relationship. Therefore, even though the man thinks he is doing a good thing by rescuing his wife in her illness, his complicity can actually make recovery more difficult for her.

Many wonder how a man can be attracted to a woman who weighs 85 pounds. The answer is that in many cases, her weight, and low sex drive, make him feel stronger.

The Knight in Shining Armor

Dally's second category of partner is actually a variation on this passive theme. The husband begins as a knight in shining armor. He wants to save and protect his wife. As he realizes that she does not really want to be saved, he loses his purpose.

"The typical pattern is he'll try and try and try and find nothing really works to help her," says Jim Schettler, a licensed marriage and family therapist at Remuda Ranch.

Without any gratitude from her, he tires of fighting dragons. She is not meeting his need to be the savior. In essence, he gets sick of his wife's sickness.

Eventually, he starts needling her about it, in a passive-aggressive way. He may make wisecracks in front of friends about how she does not eat. Perhaps he hides the toothpaste in the bathroom where he knows she goes to vomit. Or he simply recognizes his helplessness to change her and withdraws. Withdrawal can take many forms, such as an affair or an immersion in work. He may go all the way, breaking up the marriage, asking for a divorce. The overall dynamic only exacerbates her eating disorder. She feels harassed or abandoned and looks for succor where she always does, in her eating disorder. It is a no-win situation.

Macho Man: Control and Conquer

Dally's third category is marked by older men who forge a father-daughter relationship with their wives. These men may be angry and controlling or kind and loving. Either way, their wives serve as an extension of themselves. Whether they are executives, doctors, attorneys, military officers, or ministers, most of these men are accustomed to managing other people. They assign duties. They are in charge.

This is the attitude that they bring home.

Ward Keller, president and CEO of Remuda, is a multimillionaire whose 10-year-old daughter became ill with anorexia nervosa. He personifies Dally's third type.

He was the head of a company as well as the head of a presumptive model family. In both places, he demanded perfection but was insensitive to others and crushed any voice of dissent.

"If there were problems at home, then my wife was to blame," he says.

In essence, he avoided any self-reflection about his own role in exacerbating his daughter's problem by convincing himself that emotional affairs lay in the hands of women. So great was his growing sense of impunity, he was convinced that if he participated in family therapy, the counselor would send him home and focus on his wife, "the real problem."

In this case, the eating disorder played out in a father-daughter relationship, fueled by Keller's macho controlling behavior. But Keller's wife was also feeling the dysfunction. Despite attempts at family therapy, and Keller's eventual insights into his shortcomings, he and his wife later divorced. His daughter has found her own path toward healing, now working to help women with eating disorders at Remuda.

Husbands who are oppressive perfectionists, insensitive, and in denial choose a partner with an eating disorder because she will go along with this behavior. As a bonus, she may be slender and trophy-like in appearance. She may be competent because she, too, is a perfectionist. She may be childlike in her devotion to him, willing to absorb his blame. And if she is a talented, creative person, he can tap into her creativity and channel it into his own self-promotion.

In the worst cases, he is abusive—physically, sexually, psychologically. Psychological abuse by a husband is defined in many ways, including criticizing his wife's personality or deeply held values, humiliating her in public, withholding emotional support, restricting her behaviors, making all decisions, controlling whom she sees, and deciding what she is allowed to do.

The bottom line is that he does not love her for who she is. He loves her for what she can do for him. As his dominance continues, she regresses deeper into self-loathing. She feels more inadequate. Thus, under these conditions, the eating disorder gives her the only control that she feels she has.

Mr. Clueless: He Just Doesn't Know That a Problem Exists

It is easy to paint husbands as both victims and architects of their wives' eating issues. Researchers are quick to point the finger because, as noted earlier, there is some evidence the men involved with these women are mentally troubled themselves. In 1992, for example, researchers studied seventy-three partners of bulimic women and found that 25 percent of the men had psychiatric disorders such as anxiety or personality disorders, 27 percent had weight or obesity problems, and 40 percent drank excessively.

Studies such as these have created the aforementioned myth: every man who is attracted to a woman with an eating disorder must be sick himself.

However, more recently, research has provided another reason for such connections—and yet another category of partnership. This type consists of healthy men who simply do not understand what is going on with their partners. Their naiveté speaks to societal norms that say a slim partner, sometimes exceedingly slim, is an attractive one. And desiring such icons of beauty, some men may unwittingly become accomplices in the promulgation of their partners' eating disorders.

Van den Broucke's group in Belgium gave psychological tests to twenty-one men whose partners had eating disorders. Even after employing rigorous measures to evaluate depression, psychosis, and general distress, Van den Broucke could not pick up any statistical differences between the psychological health of men whose wives had eating disorders and men in nondistressed marriages. In fact, husbands of the patients seemed to be slightly *less* distressed than the norm.

"These men, they love their partners," Van den Broucke says.

And they feel as if their marriages are pretty good.

While this contrasts with what Dally and others are saying, probably all the researchers are correct. There are many different types of men in these situations and many different ways in which they relate to their partners.

But if one accepts Van den Broucke's results—that there is a healthy contingent—one has to solve this conundrum. How can a man remain healthy and undistressed when he lives with an emaciated woman, an impulsive binger, or a woman who consumes three helpings at dinner and spends hours the next day at the health club?

The answer is that she may be painstakingly careful to keep her problem secret. She may work out for three hours in the middle of the night and binge when he travels on business. She may become masterful at hiding her disorder, even from the one who is supposed to be closest to her.

"We have had more than one husband not have a clue that their partner is bulimic or bingeing," Lackstrom says. "He comes in for treatment and I can see his eyes getting bigger and bigger as he finds out the extent of her problem."

Woodside estimates that about 75 percent of women with eating disorders tell their partners up front, just as Carrie told Eric on their first date. But the other 25 percent do not tell, and their partners have no idea until far into the relationship.

One husband who was married for fifteen years never saw the signs of his wife's bulimia. Even more surprising, the husband was a detective. He found out only when she told him she was entering inpatient treatment at Remuda.

With bulimia, the ignorance on his part is somewhat understandable. But what about ignorance about anorexia nervosa or binge eating disorder, conditions in which a woman's weight problems are much more transparent?

A spouse may not fully understand what is going on. If he has actively sought out a woman with anorexia, binge eating disorder, or a subclinical form of either, he already has a different standard of weight and shape compared to many other men. The fact that his wife might be ill is less important to him than meeting his physical ideal for a partner.

In another, more likely scenario a woman had an eating disorder before she met her partner, but now she has gone into recovery, as Carrie did. When she said "I do" at her wedding ceremony, she only had an "issue with food." In her mind, this was not an eating disorder—so why bring it up? It's over. If she does bring it up, she frames it as an issue in her past. Baggage.

Eating disorders wax and wane through a lifetime, and stress exacerbates the illness. Imagine what the big stresses of life, including marriage, might do to stir up a woman's latent eating disorder. If it boils over as a relapse, she is simply too embarrassed or too afraid of losing her partner to confide the extent of her trouble. So she tucks it away, even though the concealment will threaten their intimacy.

The Ostrich: Denial and Distance

The other side of the ignorance coin is denial. Denial helps to answer the question "If you have a partner with a marked weight fluctuation, how would you not notice?"

Clinician Joanna Poppink relates an outrageous case of denial. A woman with an eating disorder was experimenting with laxatives. Periodically, she, in Poppink's words, "went over the top." In the middle of the night, she would be unable to control her bowels and soil the bed with diarrhea. She would nudge her sleeping husband, who would get up drowsily while she cleaned herself and changed the bedding. She would then tell her husband, "OK, honey, you can get back in bed."

The next morning, he would never discuss it.

Why not?

"Because it was fine," Poppink says. "His life was fine."

Brian, a professor of liberal arts at Yale University in New Haven, Connecticut, knows the meaning of "fine" firsthand. He thought his marriage was "better than real." For seven years, he had experienced his partner as "the warmest, earthiest, most affirming and supportive woman."

And then she arrived home one weekend, after a camping trip with "Amy," an old friend, and announced that she was bulimic, had been for most of the marriage, and that she was leaving Brian for Andy, a past boyfriend, the one with whom she had actually gone camping.

How had Brian missed it?

He admits that, in retrospect, there had been signals, subtle cues he might have followed. He remembers an impromptu dinner party when his wife stopped him just as he was running out for some cheese and crackers. She said that she had two boxes of unopened Triscuits in her car. Brian asked her about it, but because she gave him a benign explanation—*I forgot to unload them shopping*—he did not react at the time.

He remembers a persistent reddish stain—what he later surmised was the remnants of vomiting—in the toilet upstairs. He recalled butter in the refrigerator that was missing and then showed up again as new sticks in slightly different wrappers. He noted the empty jar of honey.

When Brian asked his wife about the condiments, she answered, "Oh yes, I made a batch of cookies this afternoon."

"Where are the cookies?" he asked.

"Oh, I took them to the co-op," she replied.

And that was that. If Brian had been a "sophisticated consumer" of eating disorder information, he might have been able to put two and two together. But he had been happy with the marriage as it was.

"If you had given us both truth serum in the middle of our marriage," Brian says, "I would have said, 'Boy, do I love being married,' and she would have said, 'I am so unhappy.'"

Obviously, the couple could not have honest communication, because Brian's wife, ostensibly open about other issues, was keeping an insidious secret from him. And that is exactly what happens in marriages with eating disorders—secrets grow like cancer in the relationship.

FROM THEIR PERSPECTIVE AS A COUPLE

Formal studies of eating disorders and relationships are scant in the medical literature. This is not surprising given that early research tended to focus on young girls, who were unlikely to be in committed relationships. One exception, again, is the work of Dally in London. He studied fifty heterosexual couples in which the female partner had an eating disorder. By gathering medical records and scribbling observations onto index cards, Dally was able to divide the couples into four groups, depending on when a full-blown illness first emerged.

Women in group 1 became ill during the engagement period. Group 2 dropped their weight after marriage but prior to a pregnancy. Group 3 patients acquired their full-blown disorder within three years of becoming pregnant. And those in group 4, the least common and least studied, emerged with anorexia after menopause.

Dally speculated as to the role the eating disorder might be playing in each category of relationship. For women in groups 1 and 2 (premarriage and prepregnancy), anorexia might have been a poor attempt at solving an emerging marital crisis. These women needed something from their mates for which they lacked the skills to ask. Even if the women had asked for support, their spouses would likely have been unable to help, given the findings about men who marry women with eating disorders. Thus, the eating disorder served to numb hurt and anger, two strong emotions that would otherwise stir an open conflict.

A typical woman in group 3 (postpregnancy) probably was feeling a lack of warmth from her partner, suggested Dally. She likely felt trapped in her restrictive world of diapers and carpools. Or maybe she wasn't getting the support she needed to balance career and motherhood. Exhausted and isolated in her turbulent emotions, she retreated into anorexia as a silent protest.

Finally, Dally speculated that postmenopausal women might have used starvation to fulfill a death wish to exert control after a loss (such as after divorce, the death of a spouse, or a child's departure from home).

Only time and further study can tell whether Dally is right. But even if he is not, he did point to an entirely new phenomenon: eating disorders have many purposes beyond simply dealing with teen identity crises.

As women grow older, their eating disorders grow with them, serving different aims. For example, eating problems can defuse marital tension. Or they can soothe a woman's loneliness in the context of a failing relationship. Dally's study says that a woman uses her eating disorder to do whatever she needs to do. This is akin to the smoker who smokes for multiple reasons—for example, to calm nerves in one moment and appease boredom in another.

How Partners Use Eating Disorders

As a Stand-in for Communication

A woman can substitute an eating disorder for talking openly with her partner. She may be afraid to state her needs in the relationship, or be fearful of bringing up topics she knows will induce a fight. She keeps silent, but the unresolved issues take their toll nonetheless. The woman takes the hit with her body.

This was the case with Maria, whose husband was transferred to a different part of Spain because of his job. Maria did not want to leave her family and friends, but she did not feel that she could say so. Her husband immersed himself in the new job, and she stayed at home in a strange town with their three children. She felt alone and estranged from others. She solved the issue by bingeing and purging. The eating disorder served to palliate the demands of her marriage and her inability to assert her own needs and develop her own interests.

As an Interpersonal Weapon

In other relationships, an eating disorder can become a way to fight back against a dominating partner. If a man usurps control, his partner may feel that she has few options for expressing herself. She may turn to a passive-aggressive tactic: she creeps into the corner and starves, broadcasting her anger at her partner through an emaciated body.

Woodside, at Toronto General Hospital, treated such a woman. She came from an ethnic and cultural background where divorce was not an option. Husbands were actually expected to have affairs, as long as they followed them with a public apology. When the patient's husband had repeated affairs and offered perfunctory apologies, she felt so enraged and humiliated that she stopped eating. An eating disorder in this case is meant to lay guilt, as the emaciated body cries out, "You bastard, look how badly you are treating me."

In a more overt drama, another woman, Lucia, used bulimia to lash out directly at her husband. The couple would fight, and the husband would try to force his wife into submission. Realizing that she could never seem to win the arguments with words, she would scream, "I am now going to binge and you will have to watch me."

And she would, winning the battle but losing herself.

In these relationships, an eating disorder acts as a weapon of assertion in a situation where other options are never tried or, when they are, they seem to fail.

As a Way to Evade the Past

Some women use eating disorders in their relationships as a replacement for past vices. What was once alcohol abuse or drug addiction morphs into an eating disorder. Researchers have long tracked a connection between substance abuse and eating disorders. Nearly one-half of individuals with eating disorders also abuse alcohol or drugs (compared to 9 percent of the general population). On the other hand, a third of alcohol and drug abusers eventually acquire eating disorders.

The connection means that a person highly vulnerable to one addiction is also prone to another.

A relationship can also be addictive. The high of infatuation is not unlike the intoxication of being drunk or in a binge state. These highs, from food, alcohol, or "love," bear one commonality: a woman is looking outside herself to feel better inside.

How does this play out in real life?

Cindy's story offers one reality. She fell into bulimia at the age of 25, shortly after she married. As a teenager, Cindy had been abused physically by her stepfather and sexually by an uncle and a grandfather. At 17, her employer raped her. Her other family members, who did not know about the incest, buried the shameful rape episode, and so did Cindy. She turned to alcohol, sex, and later drugs to keep the hurt and anger in control.

Cindy joined the U.S. Air Force to try to clean up her act. Stationed on a base in England, she met Sean, a handsome, clean-cut fighter pilot: "Tom Cruise in a flight suit."

He rescued her from the advances of another drunken pilot in a bar, and the couple fell in love. Four months later, they were engaged. Four months after that, they flew back to the United States and married.

But soon after their engagement, Cindy realized she had a major problem. The air force had not stopped her addiction. Except for the drugs, which the military forbade, Cindy had been behaving exactly as she had as a teenager. She feared that Sean would find out and leave her. So she quit her addictions to alcohol and sex, cold turkey. She believed that love would be enough.

It was not. Without alcohol and partying, Cindy felt the pangs of her past anger and shame return. To cope—and to keep her husband—she turned to dieting, exercise, and weight loss.

"I could not change my past," she says, "but I thought that maybe if I made myself look good enough, he would stay with me."

In two months, she lost 30 pounds. When abstinence became too difficult to keep going, she began vomiting as well. Cindy soon discovered that dieting and purging had the same numbing effect as drinking, albeit without the hangover. Her eating disorder went on, spawned by a desire to keep her husband while, at the same time, keeping the past hidden.

The Onset of Eating Disorders After the Wedding: A Growing Demographic

Researchers once believed that if an eating disorder festered in a relationship, the illness was a continuing problem from the woman's adolescence. But as new studies begin to emerge, eating disorders experts are realizing there is more to the story. Psychologists such as Fernando Fernandez-Aranda, head of an eating disorders unit at

University Hospital of Bellvitge, in Barcelona, Spain, and his colleague Debra Bussolotti at the University Hospital of Modena, in Italy, are breaking new ground. Their attention was piqued by a change in the demographic of women coming into their clinics. Over the years, they noticed that a growing number of women were older, and a growing number were married.

Upon digging deeper into the stories of these older women, Fernandez and Bussolotti realized that eating disorders experts might be getting it wrong. For starters, 30 percent of their married patients acquired their eating disorders *after* marrying. The finding echoes the work by Dally, who reported that 66 percent of his patients acquired their disorders after they formed their relationships. From his caseload, Woodside reports 50 percent.

While the exact numbers vary, they nonetheless explode the myth that eating disorders begin solely in a woman's youth. When an eating disorder comes on after the marriage, the problem cannot be just one person's baggage. It is their *mutual* baggage, the individual histories that bear upon all couples as they try to negotiate their partnerships.

Researchers have found that married patients with eating disorders turn out to be sicker—and sicker longer—than unmarried ones. More specifically, women with eating disorders who live with their partners report worse symptoms, more body dissatisfaction, and a more powerful drive to be thin compared to those who do not cohabitate. This finding holds even when researchers take age into account. Researchers have shown that married women are not having a harder time simply because they are older, and therefore might have had their illnesses longer. Instead, they are struggling because of the stresses implicit in their primary relationships.

The message is that marriage can start an eating disorder. In fact, one study found that marriage can do so much harm to a woman with a prior eating disorder that it predicts a poorer likelihood of recovery than if she were single.

For this reason, marital counseling may be helpful to recovery. Not only are the individual partners' own troubles causing the marriage to suffer, but so are the interactions of the couple. In other words, the relationship itself drives the illness.

Cindy's U.S. Air Force story illustrates this phenomenon. After she married, she and her pilot husband, Sean, had to relocate several times, once overseas. She gave up active military duty and tried to become a full-time mother, raising the couple's two children. This was a painful transition for her. She had trouble with isolation: new places, no friends, and no job outside the home. Making matters worse, Sean was traveling constantly. He had commitments to the military and also took on a job as a commercial pilot. When he was around, he was not the best confidant.

"He's not the touchy-feely type—more like, 'You've got a problem? Let me help fix it,'" Cindy says. "So I learned pretty quickly not to talk about what is going on inside of me, because he really didn't get it."

Cindy did not have any hint of bulimia before the ring went on her finger. But she had other vices. Those were the seeds of the eating disorder. Marriage simply added fertilizer. The eating disorder, latent before marriage, came to life when Cindy entered a stressful situation that she did not have the psychological tools to manage. One could say that this was Cindy's issue. But the stress of marriage and, later, child rearing—along with Sean's inability to offer support or emotional empathy—was the couple's issue.

In short, the new marital environment set the stage for an eating disorder's first emergence.

RECOVERY: FOR BETTER OR FOR WORSE

Recovery in situations such as Sean and Cindy's is extraordinarily complicated.

"These individuals are not static figures," says California therapist Poppink. "You are talking about different developmental stages on both sides that change throughout the partners' lives."

To illustrate what this means, at her couples workshops, Poppink asks for a show of hands to find out how many people have been married more than once. A few hands go up. When she asks, "Twice? And three times?" the numbers of hands lessen each time, until she asks, "How many of you have grown and changed in your marriage so much that you feel like you have had more than one marriage?"

Everyone's hand goes up.

The message is this: to stay together, partners *both* have to change as individuals and also accept changes in each other.

With eating disorders, however, as with alcoholism and other addictions, movement forward meets tremendous resistance. As noted earlier, eating disorders, whether subclinical or full-blown, integrate themselves into the relationship and become part of its foundation. Therapy is meant to funnel the eating disorder out of the relationship. But to a couple dependent on illness, removing it feels like tearing down bricks and mortar—even if the foundation is crumbling anyway.

Will the entire building topple?

Not necessarily. If the couple can build a new foundation using new tools acquired in therapy, the marriage can begin again. Recovery, in this case, means understanding something old has to be torn down and something new erected in its place. This is such a daunting prospect, Poppink says, that, ideally, each partner in the relationship should go to individual therapy as well as marital therapy to deal with issues the couple holds in common.

Tearing Down an Unhealthy Foundation

One of the first steps in recovery is to look at the role the eating disorder plays in the relationship. Fernandez calls these "maintaining factors"—issues between the couple that breed and keep the eating disorder going. Loneliness, imbalances of power, emotional dependency, and psychological abuse can all serve as maintaining factors for an eating disorder.

An individual therapist can help a patient tease out such issues for one partner; a marital therapist can bring to light such issues for the couple.

The next step is to bring the issues to the table and talk about what it means to let go of them. *What is the effect of cutting down on exercise? What will happen by stopping the diets?* The couple may plan for those changes, step-by-step. Ultimately, the couple will have to execute their plan in order to successfully rebuild their relationship.

Lackstrom tells the story of one couple, "big exercisers," whose intimacy was based on running. "She would run half a city block ahead of him and tell him to hurry up," Lackstrom says.

That was their relationship. They bonded around her compulsion for exercise, born out of her anorexia nervosa. However, if exercise were removed, what would they have?

"Needless to say, this did not work too well," Lackstrom says.

In another case, a woman with bulimia stopped purging and began to gain weight. Her partner noticed. He began to make critical comments about her body.

Criticism is not supporting change. And it is not helpful to say, "Let's go on a cruise, sweetie," knowing there is nothing for his recovering bulimic wife to do except lie around and eat. A cruise would be her worst nightmare—all that food and no access to her therapist.

One patient with anorexia nervosa married a personal trainer who owned his own fitness business. After she began making progress in treatment, he insisted that she ride her bike daily to the treatment clinic. Even though his wife's therapist repeatedly told the husband that unregulated exercise is one of the greatest risk factors for relapse, the husband did not understand his part in her illness. The couple could not find an alternative to exercise, and so grew distant from each other and eventually separated.

What might have helped the husband more was knowledge about set-point theory—the idea that the body is genetically programmed to weigh a certain amount. If a person rises or falls above or below that point, the body will force a return to the set point.

"We ask partners to think about what is normal eating," Lackstrom says, "what the implications of that might be for somebody's appearance."

If they can grasp the connection, they can dislodge a long-standing, destructive pattern, and the couple can move forward. But if she fails to make the changes or he fails to support them, then the couple will spiral downward. They may turn to separation or divorce.

But what may be called failure to some may not be entirely negative. In some cases, a split eventually brings relief. In his book *This Mean Disease*, Daniel Becker tells the story of his mother's long bout with anorexia nervosa. He also offers his father's perspective after the couple divorced. Following decades of caretaking and feeling responsible for a gravely ill spouse, Becker's father finally felt release. It was a matter of absolution as well as permission to have one's life back after so many years of misery.

Building a New Healthy Foundation

Couples who drag out the baggage and toss it into the trash are the ones who move on. At this stage, they are facing an open space into which they can insert a new dynamic of playfulness and intimacy. This stage of recovery can uplift and energize. Just as when they first started out together, couples involved in healing have to build a relationship together that will support them both. In therapy, they ideally work as a team.

Therapy can help partners find better ways to communicate, express feelings, role-play, or problem-solve together.

In Sean and Cindy's case, Cindy learned how to vocalize her disappointments and fears to her husband. She talked to Sean for the first time about her history of abuse. He listened and felt a mix of emotions: protectiveness, helplessness, and anger that she had in her words "lied" by omission and therefore "kept a secret for so long." But he was able to communicate with her, "touchy-feely style."

In the end, they compromised and found better ways to deal with time spent apart. For example, Sean gained seniority as a pilot and was able to control his schedule better. He took on more tasks at home. In this way, the couple created an environment where they could talk regularly and then grow in trust. Through hard work, taking place over more than a decade, the couple gradually learned how to relate to each other in an entirely new way.

What Can I Do to Help Us?

Many men ask, "What can I do?"

"What is helpful is whatever his partner identifies as helpful," says Woodside.

That may sound ridiculous, especially if the mandate comes from someone who is ill. He thinks, *How could she possibly decide what is best? She cannot even feed herself properly.*

This thinking is exactly where men often go wrong. Well-intentioned, a man may think he should take charge and "fix her," giving her advice, policing her eating, listening outside the bathroom door to prevent vomiting episodes, or putting locks on the refrigerator. If he adopts this attitude, he will lose her trust. The central theme is her need to control. The promise of that power is the lure of the eating disorder. If she lets go of her symptoms, however, and he takes control, he will effectively be pushing her backward, away from a chance for healing.

Given this reality, the first step is for both partners to acknowledge that she has an eating disorder, and that she needs treatment. Some women may not believe that they are sick and resist help. This means her partner is going to have to make some tough choices.

Jason's wife, Christine, 31, developed anorexia nervosa after the couple married. Jason knew that Christine was losing too much weight, but he had been too preoccupied with the couple's imminent bankruptcy to take time out to address the issue. Christine, malnourished, started blacking out while driving and had two separate car accidents. Later, she became suicidal. Jason tried to talk her into getting help, but Christine was too depressed to take any action. Jason called up a former therapist of Christine's and the therapist drew up papers to have Christine committed to a state institution for treatment. Both Jason and the therapist then gave Christine two options: either check herself in for treatment voluntarily at Remuda or be committed. Christine chose Remuda and stayed in treatment for two months.

When a woman enters treatment, willingly or not, a shift occurs in the balance of the relationship. The eating disorder will take precedence over her behaviors and, by extension, over their relationship. As she begins to work through her issues, they will consume her. Her partner should expect and plan for change. Big change.

If therapy is working and she is truly accepting it, she is likely to unleash a wide range of pent-up emotions: anger, fear, and vulnerability. He has to be prepared to deal with this outpouring, because some of those emotions are going to be directed at him.

Men in this situation need to stay calm and treat their partners with respect and compassion. A spouse must realize that his partner is confronting perhaps the most painful issues in her life. She is working to catch up on what she missed in adolescence and may undergo enormous psychological growth spurts. She needs feelings of stability and love to help her reach each new stage of healing. Some men can do this. Others, understandably, react with irritation. Those negative, unsupportive reactions can block her. Partners need to be aware of their contribution to an ongoing problem.

Such conflicts often play out in the sexual arena. She may lose her sex drive, for example, a common symptom of eating disorders. On the other hand, he may be afraid to approach her, thinking that she needs her space or fearing her emotional lability. Yet his backing away will only increase her feelings of rejection. She needs assurance more than anything else.

She may wake him up in the middle of the night, wanting to talk about her anxieties and insights. She may badger him. "Do I look fat?" she asks as she starts putting on the necessary pounds. She may need help with child care while she goes to treatment.

All these demands put additional stress on him. And he has to be up to the task, willing to take on enough responsibility so that she is free to do her inner work. But he must not overcompensate. He cannot take on her problem. For these reasons, he would do well to enter therapy himself.

He should not underestimate the stress on himself. Studies show that men with partners suffering from mental illness are more likely to suffer from depressive disorders themselves. On the other hand, a good relationship can help a patient. "I am feeling supported to change," she says. And so she goes the distance, potentially helping them both.

This is how Gail and Rob did it, first tackling her bulimia and then his subsequent depression. Gail, now 40, developed bulimia as a teenager. For years, she had no treatment, maintaining the secret after she married Rob when she was 28.

At first, Rob did not know about his wife's constant binges and episodes of vomiting after meals. The first inkling came eight years after their marriage began, when Rob's brother took Rob aside and said, "I think you've got a problem."

Rob confronted Gail, and she admitted the truth. She sought professional help, but without true willingness to change. After a time, she dropped therapy and simply worked harder at hiding her symptoms. She was terrified Rob would leave her but felt powerless to stop the disorder.

Rob did not probe. "Number one, I did not understand the significance or the ramifications of the disease, and number two, life was good," he explains.

Over the next seven years, the same scenario repeated twice more: people warned Rob, he confronted Gail, and she went into therapy with no signs of the disorder abating. Finally, two of Gail's friends approached Rob, this time bearing information about an inpatient treatment center. Rob did some research, called up experts, and learned what he had to do.

He sat down with Gail and said, "I know you are bulimic. I know you are bingeing and purging. I understand why you've lied about it. And we'll get help."

Gail was dumbfounded.

"I felt for the first time that he wasn't going to leave me," she says. "It was enough. It was enough."

She began outpatient therapy at the Renfrew Center, a cluster of eating disorders facilities headquartered in Philadelphia. She managed to hang on for four months, but then, two days after September 11, 2001, she suffered a relapse—after an incident in which she was prescribed the wrong medication for symptoms of depression.

At 41, Gail checked into the Coconut Creek, Florida, branch of Renfrew. Missing her family, sometimes insufferably, she began a long, painful process of learning about herself. She realized for the first time that her problem was not simply about diet and food. She revisited issues of her childhood, having nightmares and a sweep of powerful emotions.

Meanwhile, back at home, Rob held it together, commuting between their home in New Jersey and his job in Manhattan, cobbling together child care and taking out a second mortgage to come up with the $40,000 to pay for treatment.

Gail returned home a different person. She was 40 pounds heavier and feeling depressed. But, with ongoing counseling, she was able to work through her rehabilitation program and become symptom-free.

Four months after her return, Rob was hospitalized for depression for six weeks. It was Gail's turn to step up, and she did. The couple bonded more tightly, and the worst of the storm passed.

Within the next year, Gail began to ponder what she might do to help others with eating disorders. These were frightening thoughts, as she had not worked outside the home for most of her married life. She did not know where to start, but after brainstorming ideas, eventually came up with the idea of the F.R.E.E.D Foundation (For Recovery and Elimination of Eating Disorders), a nonprofit organization in Warren, New Jersey, whose mission is to raise awareness about eating disorders and, through fund-raising, help women who cannot afford treatment to pay for therapy.

Rob, through his company, had been looking for a philanthropic outlet. He joined her effort with business contacts and started annual golf outings as a fund-raiser. In less than three years, the foundation has raised more than $200,000. Gail herself has gone on tour, speaking at eating disorder events, testifying before her state congress, and helping to prod a New Jersey senator to include eating disorders in a recent proposal.

"This is the first thing I have done that I have felt intelligent and expert about," she says.

She is hitting her stride, and so is the couple.

"Gail is my best friend," Rob says. "We were united 1,000 percent."

And, that is a model of how recovery in a relationship can be done in a healthy way.

Once a couple reaches this point, they have dumped the baggage. They will feel lighter, ready to move on. From therapy alone and together they have a whole new set of tools. The couple can use them as needed to fix future marital crises, which will certainly arise.

This is intimacy in the very best sense of the term. Gail and Rob are laughing and feeling vital as a couple. And she is moving forward in her development as a woman.

4

Pregnancy

An Oasis in an Eating-Disordered Life

In a woman's passage into adulthood, weight is sometimes used as a metaphor for responsibility. When people say she is "taking on the weight of the world," they mean that she is assuming the roles and responsibilities of an adult.

With pregnancy, a woman stretches this definition of herself. As she reads her "what-to-expect" books and decorates her nursery, she is preparing for the day when she will become a mother.

A healthy woman can make the stretch. Literally. Her belly will expand and so will her identity.

This transition is so powerful that some researchers view pregnancy as a distinct developmental phase in a woman's life. They argue that women actively seek to be pregnant with a drive at once biological, cognitive, and cultural. In Eriksonian terms, pregnancy involves a crisis. It is a time of life that revives past issues and demands a groundbreaking shift in perspective.

For example, a woman may have gone through life believing that she received too little or too much attention from her mother. Maybe the mother was focused on a tenure track position or traveled for business every week, leaving her teenage daughter to run the house. As a child, the daughter may have resented this arrangement. But now, rubbing her swelling abdomen at her own faculty meetings, the daughter begins to understand. She feels the pull between the joy in her womb and the sense of responsibility to her colleagues and career. And suddenly, within that tension, she has an epiphany: *Now I know what my mother went through. It's time to stop being so angry with her.*

And then the mother-to-be adapts. She transforms herself. She invents her own image of the good mother and packages these lessons of pregnancy into her new sense of self.

That is the ideal. But if a mother-to-be had trouble transitioning in adolescence, when her hormones were also heaving and her body rounding in strange ways, she is likely to struggle again during pregnancy. In fact, she may struggle more this time around because the stakes are now higher. She has another life to take care of but no template learned in adolescence to say, *Yes, I am out of balance in my body now, but I made it through something like this before. I'll do it again.*

But, backing up a bit, this woman who has suffered from an eating disorder in the past has strikes against her efforts even to become pregnant. Hormonal and nutritional imbalances may have caused irregularities with her monthly periods. She may have a tough time trying to conceive. Other physical problems, which are poorly understood, may curtail her ability to carry a baby to term.

If she has suffered from an eating disorder in the past, her body has weathered years, or perhaps even decades, of starving, bingeing, and purging. Her bones may be weak from lack of calcium; her body salts and minerals may be depleted; the hormones and neurotransmitters that guide her feelings of hunger and satiation could also be out of balance.

In short, her body is not in the best shape to feed and support a growing fetus.

Psychologically, she is ultraconcerned with her weight and shape. Whether she has an active eating disorder, a history of an eating disorder, or the more benign "disordered eating," she has coped with her body obsessions by structuring her life around rules and rituals: She has to work out for forty-five minutes every morning and twenty minutes more every evening. She has to count out exactly twenty-four shredded wheat cereal squares into her bowl. She will eat nothing but fruits and vegetables before 5 P.M. so as to stay below her daily Weight Watchers calorie quota.

Alone, these kinds of eccentricities do not constitute a full-blown eating disorder, and a woman may actually never have had one in the past. But with pregnancy, food "quirks" can harm a pregnant woman and her baby.

Pregnancy exacerbates the anxiety that breeds these food and body rituals. To the woman with a bathroom scale in every room, pregnancy will feel like body anarchy. She might experience nausea when she works out. She might be too fatigued to do her second twenty-minute workout. She will grow hungrier and those shredded wheats will not be enough. Does she still count out twenty-four, or twenty-eight, into her cereal bowl? Or does she chuck it all in the name of "eating for two" and binge on a dozen Krispy Kreme donuts?

With this kind of anxiety, it is not surprising that many women with more serious eating problems opt out of pregnancy altogether. The issues involve physical infertility as a consequence of her eating disorder, but they also go deeper into common primal phobias about motherhood and cultural anxieties stemming from what it means to be a mother in today's society.

Generally, the course of pregnancy for women with histories of eating disorders or subclinical problems goes from wrestling with the idea of pregnancy to troubles with getting pregnant to adjusting to a pregnant body and ending up, postpartum, with a daunting battle.

The result? Each woman's experience is unique. Her story's closure depends upon the level of recovery and support along the way. If she has the foresight to amass enough resources, even before she makes the decision to bear a child, she can travel through the experience of pregnancy and delivery with more resiliency.

DO I WANT A BABY?

The question of whether or not to become a mother goes deep. On the one hand, biology drugs a woman with powerful urges. A woman's reproductive hormones ask her body and brain every month, *This cycle? Are we conceiving?* And the answer usually is no.

As time goes on, and the no's are still forthcoming, another question begins to form: even a woman in her late twenties and thirties, who seems very comfortable forgoing having children, at some point starts to wonder, *Am I running out of time?*

She may have a job or projects that she believes will fulfill her more than a child ever could. She may have dark feelings about having children based upon the way that she was reared. She may have chosen a partner who does not want to be a father.

And she is probably facing cultural currents that affect her in negative ways. Contemporary culture's views about pregnancy are complicated. On the one hand, society *seems* to revere childbearing—people offer their seats on buses to pregnant women, grocery stores have special parking spaces for new mothers and their infants, actresses show off their newborns in glossy magazines. But culture can also be cruel—conservatives lambaste unmarried women who do not practice sexual abstinence; the government has cut welfare benefits for low-income mothers; and people knowingly discriminate against fleshier women, who, for many, represent the maternal ideal.

What this means is that women who are already uncertain about whether and when to have a baby are making that reproductive decision in the midst of a confusing cultural climate.

For those with a proclivity toward eating disorders, the pressure ultimately focuses upon the body. A woman with this mind-set hears people ooh and ahh when they see a newborn in a stroller, yet, at the same time, she may imagine that they regard the lactating bodies of new mothers as "fat."

With the current slide toward ever more unhealthy standards of fashion model thinness, as expressed by a recent spate of graphic news stories—and countered by a ban in Madrid, Spain, on runway models weighing less than 125 pounds—it is no wonder. Today, the sight of a Boticelli woman clucking over her brood might evoke grimaces rather than the awe she once commanded a few decades ago. Culturally, people tend to associate fertility with fleshiness. Imagine the impact of this on a woman who comes to her reproductive years already sensitive about her body's shape and weight.

At the same time, the culture often portrays childbirth as frightening, even violent. Television shows depict women in labor, sweating, swearing, and hemorrhaging as they push out their babies. Movies, especially period films, show women in labor gripping their husbands' wrists in agony. Even classic literature and the Bible relate stories of women suffering, then dying, leaving their babies behind to bereaved or uncaring husbands. It is no wonder that women who have learned to distrust their bodies will equate childbirth with suffering, and even possibly with death.

While many women can get past these negative projections and happily give birth, those prone to eating disorders often feel that they could never accommodate themselves to the bodily changes of pregnancy.

These women's fears about their bodies' stretching and sagging mask their larger, deeper fears. A woman who is already nervous about growing up may see the birth of her child as the death of herself.

In an untitled drawing, painter Fons Van Woerkom depicts what a woman with anorexia is seeing when she thinks of becoming pregnant. It is a picture of a horrified naked woman dragging a fetus behind her by an umbilical cord. The baby looks like a ball, the umbilical cord a chain, the woman a prisoner.

It is understandable that a woman with this vision of motherhood will flee pregnancy. Her troubles often have roots in how she experienced her own mother. In a survey of female college students, those who reported the most distress about what they saw as their mothers' limited academic or career opportunities were twenty times more likely to show a depressed mood and disordered eating.

Twenty times is a lot. It could be that the daughters are simply reacting with sadness to their mothers' pain—that emotion arising from the recognition of the roles to which women were once relegated. However, if role limitations prevented a mother from self-fulfillment and, therefore, from being a good maternal role model, then her daughter may be fearful of repeating her mother's life. This fear may unconsciously influence her future reproductive decisions.

To take this thinking one step further, those women in the study who felt the most distress also developed gender ambivalence, a syndrome characterized by disordered eating, depression, anxiety, poor body image, menstrual dysfunction, headaches, sleeplessness, and sexual indifference. In short, the women who developed gender ambivalence were not sure that they really wanted to be women, at least in their mothers' enactment of the role.

Instead, they turned the ambivalence against themselves. Against their bodies. They halted their monthly periods, consciously or not. By so doing, they made the possibility of pregnancy moot.

A woman who cannot decide whether to have a baby might simply avoid the choice. By engaging in an eating issue of any severity, in essence, she is jumping into her getaway vehicle. Depending on the type of eating disorder—anorexia, bulimia, binge eating disorder—a woman focuses on starving or bingeing or purging to distract her from the decision to conceive or not.

Each disorder has its own false solutions and natural consequences on a woman's health and well-being. And possibly on the life of her child.

How Anorexia Nervosa Shuts Down the Reproductive System

If a girl has suffered from anorexia nervosa, by definition she has had trouble with her body's reproductive hormones. The body's response to scarcity is the connection between weight loss and infertility. Women evolved to stop reproducing in times of famine.

Biochemically, the body responds to a deficit of calories or nutrition by ratcheting up or down chemicals that affect the brain, the appetite, and the reproductive system. The whole system centers on a trio of body organs that orchestrate fertility: the ovaries, the pituitary gland, and a region of the brain called the hypothalamus.

At birth, a woman's lifetime of eggs are formed and wait, potent, in her ovaries. Puberty arrives. Normally, the eggs mature and send out waves of body chemicals, including estrogen and progesterone. The hormones ebb and flow monthly. Their fluctuation activates the hypothalamus, a peach pit–shaped structure at the base of the brain. The hypothalamus then signals the pituitary gland to prod the ovaries to ripen and release an egg every month.

The hypothalamus has a second function: it is a food and energy sensor. In times of scarcity, the hypothalamus senses that energy input is low. To rebalance the body, it unleashes chemicals that interfere with reproduction in order to conserve energy.

Evolution is speaking: What species would want to give birth in times of famine?

Meanwhile, body fat stores estrogen. In anorexia nervosa, body fat is metabolized and so are estrogen reserves, causing further problems with reproductive feedback circuitry.

Exercise boosts stress hormones such as cortisol and suppresses a fat-regulating hormone called leptin. If these hormones remain altered for too long, as they can be in states of chronic overexercise, they also interfere with the hormones controlling the ovaries, hypothalamus, and pituitary.

A dangerously low caloric input causes the hypothalamus and other regions of the brain to alter the production of neurotransmitters such as serotonin, which influence reward centers—appetite and mood, the building blocks of libido.

This is the basic science about how long-term disordered eating and overexercise cause a woman to lose her periods and sex drive. A woman with anorexia is not going to get pregnant without medical help. And she may want it to be this way.

While she is probably not waking up each morning and saying, "Gee, I do not want to get pregnant, so I'd better starve myself today," on a deeper level, by committing to anorexia, she is forgoing her chance to have a baby.

Whether the reasons for these behaviors are conscious or subconscious, the message is clear: some women with anorexia are using infertility to sidestep confrontation with motherhood.

How Bulimia Leads to Infertility or Unplanned Pregnancy

Bulimia can also hinder a woman's chances at motherhood. As with women who have anorexia, women with bulimia often lose their periods completely or have erratic ones. Researchers are not sure why. Some hypothesize that purging causes the reproductive tumult. But others point out that women with bulimia often starve between binges, sometimes going for several days without eating. So it is actually the starvation cycle that shuts down a woman's periods.

Stress can also play a role in this irregularity. Stress may be physical, as from vomiting, or psychological, as from anxiety about being discovered.

The bottom line is that women with bulimia also run into infertility issues.

But, unlike women with anorexia, women with bulimia may lose their periods only some of the time. When they are eating, their monthly cycles may resume, leading to unpredictable cycles. Add to this another characteristic of bulimia: women with the disorder often have overactive sex drives. According to Joanna Poppink, women with bulimia can binge on sex just as voraciously as they binge on double-fudge cookies. This connection also leads to promiscuity among women with the disorder.

The combination of irregular periods, promiscuity, and regular purging may cause a woman to inadvertently vomit her birth control pills: women with bulimia have more unplanned pregnancies than the norm.

Herzog's team at Massachusetts General observed that 54 of the 246 women in the study sample became pregnant, some several times, resulting in 82 pregnancies overall. Although the larger study consisted of women who had anorexia, bulimia, or both, only 7 of the women who became pregnant had classic anorexia, in which they starved but did not binge or purge. This makes sense: women with anorexia are not getting pregnant as often as those who have bulimia.

Now look at the psychology. A young woman who has not grown up herself, and has a desperate fear of taking care of another life, becomes pregnant accidentally. What is she likely to do? She is most likely to seek an abortion.

In the Massachusetts General study, only half of the 82 pregnancies resulted in live births, as compared to two-thirds in the general population. This was largely due to a higher rate of abortion.

The women in the study who were most likely to abort were single. In fact, the disparity between single and married women who had abortions was so striking that researchers framed single parenthood as a risk factor for pregnancy termination.

Strike one is the eating disorder, leaving the woman developmentally immature. Strike two is her fears about motherhood, born out of that immaturity. Strike three is the lack of a partner to help support her in managing the new responsibilities of parenthood.

Suja Srikameswaran, who works mainly with pregnant women with eating disorders at St. Paul's Hospital in Vancouver, British Columbia, adds another insight. The typical patients she sees are pregnant women between the ages of 22 and 42, half with anorexia nervosa and half with severe bulimia nervosa, defined by bingeing and purging so frequently as to interfere with daily functioning.

She points out that most of the pregnancies are unplanned. This fits with links between bulimia, irregular periods, and an overzealous sex drive. But in Srikameswaran's group, the majority of women chose to carry their pregnancies to term. The difference might be explained by the fact that most of Srikameswaran's group was married or had steady partners. In fact, their referral to St. Paul's clinic came because they *wanted* to have their babies. The women were stepping forward voluntarily, asking for help in coping.

The message here is that if a woman with an eating disorder becomes pregnant, she needs support, and lots of it. Every mother-to-be has fears when pregnant, especially for the first time. However, women with eating disorders often experience a fear that is paralyzing. It may be that a committed partner can help a woman with an eating disorder overcome her fears during pregnancy. If she lacks a partner, then she needs to draw from other resources, such as friends and family.

Meanwhile, bulimia and anorexia pose one more problem for women wishing to bear children: several studies have shown that women with these eating disorders tend to have higher rates of miscarriage than the norm. For example, psychiatrist Nadia Micali, at King's College in London, followed a group of more than 10,000 pregnant women in the Avon region of the UK. Of these women, 199 had a history of bulimia, 171 had a history of anorexia, and 82 had both anorexia and bulimia. These women had a significantly higher rate of miscarriage compared to women with no eating disorders.

After further analysis, Micali found that miscarriage occurred more frequently with women with bulimia: they were 1.4 times more likely to have two or more miscarriages than women without eating disorders, even those who had other psychiatric illnesses such as depression.

No one knows why the babies conceived by women with a history of an eating disorder are less likely to make it to term. The logical conclusion would be that starving, bingeing, and purging while pregnant harms a growing fetus. But it may not be that simple.

Researchers have been unable to show a clear, consistent link between severity of symptoms and likelihood of miscarriage. There are women with severe symptoms who do not miscarry, and women with no symptoms at conception or during pregnancy who do miscarry. Thus, simply cutting down on the bingeing and purging while pregnant does not ensure carrying a baby to term or having a healthy baby. A woman also has her own health history to consider—how ill she was before she conceived and what damage she had done to her body's systems, for example. And, ultimately, there are many complicating factors here that doctors simply do not understand.

Doctors say the best advice for a woman with a history of eating disorder who wants to become pregnant is to work with a therapist to stop her symptoms and work through the psychological issues before trying to conceive. And, for those with erratic periods, be sure to use birth control, particularly condoms.

Binge Eating Disorder: How Obesity Causes Infertility

Binge eating disorder does not show up often in the medical literature in relation to pregnancy. However, most patients with the disorder, characterized by regular bingeing without purging, are overweight or obese, and obesity does have known negative consequences upon fertility.

Research shows that early obesity leads not only to earlier menstruation but also to greater rates of infertility. This seems contradictory, given that anorexia and weight *loss* also cause a woman's monthly periods to become irregular or cease altogether. But too much weight tends to flood a woman's body with reproductive hormones, just as too little weight dries up the system.

The key to all this is fat. Hormones such as estrogen, in the potent form of estradiol, are normally stored in fat cells or produced by the ovaries after stimulation. At the same time, fat cells can produce a variant of estrogen, called estrone, from a weak male sex hormone. An obese woman, then, can produce too much estrogen, the equivalent of taking birth control pills, which also add estrogen to normal levels in a woman's body.

Another reason for infertility in relation to obesity is polycystic ovarian syndrome (PCOS). This condition, marked by numerous cysts in the ovary, also causes the ovaries to alter their production of sex hormones, making PCOS the cause in up to 20 percent of infertility cases. Researchers estimate that anywhere from 30 to

75 percent of the cases of PCOS occur in obese women, although physicians are not sure of the exact reasons for the link.

Women who are obese also tend to make too much insulin. Not only does this lead to insulin resistance, the precursor to diabetes, but excess insulin also worsens infertility problems by overstimulating the ovaries, forcing them to shift their balance of hormone production.

Doctors can sometimes successfully treat infertility in these cases with specific combinations of oral contraceptives. But the treatment is complicated and controversial because oral contraceptives can also worsen problems with insulin resistance and create other risks for diabetes.

At the same time, even with fertility treatment, overweight and obese women will have a tougher time conceiving. In a study of 3,586 Australian women who sought fertility treatment, researchers found that obese women were 60 percent less likely to get pregnant during treatment than women with moderate weights. The study also found that the rate of infertility for obese women paralleled that of women who weighed too little. In short, binge eating disorder, reproductively, represents the mirror image of anorexia nervosa: both cause infertility.

The Outliers: How Other
Eating Disorders Cause Infertility

In addition to anorexia, bulimia, and binge eating disorder, there are other kinds of eating problems that can affect a woman's ability to conceive. In the worst cases, women with EDNOS have symptoms that are anorexic or bulimic in nature. They are just as serious, but they do not fit either diagnostic criteria. For example, a woman who purges regularly, overexercises, and loses her periods but does not drop below 85 percent of her normal weight range cannot be classified as having anorexia nervosa. And yet she is infertile.

Elite athletes, for example, are prone to having irregular periods (oligomenorrhea) or no periods at all (amenorrhea). In fact, depending on the sport, anywhere from 3 to 66 percent of adult female athletes do not menstruate regularly, as compared with 2 to 5 percent of women in the general population.

In a survey of female athletes playing in nine different sports at three NCAA Division 1 schools, 33 percent were actively trying to lose weight to compete in their sport and 16 percent either met the full criteria for or demonstrated symptoms of an eating disorder. The message is that those athletes who lose too much body fat, and so decrease their fat-to-lean ratio, can be choosing infertility, consciously or not. They are at risk for a condition known as female athlete triad, characterized by reproductive troubles, disordered eating, and osteoporosis—all at a relatively young age.

This does not mean that any woman who is an intense athlete does not want to bear children, but these women often find it difficult to give up their passion to prepare their bodies for a successful pregnancy.

Another infertility problem arises in women with subclinical disorders. This group includes those who once had an eating disorder but recovered enough to move beyond diagnosis as well as those who never were ill enough to qualify for diagnosis. While rarely studied, this group brings a disturbing twist to the decision to have a baby or not.

A woman with a severe eating disorder tends to focus on little more than her symptoms: *What did I eat today? How many times did I binge? How much do I weigh?* However, a woman with a subclinical disorder may direct her thinking toward larger questions: *What will it mean if I have a child and that child sees my disease, which I can't control? Why am I reluctant to get pregnant?* She is facing her problem in this way, trying to get past her fears enough to say yes to having a baby. But her body may still be saying no.

Now, because of advances in medicine, such women *are* becoming pregnant. But there are ethical issues to consider if she still harbors the remnants of an eating disorder that may reemerge at the first sign of stress. What will be the consequences?

GETTING PREGNANT

A Risky New Phenomenon: Women with Eating Disorders in Fertility Treatment

On a tree-lined street in suburban Cleveland Heights, Ohio, a purple-painted house nestles in a yard littered with Little Tykes toys. This is the home of psychologist Lucene Wisniewski, who specializes in treating pregnant women with eating disorders.

She opens the door, her 11-month-old daughter on her hip. Her two sons peek from behind her legs, blueberry muffins and plastic dinosaurs in hand. To Wisniewski, motherhood has been transformative, an experience she is integrating into the treatment of her patients.

She has been studying the issue of eating disorders and pregnancy for a while and knows the history: "It used to be believed that if you have an eating disorder, you have a harder time getting pregnant," Wisniewski says.

Biology was keeping this group in check, researchers thought. But now they are realizing that if women with eating disorders are having fewer children, "it's because they don't want to have them, not because they can't," says Wisniewski.

Studies show that most women who are infertile due to weight problems (with no other complications) can reverse their infertility by simply reaching a normal weight. But with medical technology today, a woman can conceive without gaining weight; she does not have to give up her eating problem fully—what Wisniewski calls her "other baby"—in order to become pregnant.

In this way, fertility treatment, as valuable as it is for couples who have suffered greatly due to infertility issues, has become a way to bypass the work of healing from an eating disorder. For the first time, society is witnessing the rise of a group of mothers who are grappling with their eating disorders while they struggle with the challenges of pregnancy.

How many women?

According to the Centers for Disease Control and Prevention, 1.2 million women sought fertility treatment in 2002 (the most recent year for which figures are available) and 6.2 million (10 percent of women who are of reproductive age) visited a doctor about infertility issues at some point in their lives. No one has tracked on a national scale what proportion of women with infertility issues also has eating disorders. But researchers interviewed 66 women who visited a fertility clinic seeking treatment and found that 17 percent had bona fide eating disorders. In a similar study by Australian researchers, a startling 13 of 14 women who had ovulation induced at another clinic met the criteria for an eating disorder at some time in the past. And 5 women in that study were diagnosed with an existing eating disorder.

In her large-scale study in the UK, Micali found that 20 percent of the women with anorexia, 11 percent of the women with bulimia, and 20 percent of the women vascillating between both anorexia and bulimia had gone to a fertility expert for treatment—as compared to 11 percent of women without eating disorders.

In short, women with full-blown and subclinical eating disorders end up seeking fertility treatment more often than women without the disorders. And while the numbers are not comprehensive, they are nonetheless alarming because the percentage is so high.

More disconcerting, *none* of the 66 women in the first study had disclosed their disorders to their primary health-care providers.

The reluctance to speak up is understandable. If an eating disorder is not shameful enough for its own sake, it is worthy of chastisement when it might harm the fetus. Women with subclinical problems might have other reasons for secrecy; they genuinely may not think their "food issues" are worth mentioning.

Additionally, while many believe that no woman should be denied the right to have a child, no matter what her history of mental illness, fertility treatment for eating-disordered patients presents many controversial issues.

Beyond the health of the infant, there are also direct implications for the health and well-being of the mother. For example, there are physical challenges to consider. Fertility drugs stress a woman with already-compromised health and hormonal imbalance. Psychologically, she may not be able to bear the stresses of that medication. She is already a perfectionist, hypersensitive to her own inadequacies. Depending on age, diagnosis, and type of treatment, the odds are that the treatment will not be successful. In 2003, only 18 to 43 percent of assisted reproductive technology cycles—defined as all fertility treatments in which both eggs and sperm are handled—resulted in pregnancy, and only 11 to 37 percent resulted in live births.

The fertility process itself, not to mention the specter of a miscarriage, can devastate a woman with a poor self-image. Therefore, any woman with a history of eating disorders, especially one who is undergoing fertility treatment, should consider counseling. (This is also true for any fertility patient who is subclinical, perhaps even a person who is simply overly concerned with weight and shape.) She has to be prepared for pregnancy and childbirth and supported, as the highs can make her euphoric and the lows can plunge her into depression.

>>> Cheryl's Eating Disorder

At 30, Cheryl had never menstruated naturally in her life. As a teenager, she had been diagnosed with anorexia nervosa. She had gained back weight after four years of therapy. Even so, she had never had her periods without hormone supplementation.

When she later married and wanted to have a child, she was left with no option other than the "fertility drill." First came the tests: temperature taking, pelvic exams, and squirts of dye into fallopian tubes to check for blockages. Later, a semen specimen in a cup. Drugs such as clomiphene (Clomid) to stimulate ovulation. This failed. Cheryl and her husband, Mark, brushed off the loss of six months' time and nearly a thousand dollars and moved to the next level of treatment—egg-prodding hormones.

Mark manned the syringe, full of a hormone that would ripen the eggs in Cheryl's ovaries. She took the shots nightly, and the next day she'd ride her bike to the clinic for a blood test and ultrasound, the cold probe thrust into her like an unwelcome lover.

On her back, Cheryl would grit her teeth and pray as she watched her insides displayed on a TV monitor. She learned to search the screen for the mass of ovary, gray and pulpy. She'd scan the picture for disks that looked like amoeba: these were her follicles, the pods that held her maturing eggs. The technician would locate the largest ones and measure them with an electronic ruler.

"Thirteen millimeters," the technician would call out. "Fifteen. Oh, this one's seventeen."

When the measurement reached 18, Cheryl would get a prescription for hCG, human chorionic gonadotropin. The hormone, also injected, would nudge the follicles to release a mature egg.

Then she would ride her bike home, timing thirty-six hours to conception.

There was nothing vaguely romantic about the experience, as every woman who undergoes fertility treatment knows. The first cycle failed. Cheryl sobbed in the bathroom as she bled. She threw the bloody tampon in the toilet and vowed to continue trying to conceive.

As the cycles of treatment went on, Cheryl learned to associate ovaries with cold probes, a womb with a TV screen. She felt a helpless falling sensation, legs open, doctors and medical students probing. She underwent the crying jags, the emotional tension, and the bloating that hormonal interventions can bring.

And there were the bills, about $6,000 for each cycle, and more for doctor visits and tests.

As it went on, Cheryl felt heavy, physically and psychologically. This spurred a resurgence of her eating disorder behaviors—eating less, exercising more. She called a therapist and started psychotherapy again after years of living partially recovered.

It is hard to judge whether fertility treatment in cases like Cheryl's is a good idea or not. When is a woman truly ready to make the transition to motherhood? In an ideal world, a woman who gets pregnant would not have any issues with food and body. But women with active eating disorders—or the more common disordered eating—desire to and do become pregnant. Cheryl, now age 42, persevered and eventually did conceive and give birth to a healthy daughter.

Why Do I Want a Baby?

The issues of becoming pregnant extend beyond biology and fertility treatment. A woman with a history of an eating disorder should reflect long and hard about her motivations for wanting a pregnancy. The reasons abound. Some women believe that when they reach a certain age, it is "time to start a family" and that having a baby will fulfill them personally. For others, having a baby is an attempt to find unconditional love. Others may want a baby as a gift for an errant husband, or a replacement for something or someone lost. Still others choose pregnancy because they want to be taken out of the pain of their eating disorders by connecting to something larger—they want to "carry a life inside."

A woman may also want to redo or outdo her relationship with her own mother. Or pregnancy may be a means to create some distance between herself and her parents, if the relationship is too smothering.

Some women even reach a stage in their recovery where they finally welcome femininity. And they imagine that having a baby will be the vehicle to take them to a new place in their development as a woman.

As noted earlier, a woman's level of psychological development strongly factors into her readiness to let go of an eating disorder. Desperate, she may have suffered for so long that she will do anything to rid herself of this eating-disordered demon. Unfortunately, pregnancy itself may be an attempt at that exorcism.

In one study, a third of mothers with eating disorders reported that they thought having a baby would be a means to get over their eating disorder. This thinking extends to women who suffer from depression or other mental health problems.

Women who view pregnancy this way might do well to reflect a little further. None of the motivations given above take the baby into account. An eating disorder takes a great deal of attention, time, and energy. The disease often becomes a narcissistic enterprise. Even if a potential mother imagines being a life-giver, her baby will not force her out of her self-absorption with her eating disorder. In fact, the stresses of being pregnant and raising a child are likely to set her up to fail, particularly if she is expecting an infant to do something for her that she needs to do herself. Thus, a woman with an eating disorder in any stage of recovery ought to reflect upon where she is, how far in her recovery she is willing to go, and how that will affect her baby.

>>> Adriana's Wish to "Connect to Life Inside"

Adriana, 26, was hospitalized for severe anorexia nervosa. While a patient, she met a man who had been admitted for depression. They got together. Having gained weight during treatment, Adriana started menstruating again—and she became pregnant.

Adriana dreamed about having a baby. She knew that she wanted it. It would be her ticket to a kind of love that she had yet to experience. She had had a terribly conflicted relationship with her parents. Her mother was verbally abusive, and when her father found out Adriana was pregnant, he threw her out of the house. She moved in with her grandmother. Her partner, in and out of the hospital, was unreliable. He would come and go, but not help out, as she would have wished. But she remained convinced that once the baby was born, the bond between them would be enough to transform her life.

Her therapists were skeptical. Neither Adriana nor her partner had a job, nor could they hold one, partly because of the time they had to devote to treatment. In addition, there was the issue of whether or not she would make it to term. The therapists understood that pregnancy with an active eating disorder is flirting with disaster. Yet they could only offer support.

Adriana's case highlights two questions: What impact does an eating disorder have on a pregnancy? And how does pregnancy affect the symptoms of an eating disorder? The answers are paradoxical, a mix of recovery and relapse.

·

BEING PREGNANT

What Does Her Eating Disorder
Do to Her Pregnancy?

Most medical studies of pregnant women with eating disorders are chilling. Mothers-to-be who gain too much weight experience a higher risk of hypertension and gestational diabetes, conditions which, in turn, are linked to birth defects and miscarriages. Pregnant women who are severely underweight at conception or gain too little weight during pregnancy are more at risk for giving birth to premature or to low-birth-weight babies.

Neonatal doctors link low birth weight to everything from infant blindness to developmental delays to fibrosis of the lungs. Low birth weight also equates, on average, to slightly lower IQs. At the very worst, a fetus born to an emaciated mother can be born with birth defects or die soon after delivery.

Ironically, in a study of underweight pregnant rats, the pups were born underweight and went on to become obese. Being starved in the womb might program overconservation of calories, so that underweight newborns would be predisposed to obesity later on.

Since this study has not yet been done in humans, the connection between underweight moms and children prone to obesity cannot be supported scientifically. But the animal studies do add to an overall message: what a pregnant woman does to her body affects the metabolism of her child, perhaps for life.

With this in mind, consider the possible impact on the fetus from a condition known as "hyperemesis gravidarum," characterized by excessive nausea and vomiting during pregnancy. Women with this condition are usually hospitalized for dehydration, electrolyte imbalances, or worse. It turns out that women with bulimia are diagnosed with the condition one hundred times more often than women without eating disorders. So, too, are women who have induced ovulation because of infertility.

Is it possible that these women are vomiting deliberately? The phenomenon has raised the suspicions of some obstetricians. But most doctors do not know when their patients have a history of bulimia. As noted earlier, these women don't tell.

Such was the case of Lauren, 41, who had a history of bulimia as a teenager. When she became pregnant, she vomited so much that she ended up in the hospital.

Was her throwing up a normal consequence of her pregnancy or something more sinister? Lauren blamed her nausea on her pregnancy. Only she knew the truth.

Whether an eating disorder was the culprit or not, her case

shows how easy it would be for a pregnant woman with bulimia to say, "I am nauseous and I throw up every morning," and then to go on purging intentionally. In this way, she eases her guilt about getting fatter while, at the same time, keeps her eating disorder under cover.

To be fair, societal pressure on mothers-to-be can be intense and inexorable. On the one hand, our culture smothers a pregnant woman with care, support, and concern. For many, particularly women with eating disorders, such an outpouring is the first and greatest in their lives.

On the other hand, woe to the mother-to-be who does something wrong. It is easy to fall off the pedestal. Media headlines castigate mothers who smoke or drink during pregnancy. While the chastisements for these behaviors might be warranted, it is hard to evaluate how reprehensible eating disorders really are.

Still, by maintaining the behavior, a pregnant mother with an eating problem can be endangering her unborn baby's life.

Again, numerous studies show that one of the most common risks of eating disorders is miscarriage—even if the mothers-to-be are symptom-free during pregnancy.

No one can ever say that any one miscarriage is caused by the symptoms of any one eating disorder, past or present. In fact, many healthy women miscarry, especially in the first trimester. But eating disorders specialists can say that women with eating disorders tend to miscarry more often than those without eating disorders, and they suffer multiple miscarriages at a higher rate.

Even more tragic than the miscarriage itself are the psychological consequences of a miscarriage on women with histories of eating disorders: "These women are at a much higher risk of feeling shame and loss or blaming themselves," Srikameswaran says.

It is not surprising that they often turn to the eating disorder for succor.

>>> Dana's Fears, Miscarriage, and Solution

This is the story of Dana, 40, who suffered bulimia and drug abuse as a teenager. In her early twenties, Dana quit her addictions cold turkey. She substituted "fitness," a more discreet type of addiction, for her vices, following fad diets, bodybuilding, and running every day. At 34, she married and soon after became pregnant.

Immediately, she called up a nutritionist she had seen in the past. "You have to help me," she said to the woman. "Because I'm scared, you know, about gaining weight. I want to make sure that this baby is getting the right nutrients."

Sensitive to the competing desires, the nutritionist put Dana on a drink supplement and prenatal vitamins. Dana, who was afraid that if she ate breakfast she would get fat, agreed to eat three meals a day and limit daily workouts to forty-five-minute runs. Then, in her second trimester, Dana miscarried. The effect was devastating. She blamed her nutritionist, who turned out to have a history of anorexia. Dana thought that history had colored the nutritionist's advice. She blamed herself for what she had done to her body with drugs, bulimia, and nervousness about body size. She realized that the birth of a baby was something that she could not control with strict routines and food rules. She fell into depression.

"There I was in the hospital, now weighing quite a bit, and I didn't have a baby to go with it," she recalls.

But the story has a happy ending. Dana learned from the experience. As soon as she could become pregnant again, she did. She decided to stop focusing on her weight and just focus on the baby. *Just let this baby be born*, she thought. And, with that focus, she relaxed her food restrictions—drinking milk, for example, which she would never allow herself to drink before. She also toned down her exercise. Nine months later, Dana gave birth to a healthy daughter.

What Does the Pregnancy Do to
Eating Disorder Behaviors?

While researchers warn of the dire complications of eating disorders on pregnancies, the truth is that these are not what most women with food and body problems think about when they conceive.

"For pregnant women with eating disorders, the biggest thing is weight and body changes," Wisniewski says. The mothers-to-be are not thinking about possible complications.

Culture hands pregnant women an unattainable ideal. Researchers trace it to antiquity, when cultures worshipped goddesses and portrayed them as plump and fertile. This began the link, as noted earlier, between fecundity and fatness, pregnancy and obesity.

There was a time when both were desirable, but today, only one is. Women in Westernized countries are revered when pregnant, but not if they're fat.

A case in point is actress Kate Hudson, who gained 60 pounds while pregnant. According to Salon.com, the paparazzi caught Hudson on camera "stuffing her pregnancy-bloated face well into her third trimester." The media had a field day wisecracking about her body change. Inspired or shamed, Hudson did the nearly impossible: after giving birth, she lost the weight within four months. To do this, she hired two personal trainers who put her through daily three-hour workouts and cut her food intake to 1,500 calories a day. Imagine an everyday mother trying to lactate on a 1,500-calorie diet. Picture her carving out three uninterrupted hours from hourly feedings, diaper changes, and laundering.

Unlike Hudson, most pregnant celebrities have redefined the look of pregnancy, donning tight-fitting maternity clothes, navels exposed. One is actress Gwyneth Paltrow, who left her maternity ward zipping up her prepregnancy fitted jeans. Actress Jennifer Garner played a pregnant CIA operative in the spy drama *Alias*. Expanding belly in tow, the heroine climbs through tunnels and shoots bad guys.

While woman can maintain much of their former lifestyle while pregnant, eventually life will change. A pregnant heroine can save the day, climbing buildings and burrowing through heating ducts, but she cannot escape her fate: she is going to put on fat as part of that change. In a society that says, "Flaunt the fetus but not the fat," there again comes the impossible standard: the ideal pregnant woman is a stick figure with a basketball at her belly. She is a pregnant Twiggy.

The message to other pregnant women is, "You can achieve this, too." Thinness and motherhood are both virtuous. But if the two conflict, thinness wins.

So, then, how does a woman, especially one hypersensitive to weight and shape changes, get pregnant without gaining weight? She can either keep her eating disorder and go for fertility treatments, or keep her disordered eating and become pregnant, but only "in the right places" of her body

In her article "The Perfect Little Bump" in *New York* magazine, Laurie Abraham wrote about women in the grip of this obsession. Some had eating disorders and some were only on the brink of them. The mothers-to-be did bizarre things to manage their body size and image during pregnancy.

For example, one woman lived on a low-carb diet of Wasa crisps and Dannon Light & Fit yogurt. Other women toiled through prenatal sculpting, spinning, and toning classes. Still others lied about their weight gain or inflated the number of weeks they have been pregnant. One woman would not let her husband come to obstetrician visits for fear that he would find out how much weight she had gained.

None of this is life-threatening. And since the fetus will pull its nutrition from the mother, before she gets it for herself, the baby is likely to be fine.

But there are degrees to these behaviors. Many warrant concern. At the extreme, they become a serious threat to the mother and her baby's health. Wisniewski tells the story of a friend, 38 weeks pregnant, who nearly fainted before her doctor's appointment at 3 P.M.

The woman had not eaten all day because she was worried about her upcoming weigh-in.

Another patient, with a history of obesity and bulimia, was "completely beside herself" about the body changes she was experiencing during pregnancy. This problem heightened with her second child as the mother worried that her body was protruding earlier compared to her first. Obsessed, the woman kept a food and weight log and compared the data, week by week, to that of her first pregnancy. If she matched up, she ate normally; if she went over the second time, she obsessed and restricted what she ate.

Perhaps the worst was a woman who could not give up her bulimia, continuing to binge and purge three times daily when pregnant.

"She couldn't attach to the fact she had a life inside her," Wisniewski says.

And that is what pregnancy is supposed to be about. She *and* her baby. Unfortunately, women with food and body issues have a hard time realizing that this is a separate life inside them, particularly during the first trimester. In this phase, more than any other, a mother-to-be doesn't feel like she is carrying a baby; she just feels sick.

She goes through biochemical upheaval. She experiences extreme fluctuations in appetite, mood, energy levels, sensations, body temperature regulation, thoughts, and, of course, body shape. She feels as if a foreign object has settled in her belly. *This being is possessing me.*

A woman who has not worked through her issues will panic. *Get it out!*

Women with borderline eating disorders, who already have deep issues of control, may use purging or starving to deal with their pregnancy, because for them the experience of pregnancy is a mixed blessing. In this situation, pregnancy can take a woman with a relatively minor food or body issue and push her over the edge.

Pregnancy as an Oasis

On the other hand, if she can forgo her eating-disordered behaviors into the second trimester, she might just reach an escape threshold. A majority of women suspend their eating disorder symptoms during pregnancy, and even begin to experience pregnancy as an oasis from their eating disorder.

At first this seems paradoxical. Here is a woman who, before pregnancy, has been stressed by the very thought of adding a pound or an inch. How does she reconcile this need for control with pregnancy?

Women with eating disorders often relinquish their unhealthy behaviors as their pregnancies advance. While this may seem surprising, many of the medical studies that depict the worst conditions of pregnancy and childbirth tend to involve small numbers of women with eating disorders, and often the sickest ones. Thus, those women with eating disorders who fall at a healthier place on the spectrum actually represent a very different narrative.

Pregnancy forces a woman to confront her food issues head-on. She gets some help from nature: after the first trimester, she starts to look *pregnant*, not just thicker. This woman now has a virtuous excuse to explain her added weight. At the same time, she feels her baby quickening, and this helps her to accept the reality and new-found wonder of her situation.

But the most common reason that women give for their change of heart and behavior during pregnancy is that they must change for the sake of the baby. *It's OK to screw up my life, but it's not OK to hurt my child.*

For many women, thinking about the baby is the first step toward thinking more deeply about her own psychological issues. Her body is changing rapidly, the eating disorder is not working, and she is getting fatter. She is also getting more nervous about the baby, whether she will be a good parent, and whether her growing body will ever shrink. All of these considerations together prompt many women to finally go into therapy. In fact, Srikameswaran says that although many of her patients have had their eating disorders for a decade or longer, "contact with us is often their first contact with treatment."

This overturns the myth that girls with eating disorders recover and only later get pregnant. Instead, therapists are now seeing a rise in the number of pregnant woman with eating disorders, and it is the pregnancy that forces them out of the closet.

Once she's in treatment, real change can happen. While often painted in a negative light, hormones can actually coax along the healing process. During pregnancy, chemical changes in the brain often draw a woman into a receptive, opiated state. She is connecting to life and, as such, may be more accepting of therapy and its potential to help her to live more fully.

As she relaxes into this state of mind, she is more willing to ask profound questions: *What do I want from life? What kind of role model do I want to be? What do I want for my child?*

As she tries to answer those questions, her pregnancy becomes a recess, a period during the life cycle when the eating disorder wanes and, in some cases, stops altogether.

CHILDBIRTH: THE SUM OF HER BEHAVIORS

Childbirth is the pinnacle of pregnancy. Women remember and recount giving birth. It is an experience that is at once arduous, ecstatic, terrifying, primal, absorbing, and indelible. Most poignant from the perspective of eating disorders, childbirth is transforming. What a woman has nurtured for nine months comes to fruition. She sees the baby for the first time. She is ready to begin mothering.

Or is she?

Studies, including one involving 1,000 Swedish mothers with histories of anorexia, show that most women and their babies do relatively well. However, there is a common childbirth complication that, while not normally life-threatening, does bear consequences: women with eating disorders have cesarean sections more often than healthy women. Doctors are not sure why. It could be a purely physical matter; an eating disorder may render a pregnant woman vulnerable to complications that require emergency C-sections. On the other hand, it may be a matter of psychology; obstetricians know that they are dealing with a high-risk group and order more C-sections to prevent potential complications. Regardless of the reasons, a C-section sets up yet another hardship on a woman who is already vulnerable to physical problems.

Despite this and other risks, most of the women with histories of eating disorders do give birth to healthy babies and suffer few, if any, medical complications themselves.

POSTPARTUM: BACK TO THE DESSERT

But childbirth is not the end of the story. In fact, birth is the beginning. Unfortunately, pregnancy is rarely a cure for an eating disorder. More often than not, it provides merely a temporary respite. For unless a woman has internalized the motivation to change, she is going to have a tough time as she begins her new life cradling a baby in her arms.

Postpartum, she must face her body anew, which is not the pre-pregnancy body that she remembers. Her breasts are swollen; her abdomen has stretch marks. She is fat—by her standards—but now with no baby inside as her excuse.

This realization can happen soon after giving birth. In fact, some women have been anticipating the aftermath of pregnancy all along. They were able to eat with relish while pregnant, letting loose and feeling free. But secretly, they harbored a vague worry. The eating disorder beast said, *Yes, eat now, but the day will come when you will have to pay.*

That day dawns the moment the baby leaves her womb.

Cheryl experienced the first pangs of postpartum depression in the birth center. First, she felt a surge of maternal warmth and joy when she held her newborn daughter, Emily, up to her breast and Emily opened her tiny mouth and suckled. But as the baby slept, Cheryl was not lying next to the crib. She was standing sideways in the mirror, pinching her slack abdomen, which felt like a partially deflated inner tube. It was as if ice water had been thrown on her dream. *Oh my God, this cannot be happening. I'll do anything; just get me out of this body.*

On the surface, she was obsessed by her fleshiness. Internally, she held a fear, a terror, really, of having to endure and to cope with her new body, the body of a mother.

Any woman who has given birth faces enormous demands: increased weight, healing from the physical toil of childbirth, sleep deprivation, fluctuating hormones, and stress from trying to figure out what her baby's varied cries mean. *Should I change the diaper or offer milk? Should I pick her up or let her cry herself to sleep? Do I have what it takes to be a good mother?*

A healthy woman is focused on these questions. Ideally, she asks for and receives help when she needs it. When she cannot, she struggles but may finally pull together the resources she needs. And she is able to juggle the demands, get some sleep, and accept her changing body, however grudgingly; her body's form is simply not that important compared to other changes in her life.

However, when an eating disorder is still active, a new mother cannot handle the duties of her new status. She may have depleted her limited energy and nutritional reserves in sustaining her baby. She may also be dealing with the aftermath of medical complications, recovering from a breech birth, a C-section, or a bout with gestational diabetes.

Therefore, she will channel her dread into one conclusion: she has gained weight. Putting on pregnancy pounds can resurrect all sorts of competing emotions and difficult childhood memories.

Even more, a woman with a history of an eating disorder is going to experience extra stress as her desires conflict. She wants to be the perfect mother, but she also wants the perfect body. She is not only glad that the baby is out and she can go back to the gym, but also irked because for the first time in her life, perhaps, she cannot get to the gym when she wants to. *Babies are demanding.*

This mother is feeling a profound loss. Her baby was her ticket to freedom from her eating-disordered behavior. Now, with her womb empty, she, too, feels empty.

She takes her sadness, which she may be feeling intensely now, and buries herself in her old eating disorder as a means of coping. Just as the eating disorder functioned as a crutch during her adolescence, it now deters her from building a new identity as a mother.

And women in this situation struggle painfully because during pregnancy many tasted what it was like to be eating disorder-free. Studies show that most women with eating disorders return to their behaviors within nine months of giving birth. In fact, in several studies, pregnant women with bulimia reported worse symptoms after pregnancy than before.

Exactly how many suffer these reversions varies by study. In Herzog's group, 30 percent suffered from postpartum depression, compared to 3 to 12 percent in the normal population. The most vulnerable women in this study were those with histories of anorexia; two-thirds were diagnosed with postpartum depression. Researchers are not sure why, but some speculate that women with anorexia might be the most attached to the thinness ideal.

No one tells mothers how long it will take until they lose their pregnancy weight. Researchers have found that most women have unrealistic expectations about the length of time it takes to lose the excess weight. Rapid weight loss by celebrities like Kate Hudson serves to fuel the popular myths. Meanwhile, average mothers who fail to achieve these impossible weight reduction goals feel bad about themselves and are more prone to depression. As an indicator, researchers have found that 40 percent of new mothers, healthy and unhealthy, felt dissatisfied with their weight six months after giving birth.

By virtue of their extreme body concerns and habits, women with eating disorders are vulnerable to these unrealistic models of postpregnancy weight loss. Their own failure to lose weight can trigger latent depression or push an otherwise mild case of postpartum blues into a full-blown depression.

On that note, recent studies have taken up the issue of pregnancy and depression. The first, published in the *Journal of the American Medical Association*, showed that women who had been taking antidepressants before getting pregnant and stopped them during pregnancy relapsed two and a half times more frequently than women who did not stop their medication. Therefore, if a woman stops taking antidepression medication when pregnant, she may end up with a condition that is dangerous to both her and her child.

On the other hand, a study published in the *New England Journal of Medicine* shows that women who took "selective serotonin reuptake inhibitors" (SSRIs) such as Prozac, Zoloft, or Paxil during the second half of their pregnancy had a small but significantly higher chance of delivering a baby with persistent pulmonary hypertension, a condition that typically involves severe respiratory failure.

Apart from some technical complications with the second study, doctors right now are calling for more research into the topic. The message is that women with histories of depression, and those with eating disorders who are taking antidepressants, need to consult with a doctor to help weigh the risks and benefits of continuing to take the drugs while pregnant.

In the realm of eating disorders, experts have reached a sobering conclusion: "If a woman with an eating disorder gets pregnant, she needs to be in treatment," Wisniewski says. "We should not expect her to cope on her own."

As an example of how bad it can get, Lauren, on antidepressants, gained too much weight during her pregnancy. She suffered through gestational diabetes, a thirty-eight-hour labor, and a C-section. For the first six months postpartum, she "checked out," both physically and psychologically. "I just handed my daughter over to my husband and went to bed."

She emerged from this period even more overweight. Her general practitioner told her that with her diabetes she ought to lose 10 pounds. Lauren began to diet, but once she started, she became bulimic, a relapse to her adolescent problem.

Finally, out of control, she became desperate. She took a good look at her life and her eating disorder. "It was winning out over my daughter," she says.

With that realization, she went for help and was able to stop her symptoms.

WHAT ABOUT DAD?

During pregnancy and the postpartum period, a woman is likely to explore her relationship with her partner. She is probably expecting help from him. But she may learn that her ideas and his are not compatible. If there were problems in the relationship before the pregnancy, they may become magnified after the baby comes. He may continue as usual in his own world, leaving her to shoulder the extra demands of feedings, laundry, and pediatrician appointments. And she may be trying to go back to work. Or she may fail to assert herself, as Adriana did, feeling, *Well, I should be able to do all of this on my own.* The birth of a baby may reveal the cracks and rifts in their partnership.

Or the couple may come together and rally around their new roles and new values, having discovered that parenting a child is daunting, even for a couple in which both partners are healthy.

GETTING HELP: START EARLY

Lauren was able to weigh her values—my daughter versus my eating disorder—and put her child first. While it might have felt like a conscious decision for her daughter's sake, her decision was made possible by her own advances in healing. Therapists say this internal motivation has to happen in order for a woman to truly recover. She cannot keep up her abstinence solely for the sake of someone else.

Healing for women with extreme shape and weight concerns can start even before pregnancy. With a therapist or a healer as a guide, a woman who has problems with her weight and body image can set realistic expectations of what changes she can expect to occur in her body, rather than be surprised or frightened by what will take place.

Realistic, though, is not perfect—even if the idea of a perfect pregnancy is trumpeted in the media. Women prone to eating troubles should be cautious: pregnancy-related books, articles, DVDs, kits, and TV programs offer a mixed bag of counsel and prescriptions for weight gain and nutrition. *Eat this. No, don't eat that. Continue jogging. No, give up running. Gain only 25 to 30 pounds. No, that's not enough.* These contradictory messages can combine with an intense body focus to retrigger a woman's obsessive thoughts about food: *I need to control how much I eat and how much I weigh.*

Emme Aronson learned about control. One of the world's top "large-size" fashion models at 5 feet, 11 inches and 195 pounds, Emme, age 42, had struggled throughout her life with humiliation about her weight and body type. In fact, her father, who was bulimic, used to weigh her daily and then draw red Magic Marker circles on the places where her body needed to be trimmer.

She developed an eating disorder characterized by bulimia, in which purging came mainly through exercise. But with help, Emme began to accept her body. "Once I found out that eating disorders existed and there was a word for it, that is when I started to seek help," she says. "It was like the heavens opened up. I thought, 'Oh, God, I am so not alone.'"

At 38, she got pregnant. A nightmare appeared to be coming true. Even as she ate a healthy diet, exercised moderately, and minimized her stress, Emme gained 70 pounds. She was shocked, especially since obstetricians generally were recommending a 25- to 35-pound weight gain during pregnancy.

Emme talked herself through her fears. She purposely ignored society's judgmental attitudes toward weight gain and tried to accept her pregnant body as it was. She played a mental game: instead of focusing on herself, she focused on the baby, turning the idea of "being fat" into "being rounded, more filled with child."

She also explained her history and her past shame to her obstetrician. He backed her up. "I would come in and say thank you for not making me feel like an inferior person for gaining weight during my pregnancy," she says. "And he was like, 'Oh no, you are doing great.'"

Emme now wants to use her experience to bolster other women with histories of eating disorders who are contemplating pregnancy. She talks about set-point theory, an idea that an individual's particular body is structured to weigh a certain amount, which is important because deviating too high or low from the body's norm creates disease. Set point is not just about weight but also about body type. Some women are ectomorphs, naturally thin and lightly built, with flat chests and poorly muscled limbs. Others are mesomorphs, with athletic, husky, hard, muscular bodies. Still others are endomorphs, who easily gain weight in the form of fat or muscle.

Emme is an endomorph. Because of her body type, she put on more weight during pregnancy than the average obstetrical charts recommend.

Her story also illustrates that a pregnant woman with a history of an eating disorder might gain support if she tells her obstetrician about her past eating disorder behaviors, even if she no longer engages in them. The key is to look for an open-minded obstetrician.

A traditional doctor might be unwittingly adding to a woman's tension with regular weigh-ins and discussions about exact numbers of pounds to gain or lose.

Psychologists Debra Franko and Emily Spurrell, at the Harvard Eating Disorders Center in Boston, actually published a paper urging obstetricians and fertility experts to be on the lookout for patients with eating disorders. The researchers advocate routine screening through questionnaires.

Here are the questions that a pregnant woman also can ask herself to see if she is at risk:

In the past twenty-eight days, how many times have you:

1. Tried to restrict what you ate, whether or not you succeeded or failed?

2. Tried to follow rigid rules around eating, such as calorie limits?

3. Tried to avoid certain foods altogether?

4. Gone for more than eight waking hours without eating anything?

Answering yes to several such questions can indicate a possible eating disorder. Also at risk are pregnant women who fail to gain weight over the course of two consecutive obstetrician visits and those with histories of eating disorders who suffer from severe nausea and vomiting.

There is some controversy over the ultimate goal of intervention. Some say the focus should be a healthy baby, no matter what that means for the mother. If the baby is in danger, a mother-to-be should be forced into treatment, or forced to eat a certain diet, even if over the long term such intervention is not going to hold. Others support the health of the mother first because when the mother does well, so does the baby. What this means in terms of intervention is that treatment should first target a mother's comfort level.

For example, Kim Williams, a dietician at St. Paul's, works with pregnant women with eating disorders, helping them with nutritional education.

"I tell them that I am not going to push anything that they are not ready to work on," Williams says.

So instead of presenting the women with a perfect meal plan and scolding the women who do not meet it, she sets realistic goals. She might say, "Maybe you could add some more protein to your diet," or "Do you understand that your hunger really goes up during pregnancy, and that in itself might be a trigger to bingeing, which could then lead to purging?"

Then she might give a pregnant woman a journal and ask her to write down what she is eating and include whether she binged or purged or used laxatives.

In this way, she and her patient can start to understand what triggers the bingeing and purging, or the restricting—and then work on prevention.

The overall idea of a mother-based approach is first to establish a sense of trust between patient and therapist and then build from there throughout the pregnancy. The baby's well-being arises from that.

Another approach that women with shape and body issues can turn to is cognitive behavioral therapy, a kind of mind-over-matter approach that unravels faulty thought and behavior patterns and substitutes healthier ones. This can help diminish the symptoms. And since symptom-free gestation lowers the risk of subsequent complications, the woman is likely to have a more successful pregnancy and childbirth.

But a new mother has to remember that the changes she makes during pregnancy may not last.

She should stick with her treatment in the postpartum phase, even if the demands of taking care of her baby seem to leave little time for therapy. To make the changes last, a mother-to-be or new mother is going to have to learn how to interpret her feelings accurately. She has to learn what she means when she blames her body for uncomfortable emotions. For example, saying, "I feel frightened about becoming fat during pregnancy," might mean, "I am afraid that when I go on maternity leave and no longer earn any income, I am going to become dependent on my husband. I don't want to lose that kind of control."

Abandonment is often a huge issue in these explorations, especially if the new mother had a push-pull relationship with her own parents. But with effort and time, a woman can work through her past as it influences her present and future status as a mother.

This new role is her future. Ultimately, she has to ask herself the hard question: "How well does the eating disorder fit into my vision of my life and family?"

In this way, she can transform *herself* into the reason for her recovery. She discovers that she is worthwhile as a mother, in any shape or size.

5

Parenting Years

A Kind of Sibling Rivalry: When the Eating Disorder Competes with Children

P arents and children communicate through food. From the moment the nipple enters the infant's mouth, the dialogue begins. And it unfolds with each subsequent decision: what to pack for lunch, which snacks are allowed, what to serve at mealtimes. But the parent-child connection goes beyond the dinner menu. Food is an integral part of the child's psychological development, for better or worse.

I know this all too well. I remember one Christmas when I was 10 years old. My extended clan, half-Czech, half-Slovak, had grown so large over the years that this one holiday we spent more than six hours joyfully opening presents. My mother, wringing her hands on her apron, stole into the kitchen every fifteen minutes to baste her roast, long since done. Time passed. Too much time. At last, when my family finally sat down to dinner, my mother watched, horrified, as she imagined everyone passing judgment on the stringy beef brisket.

In reality, the family was oblivious. I alone noticed my mother's face, pinched and growing whiter. In my typical preteen mode of trying to make everything right, I took the platter, forced a radiant smile, and raised the serving fork to take a giant piece.

Offended, my mother lost her composure. She jerked the platter from my hands, marched into the kitchen, and dumped the meat into the trash. The room went silent. This was the moment when I learned to equate food with perfection. Indeed, the failed roast became a reference point: why the next Christmas dinner and the next and the next were so much better. Perfect. Always a perfect roast from then on. But as a family, we never laughed with such utter joy again. My mother taught us through food that perfection supersedes fun.

And I integrated that lesson into my psyche. As I got older, food again became a metaphor. At 13, I refused to eat a plate of my mother's macaroni and cheese. This was a power play, a teenager bucking up against her parents' expectations. In response, my mother erupted, picked up the plate, and shoved it into my face. As I sat stone-faced, the pasta dripping from my cheeks, I knew I had won. My mother could no longer force me to be perfect because she could no longer force me to eat.

But I also had lost. I had to struggle for the rest of my life with an eating disorder.

It is through stories about food like these that we come to understand our relationships with our mothers. It is not surprising that we associate them with food. They are, after all, our first source of nourishment. Mothers decide when, what, and how to feed us and, in doing so, define who they are—and therefore, who we are.

As a daughter, I see this: my mother is an overachiever, born a generation too early for the women's revolution of the early 1970s. She channeled a drive that had few other outlets into food and family, seeking, and not accepting less than, perfection. Unlike other members of my family, I had a unique sensitivity to her drive and disappointment. It was as if, after my birth, we kept a psychic umbilical cord through which she transmitted her feelings, often the ones that she chose to deny on the surface.

It is this sensitivity that researchers say comes from nature. We, the women who develop eating disorders, are born with a genetic predisposition for such sensitivities. But how much is nature and how much nurture? These are the questions that eating disorders researchers are asking as they begin to look at cases in which the mother has had an eating disorder and she raises her child in that reality.

In her book *The Hungry Self,* Kim Chernin argues that all aspects of development—gaining a sense of trust, autonomy, initiative, industry, and identity—are negotiated through the child's connection to food and feeding. An infant howls with hunger, and the mother provides milk. By learning that warmth and satiety are just a cry away, the infant develops a sense of trust as food needs are met. A toddler learns self-determination when she realizes that she can open her mouth—or not—to eat the spoonful of pureed beets that her mother offers.

She gets to choose. Not the parent.

"Food is so charged, so significant, so informed with primal meaning," writes Chernin, "that we might well expect the communications that take place through food to carry more weight than those that arise when a child totters about knocking into furniture or pushes a truck across the floor."

Now we mix an eating disorder into the stew. If a mother stands in the pantry bingeing, vomits in secret, or cannot bring herself to eat at all, her child will be aware—even though she may not witness her mother in these acts. The child cannot decipher concepts like, *My mother is limited by her circumstances* or *My parents' marriage is dysfunctional.* Nonetheless, the child will figure out that her mother is upset or angry, or that her parents are fighting a silent war.

Some children are more sensitive to adult emotions than others. But all children learn from the way that they are fed. Food can be withheld or given too freely, or given for purposes other than nutrition. If a child is soothed by candy, she grows up rewarding herself with that indulgence. Fast-forward to her teens, and she may be battling an addiction to sweets. As an adult, she will have a more difficult time regulating what and how much she eats.

Does the child, particularly the daughter of a woman with a history of an eating disorder, then develop an eating disorder?

Studies suggest that an eating disorder originates when a child, born with a certain sensitivity, reacts to circumstances with behaviors that she has learned from her parents. For example, if mealtimes have always been a family battleground, then the daughter might be more inclined to use food as a means to resolve power plays.

If a mother has issues around food, she probably has issues around control as well. She may not pass on the exact same food issue, but she will pass on the problem of control. That replication can become a carbon copy of her disorder. If the mother has a history of anorexia, for example, then her daughter may develop this same eating disorder.

In other cases, the mother's problem may evolve in the daughter into another kind of eating disorder. Daughters of mothers who diet excessively, for example, are more prone to binge eating and obesity compared to daughters of mothers who did not diet as much or as often. Also, therapists cite examples of girls born to overweight or obese mothers who acquire anorexia in an attempt to avoid the shame that their mothers bear.

In two of the largest and most systematic studies of eating-disordered families, researchers studied the women and then combed through their family trees for other cases.

The relatives of women with anorexia or bulimia are seven to twelve times more likely to have acquired eating disorders in the subthreshold or diagnosable form than the relatives of women without eating disorders.

Binge eating disorder also shows up more often in the relatives of those with this disorder. These mothers, aunts, sisters, and cousins are also more likely to show symptoms of other forms of mental illness, including depression and anxiety disorders.

Something is being shared in these families. What is it?

Genetics, of course. And although research is now being conducted to find the genes predisposing a child to anorexia, bulimia, and binge eating disorder, these studies can only touch the surface. Genes are not the entire story; a mother with a history of an eating disorder is interacting with her child, passing on habits and values as well from the home environment, in her behaviors about food.

The research is still ongoing. No one has traced a direct line from infancy to adolescence to be able to say, beyond a doubt, that if the mother suffers, the son or daughter will suffer, too. Similarly, no one can give a checklist to a mother with a history of an eating disorder and tell her, "Do this and your child will be fine; do that and she will not."

Instead, investigators organize studies about eating disorders and parenting into chronological segments: the first year is marked by issues of breastfeeding; the toddler and preschool years focus on mealtimes, play, and physical growth; school-age years focus on behaviors, performance, and the first inklings of body-weight consciousness; and, finally, in adolescence, where we began this book, we see either the repetition of an eating disorder or the rebellion against it.

THE FIRST YEAR

The Mother's Perspective: Eating Disorders Compete with Bonding

When a woman with an eating disorder has a baby, she gives birth to a conflict. In order to become a mother in the fullest sense of the term, she needs to give up her first baby, the eating disorder. If she does not, she will now have two babies with conflicting needs. And, in both cases, they revolve around food.

But generally, a woman with an eating disorder clings to her first baby, the disorder, even though she may try at the same time to nurture the second. This indecision leads to a perpetual rivalry, and it shows up again and again throughout the child's life.

Early on, the competition plays out in the realm of breast-feeding.

The decision to breastfeed is an emotionally loaded one. Public health practitioners are now pushing—some say forcing—the practice. Meanwhile, each woman has her own strongly held, sometimes guilt-ridden, opinion. Rather than debate here whether it is best to breastfeed or not—or for how long—we would do better to explore how an eating disorder works its way into the choice.

Studies show that many women with eating disorders or body-shape and weight concerns breastfeed less than women without such disorders, or have more difficulty with the process. When asked why, some new mothers with histories of eating disorders reported that they felt too depressed. Others, particularly those with anorexia, said that they felt "too embarrassed" by the act. Still others did try but quickly lost motivation.

What is going on?

As noted in Chapter 4, the postpartum woman with an eating disorder runs the risk of depression and, because of those strong negative emotions, she is likely to fall back into her old habits. She probably never felt comfortable with her body. She is even less likely to feel so now in the postpregnancy period. In fact, those with the highest concerns about weight and shape are the ones least likely to breastfeed.

The metaphor for these sentiments is swollen breasts, certainly part of pregnancy's legacy. Breasts mean many things. They are at once erotic and maternal. Breasts embody desirability and also sustenance. They define womanhood. And we know that a woman with an eating disorder, particularly anorexia, wants no part of this equation: mother = fertility = fat.

There are clearly many reasons not to breastfeed: Some women have infections in the mammary glands. Others cannot get their infants to suckle properly. Still others have full-time jobs that conflict with regular feedings, and they choose not to express milk and store it for later feedings. But when eating disorders are involved, a different dynamic is affecting the lack of desire or inability to breastfeed.

Many new mothers with eating disorders are simply too obsessed by dieting or engaging in their eating disorder behaviors to breast-feed. There are two forces at play here: one is biological and the other cognitive.

Where biology is concerned, starving causes a new mother to stop lactating, even if she starts out at or above a normal weight. The situation worsens for a new mother who is underweight, trying to get even thinner. Women in this situation lose their milk supply early on and so cannot breastfeed.

From a mental perspective, a woman who is purging regularly, exercising wildly, trying to get the added pounds off, is also unable to give her time and full attention to sitting down with her infant to nurse regularly. She is beyond distraction; she is obsessed with her first baby, the eating disorder.

This combination of body and mind issues played out in Cindy's breastfeeding experience. She eliminated her bulimic symptoms during her pregnancy. Immediately after giving birth, she "stopped eating." Her milk dried up within weeks. She felt guilty. She knew that by engaging in her disordered behaviors, she was choosing them over her daughter.

The result? A painful tug-of-war. The new mother really wants to mother perfectly; she wants to bond to her baby. But she cannot when her eating disorder demands the same commitment. This dynamic often builds from a fear of intimacy that then plays out, as usual, on a woman's body. Breasts and breastfeeding mean a body-to-body connection. Only the womb holds a mother and child any closer. Some women with histories of eating disorders simply cannot stand to be that close to their newborns, even though some primal part of them may respond naturally to the instincts of motherhood.

The result is that a woman feels conflicted, but this emotion expresses itself as a cold feeling of dread about her body. Barbara, who suffered from an eating disorder much like anorexia, describes the internal feelings.

"I loved nursing," she says. "But I have to say that I didn't like my breasts [after giving birth]. They were too big."

Barbara's breasts were not overly large. In fact, when she went shopping for a nursing bra, she could not find one small enough to fit her. She had to settle for a training bra.

"Still, for me, I felt huge," she says.

Her breasts felt huge. *She* felt huge. She could not erase the thoughts about her body's changes even as her new baby enraptured her. Something in her was working to sabotage her joyful feelings of motherhood.

Barbara recalls: "I got home from the hospital and was loving the connection with my daughter, in complete bliss. And then I got into the shower. I'll never forget this: I could literally lift up my stomach and let it go again."

Such disgust can be so powerful that it can sever the mother-baby connection, the same way that body disgust can damage the connection between adult partners in loving relationships. Even if a mother chooses her real baby over her eating disorder baby, at any particular moment she may find the tension unbearable. That is because her real baby is a powerful psychological force. Its demands require that she let go of her old self—her body before pregnancy—and adopt a new self.

To realize herself fully as a mother, then, a woman must make a choice—and a transition.

But a woman nursing an eating disorder is in severe conflict. How does she bake the brownies, devour them, put her hair in a ponytail, and vomit, all the while being on call for her baby? How will she sanitize the bathroom in time for when the baby wakes up howling for food? Which baby does she feed?

Some therapists say the way around this is education. The strategy is to help the woman in this situation to understand the benefits to her baby of feeding breast milk versus formula. An astute practitioner could tell this compelling information to a mother with an eating disorder. And she might understand and embrace the facts. And yet letting go of her food and body obsessions would still be enormously challenging. She may understand *intellectually* why she should stop her eating-disordered behaviors: the baby has to receive a steady flow of nutrients or it will die. This understanding, however, is often not enough to get her over her fixation: those breasts and that body that are so different—and not who she believes that she is.

More recently, studies are showing yet another dimension to the breastfeeding story. Psychiatrist Nadia Micali discovered that women with histories of eating disorders actually breastfeed their infants *more* than women without eating disorders.

More? This seems contrary to the studies mentioned earlier until we learn what else Micali found. She discovered that the kind of eating disorder the breastfeeding mothers had was bulimia nervosa, not anorexia. Previous studies focused more on women with anorexia.

Women with bulimia are more likely to be eating than those with anorexia. Thus, their milk supply is more likely to remain flowing. In other words, more breastfeeding women with eating disorders in Micali's study had bulimia, as opposed to anorexia, and therefore *could* breastfeed.

That is part of the reason for the discrepancy. Another piece of the puzzle comes from different studies, which have shown that breastfeeding can actually accelerate weight loss after pregnancy. Indeed, lactation burns up to 500 extra kilocalories a day. And public health messages have noted this as a fact when encouraging women to choose this option.

Women, particularly those with bulimia, gravitate toward purging. A desperate woman is likely to take up any purging technique that works. Putting it all together, the women with bulimia in Micali's study may be viewing breastfeeding as a newfound purging device. "Women have figured out that by breastfeeding you can keep your weight down," Micali says. In this way, they are likely exploiting this nursing benefit to avoid giving up their body image problems.

One more twist. Recent studies have shown that breastfed children are 20 to 45 percent less likely to grow up to be obese adults, and that a child's risk of being overweight drops by 4 percent for each month they are given mother's milk instead of formula. Even though further studies demonstrated that these anti-obesity effects are relatively modest, still this fact has been championed by mothers obsessed about fatness. They are using breastfeeding as a dieting strategy for their infants as well as for themselves.

The Infant's Perspective: Ravenous or Refusing Food

How does this affect the baby? An infant cannot speak. It cannot say, "Come on, Mom, get over your fat-body thing and feed me." But the infant can tell its mother it is feeling her conflict. One way is through the baby's body.

At the extreme, medical reports describe infants of mothers with eating disorders who fail to thrive or are simply smaller than infants born to mothers without eating disorders. One of the most sobering reports described the babies born to a group of 140 Danish mothers who had anorexia nervosa: more than a quarter of the infants had eating and weight problems in the first year of life, and nearly a fifth failed to thrive—defined as failure to gain normal weight and sometimes height.

Studies suggested a combination of causes for these problems. At conception the mothers of the smaller babies tended to weigh less than the mothers of normal-weight babies. In effect, mothers engaged in eating-disordered habits can indirectly endanger the health of their unborn babies.

After giving birth, the problem goes on. Case reports describe mothers with eating disorders who ration food for their *babies*, diluting formula in bottles, for example. Mothers, in these cases, are extending their eating disorder directly onto their children. And the children can suffer injury that can plague them throughout their lives.

According to the March of Dimes, there is a long list of problems linked to low birth weight, from impairments in lung function to cerebral palsy to mental retardation. The most recently reported example is a severe form of attention-deficit hyperactivity disorder and a similar malady known as hyperkinetic disorder.

Low birth weight and failure to thrive are only two problems that infants of mothers with eating disorders may suffer. Researchers have uncovered a more severe—and more indirect—illness called "infantile anorexia." Pediatricians first spotted it among feeding disorders in children who fell below the fifth percentile for their age or children whose weight was less than 80 percent of the ideal body weight for their age for at least one month.

Babies with infantile anorexia willfully refuse food, even as they drop in weight. One may wonder why an infant, who does little else but follow instinct, would choose not to eat. The key is that the child with the disease is simply reacting to his or her surroundings in the only way he or she knows how. Through food.

Studies link infantile anorexia back to parents who tend to have conflicted issues with autonomy, dependency, and control. In these situations, parents try to encourage their child to eat based on their own determinations of when to eat and how much to feed their child. However, the infant does not always comply. The parents react to the infant's rejection and become anxious and frustrated, trying to get their "picky eater" to eat more. The baby further senses the parents' anxiety, adding to its own, and so eats less. The cycle goes on until the baby becomes truly ill.

Infantile anorexia might have genetic origins. Gene makeup might cause a baby to feel full faster or to become easily upset and refuse food. But the disease also may be fostered by the baby's environment. One study of 102 children evaluated the mothers of infants diagnosed with infantile anorexia. Although the mothers did not have eating disorders any more frequently than the mothers of healthy babies, the mothers of eating-disordered children were more insecure, particularly in their relationships with their own parents.

In some way, the mothers were communicating insecurity to their babies at a time when the baby most needed to feel secure. This is the stage in development that Erikson refers to as trust versus mistrust. The baby has basic needs: food, shelter, and emotional safety. If these needs are met, the child learns to trust that the universe is a safe place. But if the child is deprived, she will not feel the necessary contentment to take the next developmental steps.

Thus, if a mother is purposefully withholding food, the baby does not have its needs met and fails to develop trust. The baby will then act out this mistrust, wailing at first, and then head-banging or sucking continually when no one comes to feed her. In severe cases, she will fail to bond with her mother or other caretakers. Her starving body is the expression of her starving psychological self.

Even if the baby is fed on schedule, this does not mean he or she is being nurtured psychologically. Psychologist Seth Pollak, at the University of Wisconsin, studied children adopted into American families after being raised from birth in foreign orphanages. There, the babies failed to receive standard emotional and physical contact from caregivers, even though they received regular feedings. This lack, in turn, affected the infants' brains. Compared to controls of American children raised by their biological families, the adopted children produced lower amounts of two hormones, vasopression and oxytocin. These are the hormones of bonding. They are associated with stress regulation and usually rise after socially pleasant experiences, such as comforting touches.

The study shows that a failure to receive typical care can disrupt the normal development of hormonal systems. This, in turn, interferes with the calming and comforting effects that normally emerge between children and their caregivers. In essence, psychologically neglected babies, even if fed, will fail to bond.

In the realm of eating disorders, this failure is significant. From the baby's perspective, infant anorexia is one extreme expression of bonding trouble. A child with the disease is refusing sustenance because of emotional duress.

At the other extreme, infants facing emotional strain can "binge"—in a loose sense of the term. This is best illustrated by studies of infant sucking rates. When researchers want to know an infant's state of mind, they often measure aspects of suckling: rate of jaw movement, head turning, and length of feeding time, for example. It turns out that babies of mothers who have had eating disorders suckle differently from the children of healthy mothers. The former suckle faster—more avidly. Further, the same babies grow up and wean, on average, nine months later—and with more difficulty when compared to babies with non-eating-disordered mothers.

What is going on? In essence, the baby is saying, "Something is wrong with the way you are taking care of me."

Let's unravel this by first taking a closer look at the study. It says something about the complex dynamics of a mother with an eating disorder and her baby.

Mother-Child Perspective: Eating Disorders Blur Bonding and Boundaries

Psychiatrist Stewart Agras and his team at Stanford University went to nurseries in the Bay Area and recruited newborns and their parents to participate in a "five-year study about child nutrition and growth."

The parents of 216 infants signed up. To the researchers' surprise, a disproportionate number of mothers (21 percent) had eating disorders. Their prevalence in the study was three times what the researchers had expected—based on known estimates of eating disorder frequency in a normal community sample.

Either epidemiologists have been underestimating the number

of mothers with eating disorders, or the Bay Area is uniquely ripe for the illness, or the mothers who want to participate in this kind of study are those most obsessed about their babies' nutrition and weight. Or all three may be true.

Many experts agree that public health officials have underestimated eating disorders in the general population. Psychologist Eric Stice, at the University of Texas, Austin, who worked on the study, says that based on his clinical experience, the Stanford–Palo Alto area has a higher-than-normal percentage of women with subclinical eating disorders. Often the women have had anorexia or bulimia nervosa but are now "stabilized" so as not to be in "medical danger." Still, the women are underweight and food-obsessed.

"That is manifest as mothers who are hyperconcerned about how their kids eat," Stice says. He calls this "residual paranoia." It plays out in the way this group feeds their babies. More avid sucking, which is true of these babies, often means that infants are hungrier and more ravenous than the controls. A clue as to why comes from the fact that the majority of the ravenous babies were girls; it turns out that the mothers with eating disorders fed their daughters on a less regular schedule compared to the mothers of boys.

The study suggests that the mothers, prompted by their eating disorders, had delayed feeding in an attempt to control their own food intake—and thereby the weight of their female babies. But the babies were hungry and communicated that dissatisfaction in the only way they knew how: sucking faster and longer to make up the difference.

This makes sense, given that most babies of women with histories of eating disorders do not fail to thrive. The babies tend to meet their developmental milestones on time. Still, the infants sometimes have to have their needs met in situations when at least one of the primary caretakers is reluctant to provide them. And so the babies have instinctively learned to get enough to eat by sucking harder and faster.

However, another explanation of the sucking rate may be genetic.

The babies of mothers with weight issues might have inherited a genetic predisposition to suck differently. This, too, makes biological sense. If a child is born with, say, a deficiency in her serotonin system, she may feel more distress than a normal baby. She may instinctually suckle to soothe that distress.

But again, the explanations all eventually circle back to the combination of nature and nurture. If a child is living with an anxious mother, the kind of mother who would sign her infant up for a child nutrition study, the infant could have inherited her mother's anxiety genes, while learning her mother's anxious behaviors.

The bottom line is that any new mother struggles. But with the vestiges of an eating disorder, the struggle can be traumatic.

"How do you figure out when the kid is hungry, when you don't know when you *yourself* are hungry?" Wisniewski asks.

The babies respond to this confusion by undereating, rapid eating, or eating for reward and comfort. In this way, the mother with an eating disorder blurs the line between herself and her baby. She projects her inner discord onto her child.

"There are pretty strong boundary issues here," Wisniewski says.

THE TODDLER AND PRESCHOOL YEARS

The Mother's Perspective:
Stress Is Mounting

To understand some of the stresses on today's mothers we need only log on to any one of 8,500 blogs written by parents about their children. The websites track every diaper change, minute of naptime, and brand of baby food. Fretting and commiserating, many parents' blogs reveal that they feel alone and terrified.

Such anxiety and venting stems partly from social pressure. As a nation, we are particularly unforgiving of parental flaws. TV shows such as *Everwood* and *Gilmore Girls* mandate the ideal: parents model extreme and perfect attentiveness to their children to inspire maturity, confidence, and achievement in them. By contrast, there are shows such as *Weeds,* about a widowed mother who does the right things but also sells drugs to try to make ends meet. Her younger son, in reaction, shoots cats, makes mock-beheading videos, and beats up other children in karate class.

The message is clear. Parents had better parent well or the consequences will be dire.

In reality, parents are often living far from extended family, losing that traditional source of support. Even new parents who had help early on with caretaking from relatives and friends will find the network begins to disintegrate when children reach toddlerhood and beyond. Maternity leave has all but ended after the first year, leaving some mothers to contend with work, day care, and child-rearing duties. At the same time, parents are cumulatively sleep-deprived. Their marriage will feel the toll; the constant demands of child rearing and readjustment will wear on both of them. Many mothers choose to stay at home, which means that they have lost the collegiality of the work environment and additional family income, and gained proximity to the kitchen 24/7.

Let's look at a mother with an eating disorder under those circumstances. She has been struggling to keep her disorder at bay. Before giving birth, she may have coped with her binges by leaving her cupboards bare. She may have dealt with a proclivity toward anorexia by avoiding meals and exercising regularly. But as her baby reaches toddlerhood—ready to eat solid food—she is going to find that her past eating disorder habits are spinning out of control. How can she stay tuned in to the demands of a toddler and find time to work out? How can she avoid food when she has to prepare three meals a day plus snacks?

Which snacks? How much? How many calories? Is my kid going to get fat?

During infancy, feeding was easier. Infant meals had fewer choices: *Right breast or left? Every hour or upon demand?* Formula added some complexity: *Powdered versus liquid? Whey, casein, or soy protein?*

Nonetheless, these decisions were far fewer than what comes next. Solid food, from pureed beets to strawberry yogurt, provides an opportunity for mothers with eating disorders to channel the normal stresses of parenting to where they have always channeled their disturbances—eating disorder behaviors.

Even though 70 percent of women with eating disorders in one study improved their symptoms while pregnant and half were symptom-free, only a quarter stayed that way throughout the first year postpartum. Other studies confirm the trend: after the first year, three-quarters of women with prior problems will have picked up some form of their eating issues again. The issues will spill out and over her baby, now growing up and demanding more complicated nurturing skills.

>>> Cindy Cannot Juggle Bulimia and a Toddler

Cindy illustrates the conflicts of a mother with bulimia and the responsibility for a toddler. She left her job in the air force after giving birth to her daughter, Maggie. At the same time, she was forced to move from England to New Mexico, and then to Wisconsin, because of her husband's job. Within the first two years of parenting, Cindy lost her career identity and her bearings. She became pregnant again and found herself nauseated, while saddled with the challenges of a toddler. She and her husband lived first in a motel for a month, and then she was alone as her husband left for eight weeks of military training. She did not even know where the nearest grocery store or playground was located.

"Anybody who had relatively healthy coping skills could get through something like this," Cindy says. "But I was nuts."

Her eating disorder, which had diminished during her first pregnancy, exploded during her second. She purged regularly. At the same time, Maggie's food became the focus of her obsessions. She did not allow her daughter to taste refined sugar until she was 2 years old. No first birthday cake. Only vegetarian foods.

Cindy controlled everything that went into Maggie's mouth. "I became a real food fascist," Cindy says.

The crux of the matter is control. Feeling out of control, Cindy attempted to order her life and that of her family with the same tight fist with which she had controlled her own renegade emotions.

A mother with a past eating disorder, one who is under constant daily stress, cannot stand in the supermarket line with a box of chocolate Teddy Grahams in her hand and feel in control. Instead, she feels wound up tight; not only is she dealing with the normal stresses of motherhood, but she also has to silence a voice in her head craving chocolate.

She is hungry because she has not eaten all day. She is thinking, *Should I buy these or not?* She wants chocolate. But she will not allow herself any. She is on a low-carb diet. She projects her distress onto her child. *Should my child have these or not?* She reads the package, tallying the carbohydrate count. Meanwhile, her child strapped in the shopping cart is getting fussy. The child shrieks and bangs her sippy cup on the plastic seat: *It has 26 grams of carbohydrates. Too much sugar. What about the cinnamon kind?* The child bangs harder.

"Stop that now!" the mother lashes out. She thinks she is yelling about the banging, but she is really yelling at her eating demons.

What does the child see? The mother believes, as Cindy believed, that she is being careful. *Maggie never sees me purge. Therefore Maggie does not know.*

But, according to Blake Woodside, the child does know. "Children as young as three or four will know that their mothers have eating problems," Woodside says. "Quite reliably."

Toddlers' and Preschoolers' Perspective:
Dependent and Fearful

Toddlers can pick up all kinds of cues that either do or do not paint a landscape of well-being. When researchers want to study children's health, they often begin with something easily measured: weight and physical health, for example. In that vein, researchers can show that, like infants, toddlers of mothers with eating disorders, on average, tend to be smaller and lighter than children of healthy mothers. In fact, psychiatrist Alan Stein, at the University of Oxford in England, studied thirty-four mothers with eating disorders and their children, aged 12 to 24 months. Eight of the toddlers had dropped below the fifteenth percentile of weight for their age. One child had fallen below the third percentile. But what was most dismaying to Stein's team was that the *birth* weights of these children had been similar to those of children born to mothers without eating disorders. In other words, the children of mothers with eating disorders did not gain the same amount of weight *after* birth as children born to normal mothers.

This lack of proper weight gain may have occurred because the mothers with eating disorders, particularly anorexia nervosa, underfed their children. If so, then the children's weight loss is about projection. A mother with anorexia, by definition, has a distorted view of her body. She thinks that she is fat, even when she is emaciated and growing thinner. She takes this same view of her child and starves him or her to keep the toddler from getting "too fat."

Examples of this situation come from case reports in which mothers with eating disorders described their children as "pudgy," "greedy," or "dawdling" during mealtimes. When doctors examined the children, however, they were not overweight, ravenous, or eating any longer than children of mothers without eating disorders. In fact, extreme cases show that the children were actually malnourished and psychosocially deprived.

Taking the child's perspective, researchers conducted a different kind of study and drew the same conclusion. They looked at a sample of children who were failing to thrive. It turns out that the mothers of the infants who failed to thrive tended to score higher than control mothers on tests that measured desire to diet and to be thin.

Tragically, the mothers of undersized toddlers seemed indifferent to their children's low weight; half of the mothers in this group were restricting their children's intake of "sweet food." A third was restricting food that in their view was "fattening" or "unhealthy."

In perhaps one of the most tragic illustrations of outcomes from such distortion, researchers found that a child whose eating-disordered mother reported him as greedy and obsessed by TV ads about food was actually underweight and malnourished. He was eating ravenously and staring at food ads because he was starving.

But some eating disorders experts also caution that these tales are the extremes, not the norm. More often than not, the children of mothers with histories of eating disorders turn out to be physically normal.

But are they normal in every way?

To address that question, it is helpful to revisit normal child development through the toddler and preschool years. According to Erikson, a toddler should be venturing out, a stage he refers to as autonomy versus doubt. What should happen is that a little girl who totters away does so solo. She falls down at first, but tries again and eventually learns that she can walk, gaining confidence.

Later, she starts taking new initiatives, experimenting with the objects in her world. Food is a big part of that world. The child flings mashed potatoes, squashes bananas, and spits out mouthfuls of spinach. She tries to pick up goldfish-shaped crackers and she does so, *by herself.*

This is one stage of child development, facilitated by a Tupperware container full of snacks.

Parents can and should offer new foods, and try hiding the spinach in the applesauce to coax the toddler to eat nutritiously. But ultimately, the choice to swallow is the child's: *It's my body, Mommy. Not yours.*

At the same time, a child, in her new adventures in food, is also experiencing new and terrifying emotions. If her mother has an eating disorder in some form, the child does not understand that. But she does comprehend her mother's unhappy face, the same mother reading the nutrition label of Teddy Grahams in the grocery story. The child takes her mother's mood to heart; the child believes that she did something wrong.

This belief, in essence, is shame, a bad feeling. Experiencing a bad feeling, the child acts out. Maybe she flings her body backward in the seat of the shopping cart. She throws a tantrum. She is attempting to deal with the scary world of emotions, those she picked up after she saw her mother's angry face. In this way, the child is pushing the boundaries just to see if they are secure. *Am I OK, Mommy? Do you still love me even when my sippy cup dumps on the floor and makes a puddle of apple juice?*

Her mother may be lost in the echo chamber of her eating disorder and not pick up her toddler's cue. The child then learns that it is not OK to experiment with new things. *Mom gets mad when I do that. Mom gets sad. Since I don't want Mom to stop loving me, I won't try anything new.*

This early experience will have an impact on the child as she gets older. Observers have seen children imitating their mothers and "learning" eating-disordered behaviors by example. Stewart Agras, Eric Stice, and their colleagues at Stanford followed 216 newborns until they reached the age of 5, sorting out the children whose mothers had eating disorders from the children whose mothers did not. Eating-disordered behaviors emerged more often in the children whose mothers had eating disorders. Over the course of five years, 34 percent of the children in the study overate; 18 percent ate in secret; 10 percent vomited after overeating; and 10 percent refused food.

What is more, the children who were most likely to eat in secret had mothers who tested as bulimic, impulsive, or dissatisfied with their bodies, and who were heavier compared to the control group.

At the same time, children who were most likely to overeat had mothers who were heavier, dieted, and felt driven to be thin.

This study unearths and solidifies a link between mother and toddler around eating disorders. The link could be simple. The mother eats in secret and so does her child. The link could also be partially genetic; a child who eats in secret might have been born heavier. The child then grows up sensitized to her own weight, in part because of her mother's attitudes and behaviors.

The training starts early—very early. Agras discovered that even a 2-year-old could be embarrassed by her weight. Again, in a combination of nature and nurture, the child eats in secret because she has learned that food goes with weight and eating equates to shame. She overeats because she has tried to diet, like her mother. But there is a difference. The little body of a toddler will not let her go hungry. She then overeats to compensate.

The Stanford study says that even if a child does not see her mother's disordered-eating behaviors, the child will still experience some echo of her mother's attitudes about food and body.

Imagine a youngster who climbs up onto the counter and pulls out a box of fruit roll-ups. She thinks she is taking the initiative, a good thing, only to have her mother reprimand her because she has taken food without permission. How does a child gain confidence and a bit of independence if her mother is overreacting about Teddy Graham nutritional values, locking cupboards, and telling the child which foods to like and dislike?

The message is clear: a child will have a hard time if her mother has an active eating disorder. The mother's own psychological development disorder is likely to affect the psychological development of her child.

But does this mean that the child, too, will develop an eating disorder?

Maybe. One other finding that intrigued Agras was the way the behaviors emerged. They started gradually, episodically. Let's say on one specific day, a 2-year-old ate too much cookie-dough ice cream, for example. She became ill. She then ate normally for the next couple of months. Later, she binged again. She did it again and again, accelerating in frequency until, at the end of the three-year study, she and many other 5-year-olds with eating-disordered mothers were at their highest levels of eating-disordered behaviors. Eating disorders sometimes emerge as early as toddlerhood and then increase in severity with age.

The Mother-Toddler Dynamic: Separation Issues at Mealtime and Play

Stein at Oxford wanted to know if a mother with an eating disorder fed her child differently than a mother without a disorder, so he videotaped the mothers as they fed their toddlers, and then compared them to normal mothers. In the end, the two groups looked profoundly different.

When they were feeding their toddlers, mothers with eating disorders fought more with their children, made more negative comments, and seemed much more anxious compared to healthy mothers. Conflicts erupted over what was being eaten and how and how much. Overall, mothers with eating disorders seemed to be overly concerned about the toddlers making messes. In fact, irritation about messes lay at the heart of almost half of their negative comments.

What do messes and negativity have to do with eating disorders? A clue comes from the playroom. Mothers in the study were asked to show their children how to use a toy. Those mothers with eating disorders—compared to controls—turned out to be more intrusive, interrupting, and distracting than mothers without eating disorders. The whole dynamic unfolded around control and who has it.

From one perspective, the mother who is ill tries to discipline her own body through her eating-disordered behaviors. She may unconsciously transfer that behavior to her child, whom she sees as an extension of herself. From the other perspective, the child is at the stage of development where she wants to experiment with auton-omy. And so she resists, with a force equal to her mother's drive to control.

Stein's study highlights the force-counterforce aspect of an eating-disordered relationship. It manifests in a physical way. Re-sults show that the mothers with eating disorders weighed less than women in the control group. The mothers who weighed the least experienced the highest level of mealtime conflict with their chil-dren. Thus, there seems to be a connection between a mother's drive to be thin and her drive to dominate her child. Perhaps the most driven mothers rear the most stubborn children. And the out-come is contention with a severity that reflects the level of initial drive.

Unfortunately, such skirmishes are at odds with what should be going on. As Wisniewski explains, parents of kids this age should follow the child's lead—unless the child is doing something dan-gerous. Their interaction should look more spontaneous, more fun. The child colors outside the lines, and her mother should applaud, not grimace and start erasing. The child eats sloppily, and her mother lets her, because the mother understands that her toddler is experimenting, seeking autonomy, learning how to use her fin-gers and, later, a fork. But when an eating disorder falls between them at the table, this healthy dynamic cannot happen. Food fights erupt, meal after meal, year after year.

As this kind of rigidity and conflict continues, one of three pat-terns tends to emerge, depending on the child.

Mother-Child Enmeshment

When a mother cannot distinguish between her needs and those of her child, the result can often be a relationship that is too close. The mother identifies with her baby, and vice versa. Their bound-aries are eroding. This means, at the extreme, that a mother starves her child when she herself goes on Weight Watchers; she projects her body desires onto her child. And the child reacts by becoming like the mother.

The enmeshment is behavioral as well as psychological. Researchers tell a story about a mother with a history of bulimia who developed an overdependent relationship with her daughter. Before the girl was born, the mother had binged on food for comfort. Once her daughter was born, the mother threw herself into her daughter's care as a pacifier for her own undeveloped emotional life. Every time the daughter uttered a whimper, the mother was there with a bottle and a gush of emotion. The mother needed to be needed.

The outcome was a 3-year-old child with eating and developmental problems. The girl was incredibly shy: she spoke only a few words and only to her mother. When introduced to other children, she cried desperately. When her mother tried to leave, the girl would comfort herself with a bottle, sucking on it constantly while rubbing her belly. The girl refused to eat in front of anyone except her parents.

Without words, the daughter had gotten the message: stay close to Mother. She also learned that "mother" means emotional comfort; "sucking" and "eating" mean physical comfort. The child never had a chance to learn how to comfort herself or discover her own autonomy because her mother was always stepping in—often with food as the vehicle.

Reversal of Mother-Child Roles

Projection and enmeshment are not the only dynamic that goes on when a mother has an unresolved problem. An emotionally immature mother may start abdicating her parental responsibilities. This may not be a conscious choice. The mother is simply focusing her energy on nurturing her eating disorder. The child, by default, compensates by parenting herself—and her mother.

Imagine the inner world of a child whose mother never sits down to eat with her. She learns, *Mommy doesn't like to eat. Mommies do not eat.* The child may think this is normal. Over time and with experience, she will start to see holes in this explanation. She sees that other mothers eat. She knows that she eats. She knows that she gets hungry. She eventually starts to question, *Why doesn't my mommy eat?* Eventually, she will do what children of this age often do to make sense out of a mother's distress: *It must be something about me.*

To compensate, the child will work very hard to make up for her perceived flaw. She starts taking care of her mother, as Cindy's daughter, Maggie, did. At the age of 2, she would answer the phone saying, "Mommy cannot come to the phone. She is crying."

Other children have learned to comfort their mothers during binges by holding their mothers' hands, drawing pictures for them, or handing them a stuffed animal. Some older children take over household chores, perhaps cooking meals for their struggling mothers.

It is one thing to give a 3-year-old a jar of peanut butter, two slices of bread, and a spoon. But when the parent progresses to such foods as macaroni and cheese manufactured and packaged in microwavable containers for parents on the go, what might be called independence for the child is really neglect. The child then becomes a parent to her parent, who, because of her eating problem, remains a child.

Mother Disengages from Child

Neglectful mothers fully ignore, abandon, or abuse their children. A woman who lives in the haze of binge episodes or the cold numbness of starvation, or the mother who spends three hours every day at the gym and comes home exhausted from working out and dieting is emotionally and sometimes physically unavailable for long periods of time. In one study, for example, a third of mothers with bulimia said that they ignored their children because they were so preoccupied with vomiting.

In one case, a mother with bulimia physically abused her son. Her illness was so severe that she binged and purged up to ten times a day. If her son interrupted one of these episodes, she yelled at him or hit him. Her son reacted to his neglect by threatening to wet himself, make himself sick, or throw a tantrum at the slightest hint of his mother moving away.

When asked about the behavior of her son, the mother replied, "He's my little man and he is protecting me."

This behavior is not protection. It is the reaction of an abused child who either identifies with his abuser by acting out or retreats into a corner. Either way, the dynamic is tragic. The mother lives her life oblivious to the damage she is causing and her child reacts to the eating disorder by cowering or lashing out against the mother.

SCHOOL-AGE CHILDREN

Mother's Perspective: Buying Too Much into Messages of Anti–Childhood Obesity

Now we reach the realm of schooling, where much of the food and body anxieties in our culture are escalating into great debates about sugar, junk food, school lunches, and childhood obesity. Women with histories of eating disorders are really struggling in this new arena.

I remember walking my daughter into her classroom on her first day of kindergarten. Amid the construction-paper apples, Legos, and alphabet letters with names like Mr. Munching Mouth, I saw a bowl of lollipops. I stopped cold. Were the teachers going to give Dum Dum Pops as a reward for sounding out M's or counting by 5's?

Indeed they were. My daughter came home with a sucker and a face full of pride: "I did it, Mom."

"Yes, honey, you did," I said.

What could I say? On the one hand, she had achieved; she had crayoned a self-portrait and written out her name: Elizabeth Ann. I knew from my work as a reporter that this was a sign that she was moving well through the tasks of the 5-year-old. Of course the teachers should reward that.

On the other hand, I had written countless stories about appetite and body fat. In reporting those, I had soaked up a plethora of public health warnings—from pamphlets, press packets, and public service announcements sermonizing about the demon of them all, childhood obesity.

Tip #1: Do not give food, especially candy, as a reward.

And so, from experience, I know this: children go off to school and parents lose control. For women with histories of eating disorders, this is a challenging transition.

A fat child in Western society is the mark of parental failure. The messages, hoards of them, say that if your child is fat, she will suffer a list of ills, including medical consequences (heart disease, diabetes, hypertension); job consequences (discrimination, lower pay, lost opportunity); and social consequences (playground teasing, isolation, ridicule). Therefore, don't let your child get fat. Stop the Coke machines in schools! Stop the junk food in cafeterias! Stop the TV ads! And, by all means, stop the suckers as rewards!

I have to admit that I, as a parent with a history of an eating disorder, have grappled with this issue for a long time. As I do, my e-mail still bulges with researchers peddling their latest schemes to prevent childhood obesity. There are petitions to chastise McDonald's for using cartoon characters to sell french fries; there are proposals for National Walk to School days; there are promotional ideas such as hiring cafeteria chefs who will make roasted salmon with green onion sauce and pita triangles topped with artichoke tapenade.

While well intended, these solutions seem to miss the mark.

Beyond the fact that my 10-year-old is unlikely to taste a forkful, let alone finish a plate of salmon with green onion sauce, I wonder how these ideas are going to solve a much larger problem in our society. In 2004, nearly one in six U.S. children was overweight or obese. The prevalence of childhood obesity has doubled in the last thirty years, and obese children as well as those who fit merely in the upper half of the normal weight range are more likely to become obese or overweight as adults. Most children do not get the recommended daily allowance of fiber, fruits, and vegetables.

Most of the national campaigns to prevent childhood obesity are not working. After evaluating sixty-four anti–childhood obesity programs, Stice and colleagues found that only thirteen—those involving the most intensive regimes—prevented weight gain. Only three intervention programs kept the participants from gaining weight beyond the three-year follow-up period.

One problem is that most programs do not address the causal factors of childhood obesity. In a survey of 1,300 organizations targeting the problem of overweight and inactive children, most provided educational material rather than helping to make structural changes in the children's environment. And most targeted children who were older than 6, long after health habits have been established. The result is that childhood obesity rates are rising, not falling.

Instead of wisdom, public health officials are bringing on confusion and worry. The messages are intimidating and mixed: *Don't let your child get fat. Her life will be miserable. But don't say things that will draw attention to your child's weight. That will bring on an eating disorder.* Adding to the chaos are business marketers who are profiting from our society's anxiety about fat while not really offering healthful, nutritious options. Instead, they are promoting their products in food pyramids that seem to change weekly as they reflect the diet *du jour.*

How does a mother with an eating disorder cope in this culture, one that is insanely obsessed with battling childhood obesity?

She probably does so in the same way that she manages herself in a culture fighting adult obesity. A mother with bulimic behaviors may first restrict her child's food and then, in a fit of craving, invite her child to dig into bowls of popcorn on "family movie night." A mother who purges through overexercising may sign her child up for soccer, swimming, and child aerobics. A mother with anorexia is likely to impose rigid dietary restrictions on her child. She will be the one going to the birthday parties and policing the amount of cake her child can eat. Or she may be the rare one who allows her child to eat all the foods that she will not allow herself to eat. Her child overeats and becomes her worse nightmare: a fat kid.

Even this mother knows that she cannot control everything

about her child's diet. But she will try. Depending on the severity of her illness, and the intensity of her drive to be thin, she will channel her desire for control into a scheme. For example, she might allege that the child has food allergies.

"That is a classic eating disorder tool," Wisniewski says.

A mother with an eating disorder simply sends her child to play dates and school lunches with an index card listing forbidden foods, everything from wheat to dairy to sugar. No one argues. Teachers, parents, even coaches have been schooled in the potential risks of allergies. She manages her child's food intake by subterfuge.* And so we end up with a culture of polarity. With children, as with adults, eating disorders rise in number commensurate with a rising epidemic of obesity. In the meantime, the campaign to stop childhood obesity is similarly dividing parents and children into two camps. The first group includes those who are growing so tired of the messages that they are simply ignoring them. The second group aggressively counters by turning to supersized, high-calorie fast foods.

To add to the confusion and panic, others, particularly those prone to binge eating disorder, have heard about a recent report by the Centers for Disease Control. It stated that people who are overweight but not obese have a lower risk of death than normal-sized and thin people. The conclusion for some is that this report gives them permission to supersize themselves with less guilt. Still other parents are fighting to change children's growth charts, that is, to change the standard so that fewer U.S. children will qualify for the label of "fat," thereby removing the stigma of that label.

Still other parents see another source of exploitation in the obesity debate. They assert that the pharmaceutical industry is behind this push, trying to expand upon definitions of obesity in order to pump up sales of anti-obesity drugs.

---

*This does not mean that any child with a peanut allergy or lactose problem is the product of an eating-disordered mom. Nor are children who keep kosher or who are vegetarians or vegans.

Many parents who do follow all the anti-obesity mandates include those women with anorexia *or* bulimia. Anti-obesity initiatives only stoke their fears. The more this group reads, the more nervous they get. They react by feeding their children tofu and greens for lunch, championing exercise, and in extreme reactions they bring on eating disorders.

While society may lament the rise in childhood weight problems, the core of the issue remains. Try as we may, we really do not control what our children eat, let alone what they weigh. Consider what could have happened when I sent my daughter off to school with her lunch box full of healthy fare: she could have eaten the food I packed, the veggie wrap and cut-up apples. Or she could have rebelled and thrown the apple slices in the garbage, opting for Cheetos from a friend's lunch. Her choice. And eventually, if she is to mature, she will have to choose for herself.

From the Perspective of the School-Age Child: Rising Body Dissatisfaction

Just what foods are the school-age children of mothers with eating disorders choosing to eat? How are they formulating their image of their bodies? It depends on the child. As noted above, toddlers of parents with eating disorders can fall into one of three camps, enmeshing with their mothers, taking care of them, or suffering from abuse. Their food choices at school, not surprisingly, will reflect the strategies at home.

For example, many children who have internalized their mothers' food attitudes or who work to soothe their sick mothers or are cowering from abuse will eat exactly what their mothers want them to eat. Fathers play into the dynamic as well, either projecting their own rules or abdicating to those of the mothers.

The parents may not realize what they are projecting onto their children. Woodside recalls a 10-year-old girl whose mother was in treatment for anorexia nervosa. The mother thought that her daughter was oblivious to her illness. And then, on Mother's

Day, the daughter sent a card. She had painstakingly re-created her mother's food diary, adding in inspirational messages to bolster her mother on her way to recovery.

"What you see at this stage are pressures from the parents for children to become extremely obedient and compliant," Woodside says. "So from age 6 to 12, you get a lot of perfect little kids."

And this dynamic plays out well beyond the lunch table.

There is evidence that children in these situations work frantically to meet their parents' goals for body size. In a survey of fourth- and fifth-grade boys and girls, researchers found that children, particularly girls, modeled their parents in terms of how they thought about their shape and weight. Elementary-age children also mimicked their parents' dieting.

Modeling to a child helps her build a repertoire of skills to get through later life. In Eriksonian terms, school-age children should be gaining a sense of self-esteem through productivity. They scribble a poem or drag and paste cutout shapes on the computer into a portrait of themselves. And they learn how to do these feats first by watching someone else and then mimicking what they see.

Children want to mimic others older than themselves because they realize that grown-ups have all the power. Kids want that power, too, as seen by their love of larger-than-life characters like Harry Potter.

But when it comes to body image, development requires more than modeling. In the study of fourth- and fifth-graders, researchers discovered that what mattered more in a child's development of self-esteem and healthy body image was not what she saw her parents do, but what she heard her parents say. It turns out that critical comments about a child's weight will erode self-esteem and make the child feel terrible about her body.

A similar finding from a British study of 379 children age 9 years old showed that the heaviest students expressed the lowest self-esteem. They also expressed the highest desire for thinness and practiced the highest levels of dieting behavior.

While the link between criticism and self-esteem did not surprise researchers, the study did give them pause because the girls with those symptoms were only 9 years old. Children, particularly girls early on, have received the message that the way to feel good about life, to feel good about themselves, to solve problems, all problems, even their mothers' problems, is to get thin. By the age of 9, thinness is *already* the silver bullet.

Moreover, this concept was not limited to the overweight girls. One-fifth of girls who were underweight also hated their bodies and tried dieting to change them.

Another study, of children in grades 3 to 6, showed that nearly 45 percent stated a desire to be thinner, 37 percent had tried to lose weight, and 7 percent scored positive on a test for anorexia nervosa. Studies of girls in adolescence found that 12 percent who scored highest on tests of body dissatisfaction and dieting went on to develop full or partial eating disorders by the time they were 18 years old. Only 2 percent of low scorers acquired eating disorders in later years.

Ironically, the current moves to *reduce* childhood obesity and the parental words that reflect disapproval with bigger bodies are backfiring. Rather than reducing childhood obesity, the large-scale anti-obesity rhetoric is leading not to thinness but to low self-esteem and body dissatisfaction, which in turn leads to attempts to diet, eating-disordered behaviors, and, ultimately, full-blown eating disorders.

Mother-Child Dynamic: Following the Thread Toward an Eating Issue

Is there truly a connecting thread from criticism of one's body to eating disorders that can be followed from school age to the beginning of adolescence? The answer is yes, but the course may not be straight. An eating disorder in a mother can manifest itself as an eating disorder in a child, although not necessarily the same category of disorder. Psychologist Leann Birch and her colleagues at Pennsylvania State University found that 5-year-old girls whose mothers most restricted their food ended up, by the age of 7, not thinner. Instead, they developed a pattern of eating when not hungry. By 9, girls who were exposed to the highest levels of restriction ironically tended to be the heaviest.

In another study of mothers and daughters, mothers who dieted the most were also the most depressed and had the greatest propensity to binge because of mood. Just so, their 10-year-old daughters were likely to experience food and mood issues. Following the connection further along the eating disorders spectrum, those same dieting and overeating girls had higher scores on a test that picks up latent eating disorders.

Thus, mothers and daughters are connecting, but in a dark place. That connection can take many forms, with the child beginning to mimic her mother's problem. But as these studies show, the child can also do the opposite, rebelling in remarkable ways.

To illustrate how meandering this path can be at an early stage of parenting, we can look to Dana, 40, who suffered from bulimia, and her two children, Haley, 6, and Austin, 4.

I meet them at their pediatrician's office in Brookline, Massachusetts. It is a typical kid-friendly place: plastic toys strewn about, *Highlights* magazines, and a shadow box table, covered in glass and filled with sand and boats. Tall, stringy Haley is kneeling beside her brother, who looks like a miniature skateboarder, green T-shirt and camouflage shorts past his knees. They are using a magnetic pen underneath the table to push the boats through the "sea" of sand.

Dana, watching them, says that she has been extremely hands-on about her children's diets, in part because Austin, days after birth, came down with a mysterious illness. Symptoms included seizures, and he almost died. Ever since, he has stayed at the bottom of the charts in weight and height. Ever since, Dana has grappled with fears about his health.

Coupled with her own history of bulimia, the concern for her children has pushed Dana toward vegetarianism. Together, they thrive on foods found only at markets like Whole Foods, including tofurky and soy milk (because of lactose intolerance). They enjoy fruits and vegetables. Dana does not buy junk food for the home. "My family does not eat chocolate," she says. Before their recent move to a Boston suburb, her children had never eaten sugar, not even in juices.

At that time, Haley entered kindergarten. "My first thought was that she was going to want me to pack all this junk stuff in her lunch box," Dana says. Concerned, Dana took time off from her job as a social worker to have lunch at Haley's new school. She was horrified by what she saw. "Candy bars and chips and all that," she says. "Why are parents packing candy in their kids' lunches?"

Dana started feeling guilty that her kids might think they were missing out. So she started occasionally baking sugar cookies with them. But her kids never ate the cookies. They typically licked off a bit of frosting, put the cookies down, and went out to play. Dana then threw out the licked cookies and, later, the rest of the batch. She could not stand to have them around her house because they would tempt her carb-conscious husband, who had been dieting on and off, Atkins-style.

However, Haley came home from school one day wanting Oreo cookies. "She doesn't even like chocolate," Dana said. "I don't get it."

Dana bought the cookies that Haley requested but, as she explained, Haley only ate the cream out of the middle. A kid not eating Oreos? I must have looked surprised, for Dana, at that moment, turned to Haley and asked, "Haley, you like tofurky, right?"

Haley, teeth split in front and blond curls framing a petulant face, looked up from the table of boats, met her mother's gaze, and said nothing.

And there in the girl's expression I saw it: defiance. It was ever so subtle. The conflict had not yet erupted. But I can envision the day when Haley is likely to look around the lunchroom and say to herself: *Other kids get string cheese and Cheetos. Why don't I?*

What will she do when she fully registers the disparity? A clue may come from another story her mother tells me. One day, the kids at school made fun of Haley's vegetarian sushi.

"Mom, they said I was eating seaweed," she cried when her mother picked her up.

"Well, you are kind of eating seaweed," her mother said.

And with that reality and the difference between her family's views and those of her friends, Haley had a choice to make. She could respect her mother's eating disorder, or she could choose the junk-food values of her friends. Which direction does such a child take?

From that day forward, Haley no longer wanted sushi in her lunch box.

TEENAGE CHILDREN

Mother's Perspective: Reliving Her Nightmare

A mother with an eating disorder wakes up to a nightmare. She sees her daughter coming of age. There are the usual mood swings, crushes, and Tampax. But this mother may also start seeing skipped meals, a diary of self-hate, and concern about how many calories are in a serving of iceberg lettuce. Too many Kit Kat wrappers in the garbage and too many empty tubes of toothpaste, and the mother, who once lived the nightmare herself, panics. *Oh no, not again.*

But there it is; her daughter is falling. And the mother wrings her hands thinking she is at fault. She could be. The line from eating disorder to eating disorder can connect from generation to generation. In a study of 5,331 adolescent girls, 3,881 adolescent boys, and their mothers, teens who rightly perceive that weight was important to their mothers more frequently obsessed about thinness and dieted.

Cassandra A. Stanton, at Brown University, followed 404 mothers and their adolescent daughters. She showed that there is a link between the amounts of fat that mothers and daughters ate, but not between mothers and sons—leading one to surmise that mothers are treating their daughters differently in areas of weight and shape.

However, the dieting link is far from complete. For example, the daughters in the same study did not eat the same amount of fiber as their mothers or follow the exact same menu. This slight mismatch implies that daughters are following their mothers' lead but also trying new ways of eating.

"Although mothers may exert a strong influence on young children, through controlling their dietary choices and availability of food," Stanton says, "maternal influence on dietary intake is reduced in adolescence, when the children have gained more independence."

And here Stanton gets to the issue: independence. As a teen, the daughter is going off *on her own,* though often not politely. The act of breaking away feels like anarchy to many parents. *Emily used to be so sweet. What happened to her?*

Now imagine how this normal transition affects a mother who has parented by enmeshment. The mother believes that she and her daughter are "best friends." And now her daughter is going away. The mother can only feel immense terror and grief because she is losing her very best friend.

Normally, a mother could lessen the impact by believing that she has given her daughter the tools to make it in the world. But when a mother wakes up to a child with an eating disorder, she sees little in this situation that can come to good. Whatever the stage in the mother's recovery, if her teenage daughter becomes ill with an eating disorder, the mother can easily regress. Beyond the normal stresses of parenting a teenager, the mother, through her daughter's problem, is reminded of her own unresolved issues and hurts. What often happens next is that the mother steps in and tries to control the daughter's illness. Then the two get further entangled, the mother trying to manage two eating disorders, the daughter unable to find her own way.

Meanwhile, the girl's father may blame the mother, leading to marital tension as well. Stress and tension, we have seen, wake up latent eating disorders. This is going to be a very difficult time for a mother with the history of an eating disorder.

Can this mother work out perhaps the most difficult part of the transition—separating her eating disorder from her daughter's—when success also means the mother will be left with an empty nest?

Barbara's story says that she can. Barbara, 54, the woman who stood in the shower mortified by her stomach after giving birth, twenty years later was horrified when she learned that her teenage daughter Emily had been rushed to the hospital after bleeding spontaneously. Emily had been taking thermogenic weight-loss tablets, pills combining caffeine and aspirin.

"That was the wake-up call," Barbara says.

Barbara knew that her daughter had been struggling with weight since the age of 16. The girl had become a professional ballet dancer, following in the footsteps of her mother, who also made a career from dancing and body movement. Barbara identified with Emily and became very involved in that struggle because she had lived it herself.

"My daughter will tell you that she doesn't have a problem," Barbara says. "As I would have told you at that age."

When asked if she felt responsible, Barbara did not even hesitate. "Oh my God, yes," she says. "The whole connection about weight has been very difficult for me because it has pushed a lot of buttons about my own struggles."

One button is the realization that Barbara may have unwittingly transferred to her daughter attitudes about body weight, attitudes that Barbara did not even know existed. "I've wondered," she says frankly, "is it easier for me to embrace my kids when they are thin?'"

Then again, Barbara has a second daughter who does not have an eating disorder. If the drive to be thin was because of something Barbara said or did raising her daughters, why didn't both girls succumb?

Perhaps one daughter escaped because, when the genetic dice rolled, she inherited her father's temperament instead. The interaction between nature and nurture is indeed complex. But figuring out the cause does not help Barbara and Emily. Barbara wants her daughter to be healthy, alive. To achieve this, Barbara had to sort out two eating disorders: the remnants of her own as well as her daughter's.

For years, Barbara found herself getting really "sucked in." Her daughter would come to her in misery, and Barbara would try to manage the girl's disease for her. She would coach her daughter about what to eat, how to set healthy body weight goals, and how to train for dancing in a healthy manner. But the approach, as kind and giving as it was, began to backfire.

"She had sort of looked to me to keep her on track and then hated me for doing it," Barbara says.

Conflicted, Emily wanted to be independent, but she also feared being off on her own. It would be better to hang on to her mother through food and body focus rather than to leave the nest. Barbara's efforts to manage Emily's disease were, indeed, those of a coach and "best friend," not those of a mother. Emily apparently recognized the nature of the dependency when she said, "I just need my mom back."

That was the tipping point. To help Emily become more independent, Barbara let go of her daughter's recovery and centered only on her own. "I had to come to terms with realizing that she just had to do this or not," Barbara says. At age 18, Emily is still dancing professionally, and she has made great strides in managing her own eating and weight. She and her mother have rebonded. But as adults.

The decision to let go is profound. It is what family counselors hope for, work toward, and celebrate. Letting go is particularly difficult for mothers who have food issues themselves. Barbara, for example, might agree that how she viewed and reacted to her own mother's need for control initiated or perpetuated an eating disorder. Having now gained that insight, Barbara is able to foster Emily's independence and also free up the psychological energy to spend on her own recovery.

From the Adolescent's Perspective:
Rebelling or Competing

On the other side of the relationship, the teenage children of a woman with an eating problem are getting saddled with two major challenges: navigating the normal upheaval of adolescence and trying to work out relationship issues with their mothers, who may still be sick.

To understand the adolescent's perspective, we need to think about a different culture. I recall a moment when I was standing with my daughter on a Boston subway train. The door opened at the aquarium stop, and a throng of teens got on. Immediately, the train was flooded in cacophony and color. We heard gum snapping, wrappers crinkling, and chips crunching. We smelled powdered cheese, synthetic grape, and french fries. We saw girls with shirts above their navels and boys in jeans with crotches hanging below their knees. We gaped at a girl's pants, cut so tight and so low that her behind, crack and all, spilled out of the waistband.

My daughter turned to me, rolled her eyes, and said one word, the word that sums it all up: "Teenagers."

Indeed. The word is synonymous with a culture, a unique and motley cult. No one but teenagers belong. At its hub is intensity, expressed through food and body. Teens convene at fast-food joints and movie theaters, reeking of butter, coffee, and nacho cheese. Teenagers wear outrageous clothing and poke and bump and rub each other in communication that is physical and overt.

So if you are a public health official or a parent and you tell a teenager not to eat junk food, to take up a sport, to stop sitting at the computer instant-messaging friends, do you think for a moment that the teenager will listen? You are an outsider, the object of their rebellion. They will listen, but only if their friends listen. They will match their eating habits to those valued in *their* world.

And what is that world like?

Teens live in a no-man's-land between a culture of junk-food values and a culture of thinness. If a teenage girl has a mother with an eating disorder, she is going to feel caught in the middle without a good role model to guide her.

With eating disorders already in the family, an adolescent is going to feel extreme tension and somehow will react to it. She is likely to choose one extreme or the other because, at her age, she lacks the developmental maturity to find a middle ground. The toddler who enmeshed with her mother and became the compliant schoolchild is likely to continue to hang on to her mother and her mother's attitudes. If she continues to identify with her mother, she is at great risk for developing an eating disorder herself.

But also, being out among young friends may serve as a wake-up call. A teen who had been relatively compliant through childhood may gradually realize that her family's unhealthy patterns are not normal.

"The child doesn't question her family patterns until she starts to hit preadolescence and adolescence," Wisniewski says.

And then she realizes: *Something is not right here.* Her friends, who see her too-thin mother, ask, "Is your mom anorexic?" And where she once would have said, "No, she just eats healthily," she suddenly opens the door to her mother's bedroom one night and asks, "Mom, are you sick?"

The Biology of Puberty Triggers the Arrival of a Latent Eating Disorder

This concept is no better illustrated than in a cluster of studies conducted by psychologist Kelly Klump, at Michigan State University in East Lansing. Her group studied 1,200 pairs of female twins, a mix of identical and fraternal. The twins, based in Minnesota, entered the study in two groups—at either 11 or 17 years of age. The studies continued for six years and tracked whether one or both in each pair of twins developed eating disorders.

Klump found that if an identical twin girl developed an eating disorder, her twin sister was 50 percent more likely to acquire an eating disorder than a fraternal twin. This finding suggests that genes may play a role in predisposing a person to an eating disorder, since identical twins share virtually the same DNA, while fraternal twins do not.

However, Klump noticed that age also appeared to be a factor in eating disorder emergence. The 17-year-old twins reported the eating disorders, not the 11-year-olds. The younger girls were, for the most part, disorder-free, although they did display the *prerequisites*—body dissatisfaction, weight preoccupation, and excessive dieting. Piqued by the finding, Klump began to wonder whether the genes that code for eating disorders became activated during puberty.

She found that a small subset of 11-year-olds did have eating disorders. And within that subset, most had reached puberty. In fact, postpubertal 11-year-olds exhibited eating disorders in the same proportion as the 17-year-olds. Meanwhile, prepubertal 11-year-olds only had the prerequisites for eating disorders, not the full-blown form.

"Something is going on at puberty," Klump says. "Something is getting turned on."

Animal studies say that the "something" might be female hormones. Estrogen and other reproductive hormones do help organize the brain. Estrogen has been linked to neurotransmitters such as serotonin, as well as a myriad of other mood and behavior regulators such as those that create body consciousness and preoccupation with self.

Could estrogen and other reproductive hormones influence the onset of eating disorders? Maybe. There is a weak link between variations in a gene that encodes an estrogen receptor and conditions of both obesity and anorexia nervosa. But the link between estrogen and eating disorders is weak. More large-scale genetic studies are now in progress to try to study that connection. Until those results are reported, it is best to say that eating disorders definitely involve genetics, but they may not alone be a matter of genes.

Here is what may happen: A baby inherits her mother's genes that predispose her to an eating disorder. In the uterus, the baby is also exposed to maternal estrogen. That could be the seed of an eating disorder, which might remain dormant until puberty, when the daughter's own estrogen levels are turned on by her endocrine system.

There is evidence that the hormonal environment in the womb does indeed play a role in the later development of an eating disorder. In a more recent study, Klump learned that the lower the level of testosterone exposure in the womb—and the higher the level of estradiol—the more likely a girl was to acquire eating disorder symptoms at puberty.

Klump hypothesized that this girl, the one with the genetic predisposition *and* the low testosterone/high estrogen exposure in the womb, was an eating disorders land mine. She was physically predisposed to be vulnerable to this disease. Then, at puberty, the dormant tendency to an eating disorder was aroused by a combination of genes, the prenatal environment, and the hormones of adolescence.

The question researchers are frantically trying to answer is: Can we defuse this bomb before it explodes? If we disconnected at least one of the components, could we prevent an eating disorder from emerging?

Maybe. One way to answer that question is to observe what happens when the teenager is a boy and does not have the hormonal makeup to create vulnerability.

>>> Ethan's Unconventional Adolescent Rebellion

Arlene, 56, suffers from alcoholism, anorexia, and bulimia. As a teenager, her son Ethan smoked, drank, and used drugs. During adolescence, this could be construed as adolescent rebellion, maybe even directed at his mother's problems. But his actions did not provoke the intended parental reaction. Ethan's mother, overwhelmed by her own issues, did not object strongly to any of her son's behaviors. In fact, she had a boyfriend who smoked dope with her son.

How does a teen rebel against a parent who already accepts and even does what are considered the "typical" teenage vices?

Ever looking for the wedge, Ethan found a way. He gained weight.

And that *did* spur his mother's ire.

Arlene was the kind of mother who worried so much about her son's weight that she would weigh him, as a baby, every day on a deli scale. At that time, she clearly had her own weight issues; at 5 feet, 7 inches she never weighed more than 100 pounds.

Ethan did not know directly about his mother's eating disorder. He understood that she had quirks: eating merely an artichoke and drinking a bottle of wine for dinner every night, for example, or working out twice daily, then binge drinking and eating at cocktail parties—and getting sick afterward. He knew that she wanted him thinner. At first, he went along with her wishes, articulated or not. He worked out. He lost weight quickly and got in shape. But after a year away at college he stopped. He became heavier again. And then his sister, Alison, told him the truth about their mother: she suffered from anorexia and bulimia.

This took a while for Ethan to accept. But eventually, he got it. The next time that his mother grew distraught about his weight, offering to hire him a personal trainer, Ethan shot back, "Mom, you only love me when I'm in shape."

"But Ethan, you look so much better when you are working out," she replied. "You're happier."

"I'm not happier," he said. "*You're* happier."

In this manner, Ethan used food and body size to rebel against his mother's eating issues. Still, he never got an eating disorder. We will never know if this outcome was determined by gender. Perhaps eluding an eating disorder in this case is simply about lacking the hormones and cultural pressures that a female experiences.

Then again, Ethan has a sister, Alison. How did she respond to her mother's problem?

The Mother-Teen Dynamic:
Whose Issues Are These?

When a girl lives with a mother who has an eating disorder, she tends to react in one of two ways: she either competes with her mother on body terms or she rebels. To illustrate the case of competition around an eating disorder, Woodside describes a teenager with a boyfriend who kept making comments about how pretty he thought her mother was. The girl's mother had anorexia. These comments fueled the girl's eating disorder as she drove herself to become as thin as her mother, to win the same adoration from the boyfriend.

When mother and daughter become intertwined around an eating disorder in this way, it is tough to separate whose issues belong to whom. If the mother has not recovered, she uses thinness as a badge for youthfulness, heightening the competition. She may even be trying to outdo her daughter. The daughter, on the other hand, is getting thinner in order to prove to her mother that she is worthy of respect and love.

As therapist Wisniewski says, "It is not an uncommon experience for me to come out to the waiting room to a mother and daughter and think, 'OK, now, who is the patient?'"

This unspoken competition says with the body: "I am the skinnier and, therefore, the better."

>>> Alison's Version of Rebellion

In the case of rebellion, the teenager may opt out of what she perceives as her mother's dangerous and miserable lifestyle. Ethan's sister, Alison, did *not* follow in her mother's eating-disordered footsteps. Alison, age 19, is fresh-eyed, long-haired, and curvaceous, dressed in corduroy hip huggers and a navel-baring T-shirt.

"I'm 5-foot-3, 140 pounds and my mom is 5-foot-7 and 95 pounds," she says. "We're quite different."

Indeed. Arlene, with a short dark bob, rich brown eyes, and hesitant smile, is ethereal, wispy. Alison is more grounded, fleshy, and vibrant. She laughs where Arlene sighs.

Alison sees the truth. She watches as her mother gets excited about fitting into her teenage daughter's clothing. In fact, Arlene goes shopping with Alison and her friends. The excursions annoy Alison. She wants her mother to be a mother. But Arlene thrives on the adoration when Alison's friends says, "My God, you are so skinny. Alison, your mom is so beautiful."

Still, Alison does not bite. In fact, she leans in the opposite direction.

"I don't know one girl my age who hasn't considered whether or not to diet," Alison says. "Having my mom has kept me from doing it because I know what she has been through. She walks around thinking she is fat. And I don't think you can be any skinnier than she is and still be able to breathe."

When asked if she has felt pressure to be thin from her mother, Alison nods vehemently.

"I think definitely she wants me to be that size-0, skinny-type person," she says. "But I don't want to. It is tough to see her and see me and think, 'Oh my God, to ever be that pretty, you have to be so bad to your body.'"

Thus, Alison, despite the hormones and family environment that might predispose her to an eating disorder, has chosen a different path. She handles her mom with blunt directness. At a restaurant, for example, Alison reached for a piece of bread and Arlene blurted out, "Are you sure you want to eat that?"

Alison responded, "Yes, Mom. You know, we are not all going to be anorexic."

On the other hand, Arlene still frets about Alison's weight. She refers to her daughter as "chunky." Arlene has hired a personal trainer for Alison and tries to get her to go to spin classes. Alison does go— but not twice daily like her mother.

Overall, Alison was the toddler who parented the parent. "I love my mom," Alison says, "Obviously we are best friends. But sometimes you need more than that."

Lacking a "parent," Alison has grown up to be a young woman who takes care of others. Woodside says this dynamic is common. So is the propensity of these young adults, the children of women with active eating disorders, to reenact their childhood dramas by choosing careers that involve nurturing: child care, nursing, and social service professions, for example.

When asked what she wants to do when she finishes school, Alison smiles. She looks into the distance for a moment and then says, "I want to become a family psychologist."

APPROACHES TO RECOVERY

Understanding the dynamics of a mother with an eating disorder can help bring awareness, and a first step toward recovery. The opportunities in each family will be unique. The mother's influence will depend on her phase in recovery, while the child's contribution will depend more on her stage of physical and emotional development.

The first step carries an implicit hope for health. It is never too late to begin.

And, to begin, there are two main ways to handle parenting and eating disorder issues. The first approach is to direct the attention to the children; the second, to the parents.

Wisniewski, who studied obesity in children, says, "I really think that lots of people don't know how to approach food with kids."

This is not because of a lack of information. There is a vast literature with advice from many schools of thought. Wisniewski lists some of them: There are the "clean-your-plate" people, who say that children should not get a treat unless they finish a plateful of the nutritious stuff. There are the "you-can-only-have-one-thing-of-sugar-a-day" people, who define moderation by rules of how much.

There is the "control-the-portion-size" group. In the book *Eat, Play, and Be Healthy: A Harvard Medical School Guide to Healthy Eating for Kids,* for example, health experts direct parents to count out a child's calories, cutting back on sugar and fat and increasing foods high in fiber, vitamins, and minerals. The eventual goal is to teach a child to identify a proper portion size, to recognize when she is full, and to stop eating once she is no longer hungry.

While these philosophies have merit, there are so many approaches to dealing with childhood obesity and eating disorders that they fall outside the scope of this book. Overall, some sound advice comes from reputable sources such as the National Academy of Sciences' Institute of Medicine. This and other sources offer tips to help parents in dealing with children in the face of childhood obesity and eating disorders.

These are some of the directives:

For infants, choose to breastfeed. This helps the infant learn how to self-regulate food intake. Bottlefeeding, while not a bad choice, does rely on external measurements, which can lead to over- or underfeeding. Also breastfeeding passes on immunity-building antibodies, which in turn prevent the additional stress of illness. And lactation does help a mother with weight loss, mitigating her weight-gain concerns.

For toddlers, accept that food jags are going to happen. A child may want only pasta for three weeks. That is normal. Meanwhile, introduce a variety of foods, again and again. If your child wants a ham-and-cheese omelet, for example, add vegetables to the omelet as well. Diversity early on can prevent picky habits later in life. But do not force a child to eat certain foods. Children are more willing to try new things when the environment feels safe and parents are relaxed about eating.

For preschool children and older, try for family mealtimes. Studies show that 15 to 20 percent of families in the United States do not eat together most nights of the week. While a mother with an eating disorder, who is promoting mealtime tension, might do well to avoid eating with her children, her absence will also affect her children, who eventually assume that Mom never eats. While parents do work late hours, and activities take up children's mealtimes, studies also show that meals can build bonds between family members, offer a means to explore children's behaviors, and establish a predictable routine. Studies also show that eating together improves a child's consumption of fruits, grains, vegetables, fiber, vitamins, and minerals as well as minimizing soda, fried food, and saturated fat. But sitting down with a toddler can be a stressful and unpleasant experience. So the goal is not about forcing meals to happen. Rather, in an age-appropriate fashion, try to create a positive atmosphere in which to be together around food.

For preadolescents and adolescents, do not push dieting, particularly fad dieting. Studies show that dieting at this age, more often than not, promotes eventual weight gain and obesity rather than weight loss. Eric Stice found that girls ages 11 to 15 years who used radical weight control were more depressed, had obese parents, and were more likely to become obese. At the same time, dieting leads to erratic eating and overeating. And it also is associated with vomiting and laxative use.

For any age, pay attention to attitudes at mealtimes. In mealtime studies with eating-disordered mothers, once the mothers saw the videotapes of themselves and learned how their attitudes about food were being transmitted to their children, the mothers were able to check their negative behaviors and commentary.

Overall, focus less on weight gain or weight loss and more on self-esteem. Children will manage eating best when they feel good about themselves. Rather than pushing a personal trainer, repeat positive affirmations to children, explaining that who they are is more important than their weight and shape.

. . .

The second strategy in managing parental and child eating disorders is focusing on the parent, rather than on the child. This may be a more promising strategy because, as cited in several earlier studies, a healthier mother will have a healthier child.

As we have seen, there are a number of techniques a mother can use if she is worried that her child will grow up fat or eating-disordered. And a mother can try to follow all the steps diligently. That is a start. So is an awareness of her own eating issues and attitudes. But what is arguably more relevant in the case of a mother with an eating issue is the state of her personal recovery. As we have seen, a child will do best when she has a healthier mom.

As one example, consider Cindy's child Maggie, who, when younger, essentially played caretaker of her mother's eating disorder. This case illustrates both the difficulties and the rewards of taking such as approach. She had to find the courage to embark upon recovery while watching Maggie and her younger sister grow up. When Maggie was 6 years old, Cindy made the decision to get treatment at an eating disorders center. She did eventually stop her bulimic and dieting behaviors, and she did get healthier.

"My kids are 19 and 21 now," she says. "And when I look at their baby pictures, I recognize them. But I don't remember a lot about when they were babies because I was so stuck in my own issues."

Years later, Maggie was diagnosed with anorexia. And this was perhaps the hardest test of Cindy's recovery. But she is staying on track.

"On the days when she is down, every five minutes I have to stop what I am doing and say, 'OK, I am going to give her back to you, God, and trust in her ability to take care of herself,'" Cindy says. "And then I get focused back on what I am doing here. My own recovery."

A mother—any mother—knows that parenting is going to be stressful, demanding, and exhausting. Parenting can also be rewarding, redefining, and transforming. A mother with an eating disorder should be aware that she is prone to relapse when under stress. She needs to prepare for that stress with ways to minimize it, seeking help from friends or a regular babysitter. She needs to nurture her marriage or partnership, because a strong relationship can help support the family. She needs to acquire the necessary tools, perhaps spirituality in some form, so that she can find the appropriate words to say to her child, even on the day when that child comes home from school crying, "Alisa said that I am fat."

I remember those tears when my daughter came back from a visit with her father's mother. "Granny told me that my belly was too big and that I needed to go on a diet," my daughter, then 8 years old, said.

It starts early. And I was ready for it. I told my daughter that she was beautiful and strong. And that strong girls can play soccer while girls who diet cannot get the energy to do sports. I stood her in front of a mirror so that she could see how beautiful her 8-year-old body is, just the way it is.

"And why do you think Granny said that to you?" I asked.

"I don't know," my daughter said. "Maybe she is jealous."

Maybe. Or just overconcerned about her own weight.

"Granny has diabetes," I said. "And she has to be careful about what she eats. But she should not treat your body as if it were hers. And we know that 8-year-old girls do not need to go on diets. You get to be the boss of your own body."

And as I said the words, I wished I had heard them from my own mother. But I understood. She was too consumed in her own issues; she was schooled in a different era, when perfect meals at holidays mattered more.

If a woman with food issues is not aware of the tension she creates and not able to make the effort toward wholeness, she will transmit something to those near her. That something, be it values or attitudes or behaviors, is unique to every mother-child situation. But the something lasts, in both mother and child, long after the child has grown and left home.

And she will be there, sitting in an empty nest, having to face herself without a child to distract her.

Thus, the time to begin recovery is now, before it's too late. An untreated eating disorder can affect not only the mother but also those she loves the most.

6

Midlife

Eating Disorders:
Millstones or Stepping-stones?

Americans have learned to live with the idea of young women, big-eyed and waiflike, succumbing to eating disorders. But society has not yet recognized a new trend: eating disorders are felling older women in their forties, fifties, and sixties, even the smartest and most accomplished among them. They are crashing harder than their teenage sisters; older women are less physically resilient. Even worse, society views an aging woman with an eating disorder as past sympathy. She is a double loser: first, because she has an eating disorder, and second, because she should know better.

Not surprisingly, then, many career-wizened CEOs, judges, and artists are disappearing quietly on sick leave; these auburn-haired grandmothers, who drive Mini Coopers and carry iPods, are forgoing the chance to take their grandchildren to the zoo. Just when they should be in the prime of their lives, confident about whom they have become and the choices that they have made, they are in trouble.

In clinical circles, midlife eating disorders are "certainly a hot topic right now," says Rachel Ammon, marketing coordinator at the Renfrew Center. "We've seen such an increase in this population that we've developed special programming." The Cambridge Eating Disorders Center in Massachusetts (CEDC) has also added two new therapy groups, one for patients 30 to 40 years old, and another for those over 40.

What was an oddity is now becoming commonplace, so much so that administrators at eating disorder clinics have begun keeping statistics. According to Edward Cumella, in the last fifteen years Remuda has tallied a fourfold increase in women older than 40 and a tripling in the number of women over 50. The bulk of that increase has occurred in the last five years, nudging up the average age of the patient population. Renfrew and Cornell Eating Disorders Program in White Plains, New York, have seen similar rises. Cornell is reporting twice as many midlife patients with eating disorders as five years ago. Other centers are experiencing similar increases in older patients.

Why is this happening?

No one can answer that question yet; the trend is so recent that large-scale studies have not yet been done. But early data indicate that the upsurge consists of three groups of older women: those getting sick for the first time, those relapsing in midlife, and those who have had a problem for a long time but have only now decided to get help.

These data suggest that something about contemporary aging is stirring up latent eating disorders. Aging acts as a millstone, dragging down a vulnerable woman. But the last group suggests that age itself can also *prompt* treatment; aging can be a stepping-stone, forcing a woman to climb out of her long-term problem.

Why does a woman choose recovery in midlife but never before?

It may be a personal decision motivated by timing; she can finally pay attention to herself after years of focusing on her partner and her children. Or she may be responding to all the recent publicity about eating disorders in midlife and naming the condition in herself for the first time.

"It is like alcoholism was thirty years ago," says Jeannie Rust, director of Mirasol. "It was so shameful that you would rather die than tell anybody."

Recent books about bulimia by older celebrities like Jane Fonda and articles in mainstream publications such as the *New York Times* might be removing the stigma.

Another explanation for the rise in midlife eating problems is demographics. With the number of women now in midlife at an all-time high, logically, the number of midlifers with eating disorders should escalate as well.

But there is more to the trend than demographics. According to psychologist Tacie Vergara, at Renfrew, the baby boomer generation is unique. This group of women—the first raised from birth with television—has been spoon-fed, schooled, and seduced by media ideals of thinness. Meanwhile, at the tail end of the boomers, women in their forties came of age with Jane Fonda's religion of excessive exercise—and an epidemic of eating disorders. Women aged 40 to 60 broke traditional roles and later paid consequences in the form of criticism, backlash, and pure exhaustion from trying to juggle multiple roles.

It is not surprising, then, that an indoctrinated woman is going to turn to the Church of the Fit Body in midlife, when times are stressful; the culture has "educated" her to project any kind of stress onto her body. *Your husband dumps you? Join the gym. You want that promotion? Get a face-lift.*

As evidence for how widely Western culture casts a body-projection imperative, Debra Waterhouse, in her book *Like Mother, Like Daughter,* and psychologist Cynthia Bulik, in her book *Runaway Eating,* assert that the *majority* of women in midlife are now experiencing some degree of eating obsession. For example, 60 percent of adult women engage in pathologic weight control, including dieting constantly and overexercising. Half of adult women say that eating is devoid of pleasure and causes guilt. And the clincher—some 96 percent of adult women worry about their weight and do not stop fretting, even as they reach later life.

Something is wrong, and it is feeding midlife eating disorders.

ANOTHER KIND OF EATING DISORDER IN MIDLIFE

While anorexia and bulimia in midlife are indeed on the rise, there is also a parallel increase in older women with another kind of serious eating problem: binge eating disorder.*

Women with binge eating disorder binge without purging. Hence, they tend to be overweight or obese. Binge eating disorder is not the same thing as obesity, which can arise from simple overeating—grazing continually, without regard to hunger. Rather, people with binge eating disorder regularly consume a glut of calories in one sitting, feeling unable to stop.

These women often do not know that they have a clinical problem, and they are falling below the radar of physicians. When most people think of an eating disorder, they envision anorexia and bulimia. A middle-aged woman thinks: *I'm not emaciated. I'm not throwing up. I'm not a teenager. Therefore, I can't have an eating disorder.*

So she does not seek treatment.

Even a woman who senses that she has a problem may refuse to get help. To explain why, eating disorders researchers surveyed the attitudes and behaviors of 125 women aged 50 to 65 years old. The women were of all weights and sizes, but none were undergoing treatment for an eating disorder. The study found that the heavier a participant, the more she strived to be thin, the greater her body dissatisfaction, and the more she tended toward disordered eating.

The simplistic societal myth is that overweight people are lazy and lack willpower. In fact, most Americans believe that personal choice, rather than genetic predisposition or marketing by food companies, is the main reason that people are overweight. But this midlife study, while involving an admittedly small sample of average middle-aged females, defies such thinking. The results show that the heaviest midlifers are the *most* body-obsessed; they feel self-loathing and so are driven to starve. Increasingly pressured, they are chan-

---

*Binge eating disorder can occur much earlier in life than in middle age. But therapists usually do not see women with the disorder until they are older.

neling their feelings of shame into body abuse, leading to an out-crop of eating disorders that develop in midlife. And when they need help, shame deters many of these women from seeking treatment.

Right now experts are estimating that binge eating disorder af-flicts roughly 3 percent of Americans. But that is likely to be a gross underestimate. James Hudson, at McLean Hospital in Massachu-setts, says that this disorder is rising even faster than anorexia and bulimia. Further, Hudson notes, women with binge eating disorder are asking for treatment much later in life. Thus, the women who binge exclusively have been hiding their problem for a long time, or they are simply getting sick for the first time, later in life.

One explanation that may account for binge eating in older women may be that this disorder simply might take more years to develop than anorexia or bulimia. Specialists such as José Appo-linario, at the Instituto Estadual de Diabetes e Endocrinologia in Rio de Janeiro, Brazil, are finding that the anatomy of the binge in binge eating disorder is different—less severe—than that in buli-mia. Appolinario recalls the case of a woman with bulimia nervosa whose binges were extreme: every day, she would take all the left-overs in her refrigerator, put them in a pot with water, and prepare a "stew." She would eat it all and throw it up afterward.

Binge eating disorder is generally not so extreme. A woman who binge eats but does not purge might consume three large meals in a day, for example. After the third, she steals away into the kitchen and quickly eats the remains of the cake. The critical difference is that she is not vomiting or dieting between these binges. Thus, her body may *more slowly* develop the kind of craving necessary to launch a full-blown disorder.

The genesis of this disorder, in part, is food deprivation. Re-searchers have shown that both purging and radical dieting can start bingeing in the first place. The body, when faced with intense hunger, believes it is in a state of famine. It does everything in its power to procure food. The body has an arsenal of biological sig-nals that push up appetite until hunger becomes an all-consuming craving. If a woman has been dieting hard, her body will not let her continue indefinitely (except in cases of anorexia where a woman wields enormous resolve not to indulge her ravenous appetite). And the moment she lets her food-restricting guard down, her body will almost force her to overeat, mercilessly and without pause.

MIDLIFE CRISES AND TRANSITIONS

Midlife stimulates a latent eating disorder because this phase of life involves major transitions. While stress and change happen throughout the lifespan, midlife adds to them. As with adolescence, midlife transitions involve shedding a familiar but outgrown body image, weathering hormonal upheavals, and discovering new identities and roles. But in midlife there is more.

Vergara lists no fewer than fifteen major transitions that can affect a woman in midlife:

Becoming a grandparent

Becoming a mother-in-law

Experiencing an empty nest

Having an empty nest filled by an adult child come home

Returning to work

Returning to school

Caring for children and/or parents

Suffering the death of a spouse

Suffering the loss of or permanent separation from a child

Divorce

Remarriage

Housing changes

Retirement

Chronic illness and disability

Growing old and facing mortality

This midlife phase, then, is truly about change, a torrent of turnover. And these midlife crises occur just as a woman is facing a profusion of physical changes as well: memory loss, decreased stamina, wrinkling, weight gain, and the hormonal effects of menopause. For some, the only factor grimmer than midlife changes themselves is the cultural pressure to deny or hide them, Vergara says.

Indeed, culture traditionally has forced women in midlife into a stereotype: she has no identity beyond her role as mother, grandmother, wife; she is happiest taking care of others. She is desexed and dried up; she lacks business or financial skills; she is a fading flower.

In essence, society forgets about her—unless she can fill in where needed: babysitting, making meals, and grocery shopping for frail parents, for example.

This is not the ideal environment for addressing a psychological crisis. According to Erikson, the overall task in midlife is to become generative, creating groups, ideas, or projects that can be passed down to the next generation. This creative spirit involves handing over the reins to younger members of society, moving on—often in the direction of exploring meaning and spirituality.

Social scientist Bernice Neugarten, at the University of Chicago, has said that a woman's fiftieth birthday is a mile marker. She realizes that the birthdays she has left are fewer than the birthdays that she has had. This brings on a period of reckoning.

"At fifty," says psychiatrist Katherine Zerbe, at the Oregon Health and Science University, "you have got to take stock. You have got to see that you have enough time to do some things. But you can't do everything."

Transition involves prioritization. And to do that, Zerbe says, a woman in midlife has to mourn. There are both literal and metaphoric deaths in midlife, the loss of youth being but one. Even at 40, a woman thinks about the bridges not crossed and asks: *What do I do now?*

Contemporary pressures push her to answer, "Get in shape" or "Lose weight." If that is her only solution, however, she is making a dangerous choice; she is setting herself up for an eating problem.

Yet many middle-aged women embrace diets or fitness quests and do not suffer eating disorders. What causes a minor midlife problem to become an eating disorder for some, but a mere "midlife crisis" for others?

Remember that eating disorders fall into a spectrum, with minor food and body issues at one end and full-blown diseases at the other. At the same time, severe eating disorders usually arise from less serious problems, gathering steam in times of stress. Thus, midlife is usually not the cause, but rather, it is the culmination of an eating disorder. It is seeded much earlier. A woman's life circumstances sow fertile ground. The eating disorder germinates, ripens over a period of years, sometimes decades.

It is truly the nature of the woman and her unique experiences that dictate what her eating problem will become when she reaches midlife. A middle-aged woman who falls near the extreme side of the eating disorders continuum probably began with the *right* genetic predisposition to set herself up. Then, as a baby boomer, she has the right collective predisposition. She also has the right set of personal life experiences, stresses, and family dynamics. Her eating disorder has blossomed.

Therefore, to understand what is going on with eating disorders and in midlife, it is not as important to explore what the stresses are that forced a woman to succumb in midlife, but rather, how she handled those stresses.

Overall, acquiring an eating problem in midlife, as in adolescence, is about avoiding the painful tasks of psychological development. Eating disorders themselves can be millstones, dragging a woman down in a swamp of stagnated personal growth, or they can become a stepping-stone to a mature self.

A Face-off Against Aging

While every woman who reaches middle age has to deal with body changes, a certain kind of woman all but refuses to accept the truth of time. She gets hooked on what researchers call "body dissatisfaction," defined as a disconnect between what a woman's body is and what she wishes it would be.

While many women in midlife are unhappy with their bodies as they age, the majority manage to make peace with their imperfections. In fact, Marika Tiggemann, at Finders University in Adelaide, Australia, surveyed women in their forties through seventies and found that the levels of body dissatisfaction did not increase as the women aged.

At first, Tiggemann, who has reached middle age herself, thought the result must be wrong: "Given all the things that happen to an aging woman's body," she says, "body dissatisfaction should worsen with age."

But the results said no. And Tiggemann realized that body dissatisfaction is a composite of two sentiments: as noted above, the first is a discrepancy between what a woman's body is and what she wishes it would be; but the second is how much she is willing to do about it.

"Everyone says, 'I'd rather be thinner' or 'I'd like to have a body that looks like this,'" Tiggemann notes. "But it matters less to a woman when she gets older."

In other words, the average middle-aged woman has grown smarter. As she ages, she increasingly dreads the changes to her skin, bones, and shape. But she is no longer willing to endanger her health to try to meet the culture's idealization of beauty.

While that holds for the majority, it is the opposite for people whose main identity comes through appearance. The most susceptible are those who have relied upon appearance to achieve rank such as celebrities, public speakers, actors, dancers, business professionals—and, of course, women with past eating disorders. These women become increasingly distraught over their aging bodies and *still* work hard, in some cases harder, to continue to meet the cultural ideal.

"Some of our older patients begin by focusing on supplements, cutting out fat and carbohydrates, and exercising more," Cumella says.

Others choose plastic surgery. *New York Times* reporter Eryn Brown writes about middle-aged career women who nip and tuck mainly to get ahead in the workplace. They comprise a hefty proportion of the 2.7 million women age 51 to 64 years old who underwent cosmetic surgery in 2005. Their pet procedure was Botox injections, which have skyrocketed since 1997. The most common surgical procedure was eyelid surgery, followed by face-lifts and liposuction. As testimony to the addictiveness of anti-aging activities, nearly half the people seeking cosmetic surgery were repeat clients.

Other anti-agers embrace "natural" interventions. For example, there are herbal weight-loss products like ephedra, a potentially lethal plant-derived stimulant that can cause weight loss. And, for the most desperate, there are illicit drugs with weight-loss side effects to ingest, inject, or inhale.

"I have had women in my practice who have been addicted to cocaine because it helped them lose weight," says Zerbe. "People do these things knowingly to drive up their metabolism."

Women in this situation become desperate denizens of health clubs, spas, and cosmetic surgery clinics, where they choose from the cornucopia of market-driven anti-aging offerings. "These things are very reinforcing, and people will do more of them, until they cannot stop," Cumella says.

>>> *Arlene: Running Nonstop on the Treadmill of Eating Disorders*

Against this aging-anxiety backdrop, add a massive midlife stress. A divorce, for example. Vergara says that separation from a partner "is a huge stressor" and, therefore, a common catalyst for an eating disorder in midlife women.

It is not hard to imagine why. In addition to feelings of loss and sometimes abandonment, a divorced woman often has to bear new financial and social pressures. She has to transition into a single woman or a single mother in the contemporary world of relationships. A woman who is back in the market today may find herself thrust into new worlds of online matchmaking or even speed-dating sessions. Even if she remarries, her new situation will undoubtedly differ from her previous marriage. Alone or in a new marriage, she will have to begin again. A middle-age woman with an eating disorder who was married for a decade or more may find her renewed focus on body image overwhelming; in fact, it may exacerbate the blow that divorce has already delivered to her self-esteem.

This is the story of Arlene, mother of Ethan and Alison.

She succumbed to both bulimia and anorexia as a teenager. She subsequently spent decades, on and off, battling symptoms of starving, bingeing, and purging, as well as problems with alcohol. But married to Michael, a Brown-educated attorney, Arlene also experienced nearly two decades of respite from her worst symptoms. Raising children and entertaining in the posh Back Bay area of Boston helped her; the roles of mother and wife replaced bulimia. Then, when Arlene reached her late forties, everything changed. Michael became involved in a money-related scandal at his business. In the ensuing financial struggle, Michael and Arlene lost their home. Soon after, their children reached adolescence, and they underwent another upheaval. And at the same time, Arlene reached perimenopause.

The cumulative tensions launched Arlene into an extramarital affair.

"It was this huge sort of tidal wave coming into my life," she says, "like I didn't have any control over it."

Infatuated, Arlene divorced her husband. A year later, her lover left her for another woman. At 51, Arlene was alone, with no children, no husband, and no prospects.

She joined a dating club. She met several uninspiring partners, even stayed with one for a year and a half. But this did not fill the emptiness, and Arlene needed something else. She began running, logging in 60 miles a week. She ran the Boston Marathon. She took up weight lifting ("pumping"), bicycle riding ("spinning"), and cardio-vascular ("stepping") classes at the gym. At 56, she works out twice a day and never skips exercise, even when she's sick.

She had her vomit-worn teeth replaced with porcelain substitutes. At the same time, the drinking, bingeing, and purging have returned, full-force.

"I tell myself not to do this," she says, "I can see myself fighting with myself and always losing."

Alone on a recent Sunday, with no one to share dinner, Arlene took a walk to buy ice cream. She could not stop at one dish. Embarrassed to buy another at the same store, she hurried up the street to the next ice cream store. And then the next. And eventually hurried back home again to purge.

"When I look back at my life and see when I didn't do this," she says, "it seemed to be when I was engaged in something emotional in my life."

The loss of her key emotional connections, in tandem with other midlife changes, burdened Arlene with loneliness, disorientation, and sadness.

It is important to emphasize that Arlene's divorce did not cause her midlife problems. It simply ratcheted up the eating-disordered behaviors that she had already cultivated. For Arlene, anorexia, bulimia, and drinking are her fallback behaviors in times of stress. Her eating disorder is a millstone that is weighing upon her more heavily in midlife, as she encounters an accumulation of stressful transitions.

A Counterpoint to Grief

Grief is another potent trigger of eating disorder. Emotions are potent instigators of eating disorders—at any phase of life. In midlife, grief is more often present; a woman's intimates—friends, spouses, family members—die more frequently than when she was younger.

The extent to which grief forces an eating disorder depends on the closeness of the lost relationship and the nature of the woman who suffers from that loss.

In general, when a friend or coworker dies, the reaction is one of fear: *I am going to die someday, too.* In this emotional context, an eating disorder may evolve as a woman tries to confront mortality. A reinvigorated exercise program and diet plan become her fountain of youth: she thinks that by getting thinner or fitter she can evade death herself.

The situation is more intense, of course, when a wife loses her husband or a mother loses her child. A widow or a childless mother can become so lost in grief that she stops eating. "It is a plea for help in the middle of unbearable suffering," Cumella says.

Or she binges as a form of escape. A woman can binge to swallow her pain, even if it is only for temporary relief.

>>> Irene: Stuffing Down the Loss of Her Sons

This is what Irene did when she lost her sons, not to death but nonetheless in a permanent way. After a divorce and a year of struggling to take care of five children, Irene was called into court. Though she fought it, a judge ordered her twin boys, age 5, to go into foster care.

That was thirty years ago. Now she is 60, and she has not seen her boys since.

In their absence, she began to gorge. She says, "People were saying I was fat and ugly, that I should stop eating. But they didn't understand. I was sad."

Three years ago, Irene's doctor finally sent her to an eating disorders clinic in order to treat her resulting obesity and diabetes. Irene was 5-foot-2 and weighed 242 pounds.

For whatever reasons, Irene chose bingeing as her crutch. Her eating problem propped her back up when grief overwhelmed her. But having relied on her eating disorder for nearly three decades, she never allowed herself to feel her grief and learn the developmental lessons such transitions may afford, skills to walk through it safely. Over time, her eating problem has evolved into a disorder. Her psychological work, now in progress, involves shedding the eating-disordered behaviors and learning other ways to manage her powerful emotions.

Late Disclosure

Studies show that nearly a quarter of middle-aged women with eating disorders have been clinically ill since they were young. At the same time, many girls begin eating disorders in adolescence and use them to stay a girl forever, at least in the developmental sense.

The situation is grave when a woman has long carried a severe eating disorder. Tired and beaten down, she does not have a recovery experience to draw upon for strength, vigor, and confidence. This forever-young girl, the *puella aeterna*, has to work from scratch, forming an identity for the first time—but in middle age.

"The eating disorder has become a lifestyle," says Seda Ebrahimi. "It is not unusual for us to get women in their forties, fifties, and sixties who talk about how they had the disorder for thirty years or so, and this is the first time they have disclosed it—or got help for it."

And these women have had long-standing marriages, sometimes raising children while clinically sick. Their families often know, oddly enough, and adapt to the illness.

"I wonder, where has the husband been?" Vergara says. "These women eat out of teeny-weeny cups and the husband says, 'My wife has never been a big eater.' The kids say, 'This is just what Mom does.' And these women go on like this."

>>> Abby: Seeing No Other Way Except Bulimia

Abby, 43, lived most of her life clinically ill. She came of age in Long Island, a "fat kid," in an oppressive Jewish family. Her mother chided her about her weight. At 16, she went away to summer camp, and while she was there she put herself on a strict diet. Not only did her weight drop from 143 to 118 pounds, but she also met a boy. His attention made her feel special, but it confirmed to her that she could only be loved if she was thin.

She returned home at the end of the summer, expecting her mother to show more approval—because Abby's weight now fell into her mother's acceptable boundaries. And her mother did praise her new body. But Abby's mother continued to make "cruel" and "critical" comments about Abby's achievements and personality. Abby, attributing this lack of approval to her weight, eventually couldn't keep it off by dieting alone. She turned instead to purging, which led to bingeing as well.

"My life became a kitchen and a toilet," she says.

It remained that way for decades, through many jobs—office temp, retail broker, and assistant to the chairman of a major corporation—and many men Abby dated, even getting engaged. But each relationship became dysfunctional. When the last one ended and she had reached a career dead end as a paralegal at a prestigious Manhattan law firm at age 40, she tried to commit suicide, one of two attempts in her lifetime.

After the second attempt, with an overdose of Klonopin, a sedative used to treat anxiety, Abby reached a turning point. She began therapy, a mix of psychological work and antidepressants. She quit her job and took a hiatus from all the stresses of her life. Awarded disability leave, she chose not to look for another job while she tried to heal.

"My eating disorder was the only way I knew, the only way I could be true to me," she says in retrospect. "It got my pain out. It was my expression."

Her task in midlife, then, was to find another means of expression. She may have just done that. Recently, she has begun trading stocks, a practice that has earned her not only income but also confidence. Abby discovered a hidden talent. At the same time, with therapy she has managed to curtail the behaviors that marked her bulimia.

"It's not gone," she says.

For example, eating lunch is still an issue. She often skips it or has to force herself to eat a small salad because she habitually liked to save her calorie quota for her dinner meal. She dogmatically practices portion control, buying foods such as M&M's in snack-size packs and only allowing herself one per day.

Her story shows that there is always hope.

Abby courageously faced a decades-long problem and reversed its course. As to her relationship with her mother, Abby, with the help of her therapist, has gained perspective.

"I get my mother's limitations," she says. "And I deal with them."

Reaching this state of mind represents what a woman who has acquired an eating disorder early on must do. She has to revisit her adolescent troubles and complete the developmental tasks that she should have addressed much earlier.

The Risk of Relapse

Eating disorders are unique to each person and require lifelong monitoring. A woman might stop her symptoms for a time, even decades. She celebrates and has every reason to do so. The danger is in growing overly confident. For if a woman has not fully resolved the childhood issues that fueled her eating disorder, she will grow up into a middle-aged woman with a latent vulnerability.

And then something happens, a midlife stress. It can push her over the edge yet again. Like cancer in remission, eating disorders offer no hard-and-fast rules about how long a woman can live eating disorder–free and consider herself "done with it."

The key is to acknowledge vulnerability and fight denial, so as not to be taken unaware. A woman with a past problem needs to understand that there is always the risk of relapse.

>>> Laura: Replaying the Past

Laura, 65, had experienced anorexia as a teenager. After dropping 45 pounds the summer between her sophomore and junior years of high school, she went through a short period of therapy. That was forty-five years ago. Treatment, then, lacked today's understanding of eating disorders. Still, Laura managed to gain back weight and only retained a remnant of her problem, a constant pressure to diet. At 5-foot-3 and 125 pounds, she remained subclinical for thirty years. She enjoyed a happy marriage and her time raising three children.

And then, at 48, Laura watched her elderly parents deteriorate. Her mother began the slide into Alzheimer's dementia. At the same time, her father was diagnosed with liver cancer. Laura began commuting from her home near Boston to New York, where her parents were living. She placed her mother in an assisted-living facility and lived with her father.

There, in the short span of weeks, anorexia hit her fast and hard.

"I was totally thrown back," she says.

Her father was constantly angry, echoing Laura's experience as a teen. "Everything I did was wrong," she says. "It was all wrong."

Stressed out, Laura stopped eating. By the time her dad died, two and a half months later, she had lost 25 pounds. She had bruises all over her body; she could not remember how she got them. She says they might have formed as she hit herself or banged her head against a wall. Her body was crying out in pain.

Her husband and son stepped in. They found a therapist, who helped her investigate long-buried issues about her father. She discovered feelings about her dad's "ambiguous sexualized affection." For example, he would pull her into inappropriate "bear hugs" from which she could not escape. As a teen, Laura's family relocated to New York City from Los Angeles. While her mother was back in Los Angeles selling the house, she lived with her father in Greenwich Village. He would take her out "on dates" to the theater or the opera.

"At some level it was absolutely wonderful and I would say that my dad and I had the best relationship," she says. "But it was also very weird."

And that ambiguity, because it was not overt, fell into a dark corner in Laura's memory, illuminated only when she had to take care of him before he died. Laura had not worked through all the issues of her childhood, probably the same ones that launched her eating disorder in the first place. Because of that, she remained bound in a childlike way to that little girl who needed her father to adore her. And when she lost her parents, and thus her identity as daughter, she went adrift. Her eating disorder served as her life raft. But, as she found out nearly too late, it had a major hole in it. Her therapy was about plugging the hole and finding a way to get back to shore.

And while her eating disorder began as a millstone, Laura turned it into a stepping-stone. The shock of losing that much weight, that quickly, brought attention to her long-buried problem. Her husband and son helped, but the change really had to come from Laura.

This is the gift of middle age: experience, wisdom, and *time*—unfettered by previous responsibilities—to transform and redirect the past for the future.

EATING DISORDERS OFTEN CHANGE
FORM BY MIDLIFE

Eating disorders in midlife, while similar to those in adolescence, also differ in significant ways. The middle-aged woman brings to the disorder both age and life experience. Her adolescent counterparts simply do not have that yet. In the context of eating disorders, this means that time changes how these diseases are expressed. Each illness—anorexia, bulimia, and binge eating disorder—tends to emerge in different forms, depending on one's life stage.

Midlife itself is a transitional life phase with its own particular stresses. In some ways, the tumult mirrors that of adolescence. Indeed, Arlene on the treadmill looks an awful lot like an older version of the teen pressured by fashion magazine cover images. Laura, under the thumb of her dying parents, appears to be a re-creation of an overly dependent teen.

"These problems have to do with identity," Cumella says. "They have to do with dependence versus independence. They have to do with belonging. These are the same issues that fourteen- and fifteen-year-olds are dealing with, but in a different way."

Anorexia Becomes Bulimia or a Subclinical Illness

What differs most is time. It changes the nature of the disorder. Most women with anorexia nervosa do not maintain the severe form of their illness into middle life. The 10 to 20 percent who do often die. In his book, *This Mean Disease,* Daniel Becker tells the story of his mother, Carol, who was diagnosed with anorexia at 34 and spent the next thirty years in and out of hospitals until her death.

Because the worst cases die off, those who survive tend to be relatively better off. Still, within that group, about half of those diagnosed early on with anorexia nervosa and a third with bulimia carry their eating problems with them into the early and midlife stages of adulthood.

The difference is that the form of the disease changes.

For example, specialists have found that many women with anorexia, perhaps the majority, partially recover. As a woman gets older, she gradually eats a little more and gains a little more weight. She reaches the point where she is not diagnosably ill.

But she has not eradicated her disease. Instead, she has bargained with it: *I'll allow myself to be heavier in exchange for a respite from this*

600-calorie-a-day regime. But not that much heavier. Putting herself on 900 or 1,000 calories a day, she still gets the perceived benefits of a relatively low weight but without such grueling work.

In a variation on that midlife shift, an estimated 15 percent of women with anorexia nervosa cross over into bulimia. (Rarely do women with bulimia cross over into anorexia.) Herzog explains this phenomenon as a kind of exhaustion; an older woman simply grows tired of starving. At the same time, she may not want her children to see her bad habits, or her husband may be pressuring her to eat more.

But having no practice at moderation, she overdoes it. She behaves like a person coming off a fad diet—indeed, that's exactly her situation. Faced with the taste of something long denied, she binges. Ebrahimi has seen many patients with anorexia go the other way, with total undercontrol of portion size. "The starvation sets her up for a binge-purge episode. It becomes a trap."

Mortified by her overconsumption—the natural consequence of her body responding to starvation—a woman in this predicament feels compelled to purge. So she switches from anorexia to bulimia nervosa, or a combination of the two.

Bulimia Changes:
Overexercising Substitutes for Vomiting

Women diagnosed with bulimia early on in life run a different life-time course. An estimated 70 percent have been able to curb their symptoms, at least for a time. A woman in this situation is, rightfully, proud of her progress. Reaching midlife, she knows better than to force herself to vomit willfully. She has learned through experience that it is not safe to binge and purge five times a day or take packages of laxative tablets in the hopes of prompting weight loss. She may not want to ruin the thousands of dollars of dental work that she needed because of her past vomiting.

But she may not be aware that she is still vulnerable.

At 50, such a woman may notice a thickening of her waistline. Listening to the health experts' advice, she begins to embrace the elliptical trainer, a "safer" weight control device. Even women without a history of bulimia, or who have crossed over from anorexia to bulimia, turn to exercise in midlife. Each perceives vomiting as "bad" and exercise as "good."

There it starts. And there it could end, with a healthy routine of physical activity. But certain women keep going. Exercise becomes an addictive form of purging.

Binge Eating Crosses the Line into a Disorder

A woman with bulimia who stops vomiting can also cross over into a binge eating disorder; she stops purging but not bingeing. Or a woman who binges may never have purged. This woman reaches midlife, not crossing over into another form of eating problem, but rather, crossing the line. Her binge eating disorder evolves into a full-blown disease.

Research shows there are two reasons why binge eating occurs. In the aftermath of rigid diets, the body thinks it is starving and responds biochemically with an increased urgency for food. Another cause of bingeing is unbearable emotional pain, as with Irene's loss of her sons to foster care.

Binge eating, repeated over time, becomes addictive. Food can tap pleasure centers in the brain, the same ones that respond to exercise, sex, and drugs like cocaine. People who binge say they do so not out of hunger, but rather, out of pain. Food strokes the wounded self; it functions as a narcotic. This may be one reason why binge disorders often accompany depression, anxiety, or other mood disorders.

No one has demonstrated better the connection between bingeing and addiction than neuroscientist Mary Boggiano, at the University of Alabama in Birmingham. She showed that rats can learn to binge eat, but it takes time. While rats are not people and her experiments have not been reproduced in humans for ethical reasons, her findings do a great deal to elucidate the biochemical impact of dieting upon bingeing. Rats do not act out eating anomalies because of cultural pressures.

Boggiano found that female rats need three things before they will binge: a severe diet, fatty or sugary food, and stress. For five days, Boggiano put the rats on diets, feeding them only two-thirds of their normal caloric intake. Two days after that, the rodents were given access to unlimited rat chow and Oreo cookies—which, because of the high fat and sugar, function like comfort foods to people. For the next three days, the animals were given chow alone, to allow them to gain back the weight they had lost while dieting. At this point, the animals had reached normal weight. If given chow or cookies, the rats would eat at normal levels.

But if the animals were also stressed, their eating would go haywire. One way to stress a rat is to give it a shock on the foot, much like the static energy that shocks people when they touch something metallic after shuffling on a carpet. Boggiano took some of the rats and placed them on electric grids. Then she flipped the switch; the animals, foot-shocked and stressed, began binging. Over the next twenty-four hours, they gobbled down 156 percent more than the control groups of rats that had only been on diets, only stressed, or left alone.*

In doing these experiments, Boggiano is hypothesizing that binging shares characteristics with alcoholism and drug addiction. It is known that upon exposure to cocaine or alcohol the brain unleashes molecules such as endorphins, also known as opioids. Intense exercise also stimulates this system. And now Boggiano and others are showing that certain foods, when eaten a certain way, create the same effect.

---

*The bingeing animals in Boggiano's study also developed "preferred foods," cookies or Froot Loops, as opposed to rat chow. When Boggiano gave these animals normal chow, the rats would turn it down and instead run down a foot-shock alley to get to Froot Loops at the other end. This mimics the behavior of women with bulimia nervosa or binge eating disorder who routinely drive from store to store in order to get their preferred "binge foods."

To test if binge eating is addictive, Boggiano injected her binge-ing rats with a drug called nalaxone, which blocks opioid action in the brain. If bingeing did trigger the opioid system—as other addictive substances do—blocking opioid action should cause the animals to lose their urge to binge. Sure enough, animals given nalaxone cut their binges by more than half. Conversely, a drug that *stimulated* opioid action, causing binges to feel more rewarding, made the animals binge with even greater zeal.

Bingeing is a legitimate addiction. But it takes time to become so. Boggiano had to put her rats through three two-month cycles of diet, refeeding, and foot shock in order for the animals to become avid bingers.

Three cycles over six months of rat life is the equivalent of eighteen years in human time. Thus, Boggiano's work shows that binge eating, at least for rats, does not suddenly become a runaway problem. A woman entering midlife has spent years perfecting her setup. Typically, she has dealt with her life stresses by using food to numb them out. Then, in midlife, she suddenly gets a mighty "foot shock"—a bitter divorce, for example. That makes her cross over into true binge eating disorder.

LONG-TERM CONSEQUENCES OF AN EATING DISORDER

Eating disorders are dangerous. When they are allowed to extend into midlife, they can be more serious than those of adolescence because the medical complications are far greater for older women.

"The body is amazing in that it adapts and adapts," says Vergara. "But after a woman has been suffering for more than twenty years, something finally happens."

"Something" can be that she starts passing out; or her elec-trolytes become unbalanced. "Something" can be gastrointestinal problems, heart attacks, and kidney problems, to name a few.

Researchers have yet to study the effects of a short, sudden burst of compulsive exercise, dieting, or bingeing by a 50-year-old body. It is known that sports-related injuries in baby boomers have risen by 33 percent since 1991, and evidence has shown that increased stress during aging—and depression arising from those stresses— are linked to faster progression of breast cancer, higher risk of heart-related deaths, and poorer brain function. This supports the idea that by engaging in an eating disorder for any amount of time, an older woman is adding new damage to the normal wear and tear of aging.

There are at least three medical problems born of eating disorders that intersect with the problems of normal aging: osteoporosis, diabetes, and mood disorders such as depression.

The descriptions that follow are meant to help a woman who has neglected her body learn about the potential impacts of her eating disorder. If she can respond to her body's pleas for respite from abuse, she might be able to reacquire her health.

Osteoporosis: A Complication of Anorexia and Bulimia

Whether an eating disorder is present or not, middle age in women marks a time of increased risk for osteoporosis due to menopause. For reasons only partly understood, regular monthly cycles protect the strength and pliability of bones. Thus, when a woman's periods stop, she loses bone. As she does, she may join the growing numbers of postmenopausal women who collectively experience 1.5 million osteoporotic fractures each year.

Women with a history of either anorexia nervosa or bulimia experience a higher risk of osteoporosis in midlife. The main instigator is lack of normal monthly menstruation. By the age of 3, girls have already acquired a third of their bone mineral. At puberty, the body adds another 20 percent. Adolescence marks the peak; the body lays down and stores up the remaining 45 percent of bone mineral. After menopause, a woman can only maintain or lose the bone density she has. If a woman had anorexia or some form of bulimia during puberty or adolescence, she did not acquire the necessary bone density that she should have.

How much higher is a woman's risk? That depends on when the eating disorder began, how severe it was, and how long it lasted. Studies show that patients who develop their eating disorder before puberty fare worse than those who acquire their eating disorder after their first period. Also, those who recovered and resumed their periods were healthier than those who recovered partially and did not regain their periods. In fact, women who recovered and began menstruating again increased their bone mass by 20 percent. Those with a subtype of anorexia, in which they do not binge and purge, also lost less bone than those who did. In one study, those with anorexia who vomited the most had the lowest bone mineral density of all.

Current technology can measure bone density through dual-energy X-ray densitometry (DEXA) to show whether bone composition is dense like a tree trunk or thinning and gap-ridden like phyllo dough. Women in midlife with histories of eating disorders have implicit risks. In one study, researchers measured the bone density of nineteen women with histories of anorexia nervosa, twenty-one years after recovery. The women still showed reduced bone density in their thigh bones.

The physicians could not prescribe exercise, as is the norm for postmenopausal women at risk for osteoporosis, because women with histories of eating disorders are prone to compulsive *over-exercise*. These doctors also could not reverse the bone loss with estrogen, calcium, or mineral supplements. In fact, more recent evidence, coming from a study of more than 36,000 middle-aged women, casts doubts on the long-held belief that calcium supplements work to prevent osteoporosis in even healthy postmenopausal woman. Thus, if a woman has had an eating disorder previously or if she is suffering from one now in midlife, she would do well to take steps to prevent bone density loss. A good place to start is a heart-to-heart talk with her doctor about the eating disorder. She can first ask for a bone density test. The results produce a measurement known as a T score: the lower the number, the bigger the problem. A T score between −1 and −2.5 means osteopenia, the forerunner of osteoporosis. Below −2.5, the diagnosis is osteoporosis.

Based on this number, a doctor will choose from a spectrum of treatments, from aggressive use of drugs such as Fosamax to simple monitoring of her bone density over the years to see if there is a loss of bone mass and at what rate.

Researchers do not know if the standard treatments for osteoporosis will work for women with a history of eating disorders. There is hope on the pharmaceutical horizon, however. Doctors are experimenting with a hormone called leptin, which is involved in body weight regulation and appetite control. Leptin is made by fat cells. When those shrink, leptin becomes scarce and the body signals hunger, slows metabolism, and shuts menstruation until an individual eats. For women with eating disorders, who make scant leptin supplies, doctors hypothesized that leptin supplementation, while possibly suppressing appetite, would nonetheless stimulate menstrual cycling. The hormone did. After receiving leptin injections twice daily for up to three months, three of eight premenopausal women, who had not been menstruating due to eating problems or excessive exercise, began to ovulate and menstruate. Two others showed signs of egg development in their ovaries; and all eight women increased their reproductive, thyroid gland, and growth hormone activity. While leptin has not been tested in women with a history of anorexia who are now of peri- and postmenopausal age, it may have some benefit on the health of their bones. As evidence, the younger women in the study did show a marked increase in biochemical components involved in bone formation.

While studies such as these continue, eating disorders experts say the best advice for underweight, middle-aged women with histories of eating disorders is weight gain and sound nutrition. Of course, recovery from the eating disorder can address these goals. As always, the quicker the recovery from symptoms, the less severe the damage to the body.

Diabetes: A Complication
of Binge Eating

Doctors once thought that type 2 diabetes was mainly an adult disease because people tend to get it in midlife or later.* Nearly 21 million Americans are now suffering from diabetes and 41 million more are prediabetic, with blood-sugar levels well above normal.

Binge eating lurks behind a disproportionate number of type 2 diabetes cases. A team of Brazilian researchers led by Marcelo Papelbaum surveyed seventy type 2 diabetics aged 40 to 65 years. The researchers found that 20 percent of their patients, mostly female, had an eating disorder: mainly binge eating disorder, but also bulimia and EDNOS. This percentage was more than three times higher than in the general population. Researchers have found a similar problem in the United States, where as many as a third of patients with type 2 diabetes are also plagued by an eating disorder. The connection between binge eating and diabetes seems simple: binge eating causes obesity, and obesity is linked to diabetes. But there may be a more direct link.

Susan Yanovski at the National Institute of Diabetes and Digestive and Kidney Diseases in Bethesda, Maryland, suggests that some diabetic patients, perhaps those with a certain predisposition, might be indulging in regular binges to rebel against the strict dietary restrictions needed to control their diabetes.

Bingeing is dangerous for anyone. But a middle-aged woman who binges and has diabetes is endangering her life. She has three factors working against her: diabetes, an eating disorder, and obesity.

Midlife aggravates all three ailments.

Studies show that after a woman reaches 40, she will gain more fat because her basal metabolic rate declines with age. But when a

---

*Type 1 diabetes shows up in children and young adults. In type 1 diabetes, the body does not produce insulin, a hormone that converts sugars and starches into energy. With type 2 diabetes, the body produces an inadequate amount of insulin or the body cells are resistant to insulin uptake. With childhood obesity on the rise, even children are now being diagnosed with type 2 diabetes.

woman at this stage in life tries to diet and lose what normal aging has brought on, she often makes the problem worse. Statistics say that she eventually blows her diet. Now, with a sluggish metabolism, she resumes her normal eating habits—or she binges after having denied herself during the diet. Her body suddenly has to digest and store a glut of calories just when all its systems are tuned to managing on a minimum. Thus, she gains back the weight she has lost, and then some. She becomes *more* overweight.

Disgusted with her "failure," she may diet on and off again, picking up all the traps of a binge eating disorder.

Weight gain also heightens her risk for diabetes. She can cross the line from prediabetes to the classic disease.

She has three problems to treat, but treatment for one often worsens the symptoms of another. Studies show that the loss of 5 to 10 percent of body weight can significantly delay or prevent type 2 diabetes in persons at high risk. But if the doctor puts the woman on a diet, the diet may prompt more bingeing. If she does not lose weight, she increases her potential for complications from diabetes and obesity.

Consequently, eating disorders experts have realized that they cannot simply embrace the traditional approach: diet in combination with one or more antidiabetes drugs. When a woman has binge eating disorder, the weight-loss strategy has to be a second priority.

"Treatment for binge eating is very unsatisfying in that regard," says Hudson. "Because you can get people completely better from their binge eating. And they sit there and they say, 'You know, I've only lost five pounds.'"

And yet that is better than a radical diet, aided by faddish weight-loss pills. Dieting, while necessary to impact obesity and diabetes, needs to be done very carefully—and with the guidance of a physician, preferably one experienced in eating disorders. Medication may help, but again, caution is advised. Most studies of weight-loss and related drugs for binge eating disorders are still in experimental stages. (See Chapter 8 for a more detailed discussion of these drugs.)

Overall, physicians recommend regular blood-sugar screening to assess the risk for type 2 diabetes. And if a middle-aged woman with binge eating disorder really wants to recover, ultimately she is going to have to face the reasons why she is bingeing.

Brain Changes and Mood Disorders: A Complication of All Eating Disorders

Doctors used to associate mood disorders such as depression with psychological factors. But when researchers began to explore the biology, they found that there is a mind-body, cause-and-effect relationship behind these mental illnesses. For example, hormonal changes at menopause can spur mood disorders. In midlife, women are at a higher risk for experiencing hormonal imbalances. These can trigger psychological changes, which then reinvigorate dormant conditions.

In the context of eating disorders, a woman's food behaviors influence her thinking and the circuitry of her brain. To understand this connection, enter your body for a moment in *Fantastic Voyage* fashion. Imagine you are standing near the lining of your stomach. Normally, hours after a meal your gut will be making appetite-stimulating peptide called ghrelin, which feeds back to the brain to spark hunger. "Hunger," in biochemical language, is nerve cells reacting to ghrelin by releasing transmitting molecules that stimulate the appetite centers of the brain. Your body is feeling the urge to eat.

If you eat, your intestinal tract will be telling your brain, through biochemical feedback mechanisms such as cholecystokinin and glucagon-like peptide-1, to damp down appetite. You will eventually feel full and stop eating.

Now, imagine that you are starving. Inside the gut, you are witnessing a molecular crisis. The cells of the brain, far away from your gut, know that they are lacking food. Without it, they will die. And so they send out an alert to get you to eat. *Now!* It's a molecular siren involving many neurotransmitters, among them serotonin, which is tied to feelings of satiety and fullness.

But if you have an eating disorder, you ignore your brain messages and refuse to eat. The brain sends back to the stomach more chemical signals, more ghrelin, a louder molecular scream, *Eat!* But still, you override the message.

If this is done enough times, you will break your body's mechanisms for sensing hunger and fullness. You will upset the sensitive serotonin balance in your brain.

What does it mean to be broken in this way?

Boggiano gives answers with her rats, where culture is not an influence on thought patterns and therefore behaviors relate to biology alone. She showed that after twenty cycles of dieting, foot shock, and bingeing, her rats' brains started making less serotonin, particularly in the brain regions that regulate appetite, body temperature, and reproduction.

"This is neuroadaptation," she says. "There is something changing at a fundamental level in the brain."

The results translate to people. Researchers have scanned the brains of women with anorexia or bulimia. Women with eating disorders literally lose brain matter over time, enlarging cavities called ventricles, because of their disease. By eliminating their symptoms, they are able to reverse much of this damage—but not all of it. Some of these changes, if left to go on for decades, become permanent.

Psychiatrist Walter Kaye, at the University of Pittsburgh in Pennsylvania, looked at the serotonin systems of women with eating disorders. He measured alterations similar to those of Boggiano's rats. Older women with anorexia make less serotonin than normal women. And the afflicted women also lose their ability to respond to what little serotonin there is, particularly in brain regions that control feeding behavior as well as brain areas identified with fear, depression, memory, flight, motivation, libido, and spatial perception.

Women with bulimia nervosa also have faulty serotonin systems. This may explain why antidepressants such as Prozac, which enhance the effects of serotonin, sometimes help a woman with bulimia to curb her bingeing. It also clarifies why the same drugs do not work in the treatment of anorexia nervosa: starving women do not make enough serotonin in the first place. Prozac has little available to "enhance."

Such changes in these and other neurotransmitters may also underlie the depression, anxiety, and impulse control problems that normally plague women with eating disorders.* In midlife, women whose faulty serotonin systems already are trying to weather the normal stresses of loss and slumps of menopause are increasingly susceptible to breakdown.

RECOVERY THROUGH BIOLOGY AND PSYCHOLOGY

Particularly in midlife, higher risks of osteoporosis, diabetes, mood disorders, and other medical complications of eating disorders show that it is imperative to treat both the biological and psychological sides of an eating disorder.

"Insight is not sufficient for change," says Ebrahimi. The search for medications to treat these illnesses is at full throttle (see Chapter 8).

While promising, drugs are not cures, says Hudson, especially with anorexia nervosa. No medication thus far has any proven effect on reducing its symptoms.

What begins healing in anorexia is weight gain. What begins healing in bulimia is halting the purges. What begins healing in binge eating disorder is curbing the bingeing. Thus, all treatments, directly or indirectly, need to address symptoms. Often that begins with putting a tight lid on dieting, which seeds so many disorders. Just as overriding one's hunger weakens important body-brain circuitry that controls hunger, body temperature, reproduction, and mood, sound nutrition can repair much of the damage that eating disorders create.

---

*Researchers do not know whether a woman is born with a serotonin problem that causes a predisposition to an eating disorder or the eating disorder behaviors cause serotonin imbalance. Either way, neurochemical imbalances suffuse the brains of women with eating disorders, making treatment more difficult.

Many eating disorder treatments first work hard to convince a woman to eat three healthy meals and two snacks a day before trying to undertake psychotherapy.

"You cannot do talk therapy with someone who is eighty pounds, malnourished, and starved; you don't have the person to work with," Ebrahimi says. "When someone is bingeing and purging three times a day, they are very numb."

She equates treatment for eating disorders to treatment for addiction: if someone comes into her therapist's office drunk, the therapist is not going to say, "Let's figure out why you are drinking." Instead, she will say, "You have to stop drinking first."

Diet and psychological healing have to work in tandem to get at the biology behind these diseases. But psychology, too, can have a biological effect. Psychological treatment means applying better strategies to deal with midlife stresses. It demands increasing self-awareness about how a woman feels in the moment when she is engaged in damaging eating-disordered behavior. And it means discovering faulty thought patterns through cognitive therapy: *I ate a piece of cheesecake. I am a failure.* And then learning a new and better thought pattern: *I ate a piece of cheesecake. I am a failure. No, I am feeding the cells in my brain.*

Psychological treatment is about changing the mind in order to change the body, and vice versa. This means honoring the mind-body connection in a very scientific way. The potential can be illustrated by recent studies about body image.

Brain researchers have learned that body image is not static; rather, it is an abstraction, slipping and sliding over time based upon experience and sensation. It is a *process,* born out of an ellipse of brain tissue called the posterior parietal cortex. This region receives visual and sensory impulses and transmits instructions for action.

To understand body image, put your hands at your waist and squeeze. Run your fingers up and down your hips. Your brain will juggle the feelings of fleshiness and contour and organize them into a definition of your shape, be it pear, apple, or hourglass. Based on cultural ideals, your brain may enhance the image with input from emotional and memory cues coming from other centers of the brain.

You end up with a feeling about yourself, your body. It might be elation or disappointment. This fits together with all the other feelings arising from your sense of your physical body.

If you had a brain injury in your posterior parietal cortex, your experience of body image would be distorted. If you had an eating disorder such as anorexia nervosa, similarly your body image would be warped. Recently, a study team at University College in London was able to simulate this distortion. The investigators outfitted seventeen people with electronic gadgets that stimulated the tendons in each wrist. The stimulators created the sensation that the subjects' hands were moving inward.

Next, the subjects were asked to place their hands at their waists while wearing a blindfold. Researchers flicked the switch on the stimulator, and voilà, the subjects perceived that their waists were getting thinner. Virtually, of course.

Meanwhile, team members were simultaneously scanning the subjects' brains by magnetic resonance imaging. When the deceit took place, the subjects' brains showed a change. They demonstrated increased activity in their posterior parietal cortexes. This illustrates that even when body shape and size do not change, the perception of it can.

Working in reverse order, changing perception can change behavior.

How?

RECOVERY THROUGH MIDLIFE TRANSITIONING: EATING DISORDERS AS STEPPING-STONES

A woman in midlife who has had an eating problem for years, maybe even decades, reaches a crossroad in her life. She has to make a choice. Either she yields to social pressure, laments her loss of a youthful physique, and holds on to her eating disorder, or she confronts these pressures and mobilizes her resources to take the path of health.

If she chooses health, she takes charge of her life. She will make the midlife transition, despite the pain of loss and new roles thrust upon her. She can become the lead actor in her own drama. She can become an authentic, mature woman.

Psychological treatment for a woman in midlife might be likened to a walk into one's personal life ahead. The goal is for her to envision her future and reflect upon what in her future has meaning for her. She has to discard what is outdated and outgrown, even though she may be reluctant to abandon her desire for her once-toned skin or her past identity. Eventually, she has to cobble together a new view of herself. In short, she changes her perception of herself.

She does not have to do this alone. A person taking the walk would do well to get help through a friend, partner, or therapist who can hold her hand along the way, offer guidance and support. Very often there is a spiritual quality to such a journey, a quest for meaning. Therapy is meant to help a woman with an eating disorder transcend her loss and find meaning in the events of midlife.

>>> Rachel Decides More Than Thirty Years of Bulimia Is Long Enough

Rachel, age 60, did this. She lived for nearly four decades with bulimia. At the age of 47, Rachel reached her personal tipping point.

"It was like, listen, enough of this already," she said. "Am I going to be doing this when I'm eighty?"

She confessed to her husband about her longtime bulimia. Then she worked to find a therapist in a location where she could have sessions several times a week. She took a deep breath and bravely plodded through four years of therapy. First, she stopped the purging. Curtailing the bingeing came later. She had slipups: "Sometimes I still stuff myself," she says. "But I don't throw up. I live with it the next day and pay the piper."

Now Rachel's healing has moved beyond discussions of the symptoms. She is at the level of "transitional work," finding out what is most important to her now, not what was important to her as a teenager. She and her husband are gradually turning over a family real estate business to their children. She has recently begun reading the Torah at her synagogue, a practice she would never have dreamed of doing when she was younger and suffering severe anxiety attacks. She has taken up projects in philanthropy. She has become a spokesperson for the National Academy of Eating Disorders. She is talking about personal issues to other women like herself, who have kept their eating issues secret for far too long.

"What is valuable and meaningful to me are my family and my children," she says. "And some of the work that I am involved in where I would like to try to feel like I can help make the world a better place."

Rachel is like many older women with eating disorder symptoms who, upon reaching midlife, decide that enough is enough. She turned her eating disorder into a stepping-stone to health.

"Women age forty and above are my favorite patients," Zerbe says.

These women have life experience and the capability for this kind of therapy, something adolescents often lack. In fact, experience with a previous recovery can help shorten a relapse. Rachel only binged once or twice and then got back on track. That is a huge success for a woman who binged and purged at least three times a week for more than thirty years.

>>> Ruth Dusts Off Her "Recovery Toolbox"

When a woman enters therapy, she slowly accumulates recovery "tools." If she slips, she can fall back upon her healing tools at any time. Ruth, age 45, figured out the value of a well-stocked toolbox. She had bulimia throughout her teens and into her thirties. Through therapy and antidepressants, she was able to curtail her purging and maintained a subclinical disorder for the next decade.

At 43, Ruth learned that she had grapefruit-sized fibroids. They caused such heavy periods that "it was like chunks of my body were falling out." She had surgery to shrink the fibroids, but after the operation, Ruth had to come to terms with the loss of her childbearing potential.

"I was perceiving myself as somebody who can have kids whenever they wanted," she says. "And suddenly, my biology was saying I couldn't."

Ruth had always wanted children. But her husband, Tom, had not. She did not press the issue because, in the aftermath of bulimia, she doubted her ability to be a good mother.

Four months after the operation, she conceived. Tom was shocked, but he accepted the pregnancy as fate. After missing the first few obstetrical appointments, during which Ruth's fibroid status was simultaneously monitored, he became excited by the prospect of fatherhood and finally went along to witness the heartbeat for himself. Upon the visit, the couple learned that the 10-week-old fetus had died.

A year later, Ruth's back pain and uterine bleeding returned and her doctor scheduled a hysterectomy. As she prepared for the operation, she lapsed into depression. But unlike her previous depression in the context of bulimia, her current state was not about feeling fat or looking perfect.

"Now I'm just goddamn, midlife depressed," she says.

Today, she knows she could return to bingeing and purging. She knows the urge, the monkey on her back. But because of longtime therapy, she is holding her own with a kind of compromise: she does not eat all day, keeping her hunger at bay by keeping busy at work; then she eats two or three helpings for dinner. But she does not purge. In the meantime, her therapist has increased her dose of Prozac. She is coping, managing as well as possible under the circumstances.

"I've made peace as much as I can," she says. "It's not about food anymore. It's just not. It's about trying to take better care of myself, trying to have a healthy attitude, healthy relationships, because I never really did. And to try to use the time that I have left properly."

Indeed, this stage of life is all about time and the many opportunities that are still left. In fact, midlife can offer the time, and therefore the opportunities, that previous life stages did not.

Midlife is the pause between the first and second half of life. It can be a long pause. But a woman in midlife is allowed to take this time for herself. Time, honored and used well, can allow recovery to happen, even at this stage of the game.

7

Late Life

Never Too Old to Be Too Thin

S he died of pneumonia. At least that is what the doctors said. On a Sunday evening in March, my grandmother, 87, threw up so violently that she aspirated her vomit and infected her lungs. Her death was an unfortunate accident.

But was that really how it happened?

Before she threw up on that fateful evening, G.G.—as we called her for "great grandmother"—attended a party. She "stuffed herself," as she often did upon these uncommon occasions when she went out. Then she stuck her finger down her throat. "Every so often you just have to have a good upchuck," she once told me.

Relatively few women in later life are seeking treatment for eating disorders. There are a handful of scattered medical reports of women in this age group with anorexia, fewer about those with bulimia, and none about binge eating disorder.

But this simply does not make sense. Study after study has demonstrated that these diseases linger, sometimes in active form, for decades. Therefore, why would we accept that a woman who had been ill for a long time would wake up on her sixty-fifth birthday, suddenly free of her eating disorder?

Some explanations for this apparent discrepancy include a simple misinterpretation of the facts. People just don't think that an eating disorder is an eating disorder in a woman who is entering the last third of her life. Because those who are close to these women, and the women themselves, do not understand the intractable nature of the diseases, they fail to recognize the seriousness of the problem.

To give an example of how easy it is to mistake habit for disease, I remember seeing some boxes of Ex-Lax in my grandmother's medicine cabinet and bottles of prune juice on her refrigerator. Many people in late life have trouble with their bowels and take anti-constipation medicine. Thus, neither my mother nor I recognized these pills as flags for an eating disorder, which we might have done if they had been in my preteen daughter's bathroom.

My grandmother seemed "too old" for such a disease. Besides, we thought, "that's just something G.G. does." We were willing to tolerate most health eccentricities because we thought they belonged with aging.

Indeed, according to geriatrician John Morley, who was one of the first researchers to study eating disorders in older patients, it is not uncommon for a person in later life to overuse purgatives.

"You get a few true laxative abusers," he says, "but it is usually because they have a fear that they are not going to have a stool rather than a desire to lose weight."

A second, possible explanation for why it seems there are so few elderly women with eating disorders is that they are misdiagnosed.

Anorexia in later life is typically *not* about the desire to look like a 20-year-old fashion model. It is based more on habit, control, and power-seeking than appearance. For this reason, researchers have classically called the most common eating disorder in this age group "anorexia tardive" (meaning symptoms long after the onset of a disease) to differentiate it from the anorexia nervosa defined by the DSM-IV.

Morley says that his group at St. Louis University in Missouri sees three general types of patients. The first, and most common, acquire eating disorders secondary to another physical or mental problem. Next in number are the women with anorexia who have been weight restrictors all their lives; an eating disorder in this case is merely a continuation of a lifelong problem or a relapse from a previous one. The smallest group involves women who are sick for the first time in later life; illness here is "an adjustment problem" to the difficult circumstances of this life stage.

WHO IS GETTING SICK

When the Eating Disorder Comes Second

Later-life eating disorders are diagnostically slippery: they tangle up with other ailments such as rheumatoid arthritis, cancer, heart failure, pulmonary disease, AIDS, Crohn's disease, anxiety, and depression. One reason for this diagnostic complexity is increased longevity. More than ever, people are living longer. In fact, the annual number of deaths in the United States dropped in 2004 by 2 percent, the biggest decline in nearly seventy years.

While on one hand this is a testament to the successes of modern medicine, on the other, even state-of-the-art treatment cannot guarantee that all those extra years will be salubrious. In 2003, for example, nearly a third of noninstitutionalized U.S. adults older than 64 reported that they were experiencing physical problems that limited their ability to handle personal care. Topping the list were arthritis and muscle and bone conditions. Next came complications of heart disease, stroke, and other circulatory problems. These physical problems only worsen with age. Two-thirds of people older than 85 are now suffering from personal activity limitations. This group may also be experiencing the onset of senility, as well as loss of vision, hearing, and libido.

Any number of medical problems can feed into an eating disorder. Geriatric physicians have long known about a problem called "late-life paranoia." A person with that condition believes that he or she is being poisoned and refuses to eat. Morley says that his medical team sees quite a few patients who acquire the condition in the early stages of dementia and Alzheimer's disease.

Again, people with this condition do not get an eating disorder first. Nonetheless, they end up with a serious problem that can be fatal if left untreated.

Late life also abounds with mood and emotional troubles. According to Stephanie Townsend, program manager and policy analyst for the National Mental Health Association, an advocacy group based in Alexandria, Virginia, nearly one in four adults older than 65 suffer from a significant mental disorder. Anxiety and depression head the list.

"Mental illnesses are very underdiagnosed in this population because of stigma and discrimination," Townsend says.

When a woman in later life worries, feels blue, or loses an alarming amount of weight, people just "chalk a lot of things up to, 'Oh, they are just getting old; oh, this is just a normal part of aging,'" Townsend says.

But mental illness is not an old-age certainty. People can live full lives until the end, and with more sophisticated treatments, older adults can mitigate their suffering just as adeptly as if they were younger.

Ironically, even family practitioners are missing the eating disorder diagnoses in these patients. The most common scenario is that an older person shows up at her physician's office, complaining about what she thinks is a physical problem—weight loss. The doctor, of course, looks for a medical explanation. And if there is one, say, diverticulitis, an infection of the intestines, the doctor prescribes an antibiotic. Meanwhile, the anorexia, tucked away behind the gastrointestinal problem, goes unnoticed and untreated.

However, depression is the most common diagnosed cause of unhealthy weight loss in older persons. While a physician may probe a health history for evidence of depression, he or she may not consider the more sinister reason for weight loss: an eating disorder. But a third of older people who get severe anorexia are also depressed. So which came first, the depression or the eating disorder? The answer is critical. While antidepressants are effective in treating many cases of later-life depression, they do not work in cases of anorexia.

Therefore, if an older woman with anorexia goes home from her doctor's office with nothing more than a prescription for Prozac to combat depression, she is headed for trouble. An aging body cannot withstand starvation for too long. Her anorexia, now more than ever, is likely to develop into a case study, a statistic that will appear, as others already have, in a medical journal.

>>> G.G.'s Physical Problem Masks a Psychological One

My grandmother's story is a testament to what can happen if a physical problem is addressed while a psychological need is ignored. Before she became ill on that fateful Sunday evening, she had had a bout of diverticulosis, a common ailment characterized by inflammation of the intestinal wall. Along with its cousin, diverticulitis, it afflicts 10 percent of Americans older than 40 and its incidence increases with age. Diverticulitis can cause nausea and vomiting.

But, for G.G., diverticulosis was more than a physical condition. It was a catchall for each of her aches and pains, physical as well as mental. Over the years, diverticulosis became the name she gave to all of her negative feelings.

G.G. was a member of the Greatest Generation, born between 1900 and 1925. This group came of age during the Depression and World War II. It prided itself on a can-do optimism that won a war, built up the country's infrastructure, and put a member of their own in the White House for thirty years. But as adeptly as this group built dams and powerful leaders, it did not have time for emotional indulgence. In fact, this generation, one that grew up on deprivation and sacrifice, learned that feelings were contrary to survival. *Crying does not put bread on the table.*

Characteristically, when G.G. suffered the loss of her husband after sixty-five years of marriage, she would not allow herself to grieve. The day after her husband's funeral, she tied on her can-do attitude like an apron. She Spic-and-Spanned the house, donated his clothing to St. Vincent de Paul, and tried to obliterate any memory of him. She was only partially successful.

Without a direct release of her grief, G.G.'s loneliness and worry about being on her own for the first time ever sickened her body. My grandmother had developed diverticulosis ten years before her husband's death. Missing him, therefore, did not cause her to acquire an intestinal ailment. But when she projected her grief and worry onto her body, the symptoms of her diverticulosis worsened. That triggered an eating disorder.

How? The diverticulosis and the eating disorder collided when she felt alone. It was then that she turned to comfort foods to appease the negative feelings. Food was one of the few indulgences that she allowed herself after she lost her social life in her husband's absence. But these binges irritated her diverticulosis. She compensated by making herself throw up, prompting hunger and another binge. The eating disorder then emerged. Amoxicillin, taken daily for years, could do nothing to treat the secondary problem.

Many people in later life lose their spouses but do not get eating disorders. As in midlife, the woman in later life who succumbs to a disorder likely has a predisposition, both genetic and collective. G.G. had the anxious nature that marks a woman at risk. She also had the collective setup: she was a member of the generation that celebrated hard work at the expense of personal pleasure. Hers was not a generation comfortable with freely expressing personal emotion.

"When this generation was younger, mental health treatment was still pretty primitive," Townsend explains. "It was 'We will send you off to an institution for a little bit and then maybe bring you back.'"

Not surprisingly, when my mother suggested that G.G. attend a bereavement group to discuss her feelings, she quipped, "That kind of thing is not for a person like me." And she suffered in ways that I can never imagine. I will never be able to get my mind around what she might have felt when she bent over the toilet for the last time.

When the Eating Disorder
Comes First

While the majority of eating disorders in late life arise secondary to other illnesses and, therefore, have little or nothing to do with appearance and thinness, there are cases in which an eating disorder occurs at this time solely because a person is trying to maintain a low weight. This is usually a continuation of a lifelong eating disorder or a throwback to an eating problem of the past.

"Those who suffer even a single, successfully treated episode in their youth, and therefore appear to have made a good recovery, may remain vulnerable to relapse even 50 years later," write Paul Cosford and Elaine Arnold, in one of the few medical reviews of the issue.

One might say that weight loss for these women is a cultural statement: even in their later years, they equate extreme thinness with youth and beauty. This is a contradiction for a generation that came of age with Marilyn Monroe and Jane Russell as ideals of beauty. Still, contemporary culture with its ultrathin standards of beauty has also caught hold of this older group and made these women sick.

Demographically, one reason why there are so few later-life eating disorders in the medical literature is that there are fewer women in this age range who are sick enough to qualify for a diagnosis. At the same time, because these women are of a generation that is typically not comfortable about admitting to mental illness, they may be extraordinarily tight-lipped about admitting to a long-term eating problem.

"We are just getting women to come out of the closet, metaphorically, about having an eating disorder in midlife," says psychologist Tacie Vergara. "I can't imagine how hard it would be to talk about sixty years with this as a coping mechanism."

And many women in this situation simply don't.

>>> A Grandmother Measures Her Worth with a Bathroom Scale

Writer Abby Ellin portrays how the bathroom scale can govern a woman's life at any age. In a story about her grandmother in a *New York Times Magazine* article entitled "The Measure of a Woman," Ellin starts with a fairy tale: Grandmother takes her young granddaughter on outings. They go swimming, shopping, to the movies, to have manicures, and to eat lunch. But as the tale unfolds, we learn that Ellin's grandmother is no storybook character: she insists that granddaughter Ellin participate in weigh-ins on every Girls' Day Out.

As she matures, Ellin's body begins to change. She becomes "a muscular gymnast" and, unfortunately for her, does not possess her grandmother's lithe body type. In adolescence, she gained 20 pounds, causing her grandmother great consternation. The older woman began to curtail Ellin's annual Florida visit until the teen lost weight. "Because the world judges on first appearance," the grandmother said.

Fast-forward to the grandmother's last months in the hospital. She was emaciated but still wanted the nurse to weigh her aging body daily. In fact, Ellin remembered the ritual: the nurse administering the grandmother's medications, securing her catheter, and helping her onto the scale.

"All I do is lie here and eat," moaned the grandmother, now sinking to 80 pounds. "I don't want to be fat when I get out of here."

Tenaciously, the grandmother hung on to the one constant throughout her life: her scale. The obsession was not necessarily about appearance, even though it may seem so. Trying to keep weight down in late life, as opposed to adolescence, is a coping pattern, cultivated over decades of experimentation, as much as it is a measure of personal value to the world.

Is It Really a First-Time Disorder?

In addition to women who all their lives have had eating disorders, or their vestiges, there is a rare group that does acquire a primary eating disorder for the first time in later life. These problems usually do not come out of the blue. One of the first questions that geriatric psychiatrists ask when they see a woman with what appears to be a first-time problem is, "What can you tell me about your past?"

For example, a classic risk for an eating disorder at any time in life is a history of depression. Case studies show that the depression does not have to come at the same time or even just prior to the appearance of the eating disorder.

For example, there is the case of a woman named Mrs. K, who had her first episode of bulimia at the age of 62. She was raised by an alcoholic and abusive father and suffered through an unhappy marriage of forty years. "Family and marital problems" forced her into the hospital three times over an eighteen-month period in the middle of her marriage. She was diagnosed with acute depression and paranoia.

Twenty-three years after the last episode, Mrs. K's husband died. Soon after, she was embroiled in an argument with family members at a wedding reception. Following that, Mrs. K lost control of her eating at the event itself. She felt so uncomfortable that she went to the ladies' room and vomited. That began her problem with bulimia nervosa. For the next two years, bingeing and purging increased until she finally sought treatment. Mrs. K, now in late life, was vomiting up to three times a day.

It may be that the family fight triggered Mrs. K's late-life bulimia, but the "cause" of her eating disorder, that complex juxtaposition of intertwining factors, happened much earlier. She had dieted most of her life and, more important, she had a history of depression and abuse. Therefore, it may be more accurate to visualize late-life eating disorders as latent beasts lying in wait in a woman with a particular set of vulnerabilities.

ANTI-OBESITY PRESCRIPTIONS DON'T
CARRY OVER INTO LATE LIFE

Semistarvation tactics, whether newly begun in late life or a carry-over from a younger age, have very grave long-term consequences. Studies show that significant weight loss in later life can shorten a person's life. The truth is that in later life people are *normally* going to lose weight. This seems counterintuitive: the general public has heard a barrage of anti-obesity messages, cataloguing the risks of gaining weight with age, but this only applies to people in midlife and younger, says Morley.

As a woman ages beyond 65, her sense of taste and smell will start to weaken. In addition, her stomach will lose its stretch and, therefore, its ability to accommodate a large meal. Adding to that, her gastrointestinal tract will start increasing biochemicals, such as cholecystokin, which makes her feel full. As a consequence, a woman is going to start losing weight after she crosses from midlife into later life, about the age of 70.

"Older people who all their life have wanted to be skinny suddenly realize it is really easy to be skinny," Morley says, "because they now have this 'physiological anorexia'; they are not as hungry as they used to be."

This is not good news. Studies show that losing weight in later life, beyond what is normal for one's age, doubles the chances of dying. In addition, Morley notes that intentional weight loss in women older than 60 can hasten hip fractures and increase the odds of having to go to an institution for care by 1.6 times. Weight loss in later life also lowers immune function, leading to susceptibility to infectious diseases such as pneumonia. And Morley says it does not matter if a person enters late life overweight or obese. Dieting is starving. And that, in later life, puts too much stress on the body.

"Even if you were 250 pounds and suddenly, in later life, you weighed 220, there is something radically wrong," Morley says.

Morley grew up in Africa and has seen the problems associated with too much weight loss. He says that Americans have trouble keeping two opposite ideas about weight in their minds. Whereas in adolescence and midlife a person should heed anti-obesity messages and modify their diet to keep from getting too heavy, she has to reverse that strategy in later life.

In fact, recent studies support the notion that some degree of extra weight, so long as it is not obesity, is associated with longer life. The problem with too much weight in late life is more about disability than about shortening life. But even doctors have trouble dealing with this complexity.

"Physicians examine an older person who is overweight and immediately think that the patient should lose weight," Morley says. "They tell the patient that weight loss is good for them. But it isn't."

In essence, by not understanding the special issues of the late-life patient, doctors are unwittingly "conspiring" with some of their vulnerable older patients to help them reawaken or develop an eating disorder.

For a woman who has been restricting weight all her life, as was Ellin's grandmother, the consequences can be even graver. She had little body mass as it was. As she continued to diet, she lost even more weight and, as a consequence, stressed her immune system and impoverished her bone density. A woman in this situation becomes prone to broken hips, bedsores, and recurrent infections—like my grandmother, whose pneumonia and blood infection within a week after inhaling her vomit led to her death.

The salient message, says Morley, is weight *stability*, rather than loss or gain.

WHY WOMEN GET SICK IN LATE LIFE

Über Anti-Aging: A Growing Trend

A woman who is 65 today rarely considers herself a "late-lifer," any more than she thinks that she is "elderly," "a senior citizen," "aged," or "old." She feels young, active, and vibrant. And she is, jetting off to Kenya on safari or spending weekends running after her grandchildren. Because of her youthful outlook and the fact that she and others like her are living longer and better, researchers are now beginning to classify her as a "young-old." Margaret Norris, a private therapist in College Station, Texas, who focuses on the psychology of aging, uses this term for the active old, as opposed to an "old-old," who becomes infirm.

The former are retired, relatively healthy, financially comfortable, independent, and actually living some of the dreams they were not able to fulfill when they were younger. This group is thriving in their golden years.

"Some people are very lucky, and this phase lasts a long time," Norris says. "But then illness or a life event strikes, and the golden years become much more burdensome."

When a young-old is forced to become an old-old, mental illness can emerge in the transition. Townsend notes that adults 65 and older have the highest suicide rate of any segment of the population, twice the national average. Suicide expresses depression in its most tragic and severe form; an eating disorder is also a form of slow and very painful suicide.

A predictor of whether that slide will occur relates to how the shift to old-old happens:

A life event, not chronology, is what propels a person into an eating disorder. It is important to note that there are 85-year-olds with the health and mental perspective of typical 55-year-olds and there are 65-year-olds behaving like 85-year-olds.

Gail Sheehy, in her book *New Passages,* says that aging, in a negative sense, happens because of a convergence of factors, rather than number of years lived. In later life, especially, everything compounds: genes, race, class, marital status, income, and preventative health. They all forge the reality we term "longevity." Ideally, living a long life means not only living the greatest number of years possible, but also living the highest quality years possible.

Sheehy presents two types of aging. The first is the "wise woman-in-training," who accepts her limitations, focusing on what she *can* do. When faced with obstacles, she alters her life and still lives vitally, sometimes in very unconventional ways. She banks a positive attitude and withdraws her behaviors from it. Sexuality abounds for her, now freed from the shackles of pregnancy and child care. She steps out, wearing purple, taking a lover at 72 or starting a philan- thropic enterprise at 80. She is the ideal for how every woman wants to age.

But she is "the inspiration, not the norm." A sister to her is the one with an eating disorder; she is anything but liberated in her atti- tudes and behaviors. Shrinking away from life, she takes the final steps with white-knuckled fear.

Another way to look at this is through a generational perspec- tive. For lack of a better way to distinguish young-old from old- old, some researchers are turning to chronology. They classify those aged 65 to 79 as young-old, and from 80 and up, old-old. This divide falls right between two generations of Americans: my grand- mother's generation and the one behind her, known collectively as the Silent Generation.

The latter is a group of individuals born between 1925 and 1945. They have lived during a period of rising affluence, a booming economy, and an abundance of jobs. Stereotypically, they married young, moved to the suburbs, and lived as devoted par- ents to large broods of boomer kids. But, sandwiched between the Greatest Generation on one end and the explosive baby boomers on the other, they are looking to their elders for leadership and to their juniors for cultural guidance.

And how are baby boomers handling aging?

As noted in Chapter 6, the boomers, now reaching 60, are moving through their midlife years hanging on to their thinness, fitness ideals, and regimes. If demographics hold their patterns and eating disorders remain intractable illnesses, then some of what is going on now in the midlife group is bound to start spilling over into late-life anorexia, bulimia, and binge eating disorder.

"Eating disorders are in small numbers now in the elderly," Norris says, "but certainly in the future they are going to demand a lot of attention."

And not that far into the future. Members of the Silent Generation are now picking up boomer values and emulating their anti-
aging behaviors. As evidence, Morley points to yet another subgroup
of women, those who are emerging with true first-time eating disorder in late life. These women are developing what is being called
"cholesterol phobia," a problem that occurs when a person goes too
far in trying to lower her cholesterol.

Typically, a woman hears that high cholesterol is bad for her and
then sets about dieting and exercising. She is successful in losing
weight and lowering her "bad cholesterol" levels. But she does not
realize that too low a cholesterol count can be just as bad as too
high a value.

Cholesterol provides the woman's body with some vital services.
Biochemically speaking, the membranes of her body's cells and the
coatings of her nerve connections need cholesterol to function.
Ironically, in the spirit of public service, doctors have embraced the
scourge of high cholesterol. As with weight loss or gain, with cholesterol the message should be balance: too much and a woman increases her risk for heart disease; too little and she can damage her
immune and neurological systems.

Morley recalls a 75-year-old patient who was told by a cardiolo-
gist to lower his cholesterol. He did, by near starvation and exercise.
The man ended up in the hospital with severe pneumonia and poor
immune function. Yet the man was "very happy because his cholesterol was now down at eighty," even though he almost died.

This is not unlike a recent trend toward calorie restriction to
prolong life. There has been a spate of stories recently in the medical journals and the media singing the praises of extremely low-cal
diets. The claims are based upon animal studies in which young
mice fed about 40 percent less than normal live up to 50 percent
longer than mice fed normal diets.

Recently, researchers asked forty-eight people to cut back on
their daily caloric intake by 25 percent, some exercising, in tandem,
and others, eating as little as 890 calories a day for two to three
months. The widely publicized results celebrated decreases in blood

sugar and insulin levels, body temperature, DNA damage, and other signals linked to longer life. Even though the researchers cautioned against overhyping the results or concluding that cutting calories long-term will allow a person to live longer, people are jumping on the bandwagon, forming groups such as the California Restriction Society, which promotes a Spartan diet for long life.

Meanwhile, studies like this alarm eating disorders experts. They counter by saying that these studies have never been done on people long enough to conclude that eating scant diets will lead to longer life. Mice are not people. And in fact, Morley points out that when the researchers conducted the same calorie-restriction studies in older mice, dieting did not protect the older mice against age-related declines.

Until those studies are completed, the message in late life is still: "If you want to die, lose weight," Morley says.

Living healthy does not mean desperately seeking immortality with every new gimmick. A woman who is trying to tack on a few more years should pause long and think hard before rushing into a weight-loss plan. Otherwise, she may end up achieving the opposite of what she wishes.

Death of a Loved One

Just as grappling with mortality can spur a late-life disorder, so can grief. The reported number one instigator of late-life eating disorders is the death of a spouse or loved one. In one survey of the topic, bereavement precipitated more than half of the late-life eating disorders.

This response is understandable. When a partner of decades passes on, a woman feels abandoned. At the same time, she may already be experiencing her own physical ailments and disabilities. With the death of her partner, she suddenly realizes that she will have to age alone: *Who will take care of me now?*

Making matters worse, such a woman has often spent a lifetime relying upon a man to make her complete. She may feel like a fifth wheel if she tags along with other couples. She may have to learn to handle the finances or make life decisions for the first time. Just when she is grieving, she is forced to learn an entirely new set of coping skills.

The entire experience can be devastating in its impact. If she is a certain type of women, she may abuse her body. She may not talk about the grief or loneliness but channel her fears into thinking about her arthritis or the spot on her mammogram that might require a biopsy. She may become obsessed with aging, not so much because she is losing her looks, although that may be a factor, but because she worries about losing basic body functions. It is one thing in midlife to lose the ability to jog due to a knee problem. It is another to lose the ability to control one's bladder.

From a clinical point of view, a woman who loses her life-long partner is at risk for depression and anxiety. This does not mean that all grief is clinical depression or that all worries are anxiety disorders. But geriatric physicians agree that symptoms of depression and anxiety do rise up more persistently in later life, the gnat buzzing forever in the ear. If a woman is already at risk for either of these mood disorders, the death of a spouse—along with other late-life losses and issues—can expose her low-grade problem and exacerbate it.

>>> Martha's Grief-Coping Strategy: A Health Regime

Martha's story illustrates how this can happen. Her husband of forty-seven years died from colon cancer. Months later, Martha, at 77, began experiencing inexplicable aches and pains in her abdomen, hips, legs, and shoulders. The doctors found nothing wrong. Terrified, Martha imagined that she, too, was dying. So she channeled that fearful energy into a health regime. At 140 pounds, she dieted and began walking several miles daily. Over the next eighteen months, she gradually cut entire food groups our of her diet, including sweets, dairy, red meat, and fat. She began a regular exercise routine in her bedroom.

This was healthy, right? Exercise and good nutrition are exactly what public health announcements say older people need to maintain longevity. Martha read the health advice. She followed it, to the letter and beyond.

But she also dropped to 88 pounds. Something went wrong in her body and she could not stop the regimen before she picked up the symptoms of classic anorexia: she worked out daily; tossed meals brought to her by her daughter into the trash; cut her food into small pieces and chewed and chewed and chewed, then, dabbing her lips primly with a napkin, complimented her hostess, saying that she was "stuffed." She dressed in four layers of clothing, complaining that she felt both cold and "fatter than Marilyn Monroe."

Understandably, her doctors first diagnosed her with refractory depression in the context of bereavement. But four courses of antidepressants and related medications did not make a dent in the problem. And Martha stopped taking each one because either the side effects were "intolerable" or the drugs simply did not work.

This behavior went on for seven years. Finally, eating disorders experts figured out that Martha was suffering from anorexia nervosa first, and depression second, as a consequence of the anorexia. With this diagnosis, doctors decided that they needed to move aggressively. They gave Martha nine treatments of electroconvulsive therapy, after which she gained 4 pounds and ate "full and regular meals." She seemed to be cheerful. The combination of weight gain and improved mood allowed the hospital to discharge her.

These therapists just might have intervened in time. If so, this story shows that there is hope at any stage of life. But it is also important to note that the trigger for Martha's first-time disorder was a combination of at least two late-life crises: the loss of her spouse and the fear of her own mortality. In later life, treating eating disorders, more than at any other time, involves dissecting and treating a complicated set of problems.

"Before I was a geriatrician, I was working with anorexia nervosa in young girls," Morley says. "And even that was relatively easy in comparison to what we see in later life."

Eating Alone

Another common late-life issue linked to eating disorders is isolation.

"It's the English tea-and-toast phenomenon," Morley says. "Once you are isolated, meals become too difficult to prepare and you eat less."

As a testament to this concept, Morley's group conducted a Meals-on-Wheels study. Food delivery people sat for twenty minutes with half of the food recipients while they ate. For the rest, the delivery people simply dropped off the meals and drove off. It turned out that the simple act of companionship during a meal boosted the amount of food eaten and general happiness in the group of older adults.

Other studies support this same dynamic. Researchers have shown that at any age a person will eat 33 percent less when he or she eats alone. While this may not be surprising, what is notable is that people tend to eat incrementally more with the addition of each new person joining in the meal. Eating with three, a person will eat more than eating with two; four more than three, and so on, until it levels off at seven people—each diner eating 90 percent more than if he or she had eaten alone.

Eating with familiar and friendly people makes meals relaxing, more enjoyable, and therefore longer. In such group situations, diners forget how much they are eating; they are not parsing out a portion, particularly when the food is served family-style at the table.

Thus, when an older person is eating alone, she is likely to eat less. Additionally, food preferences and tolerances can change with age. Spicy food begins to cause indigestion; beans, flatulence. Salivary glands start to secrete less, which may be why many older people prefer to dunk donuts or biscuits into their coffee or tea. And taste buds dull, especially as a side effect of some medications. Food simply does not taste as good as it used to. Meanwhile, the stomach and colon may also be developing sensitivities from the physiological changes of aging. Eating the wrong foods can have dire consequence. The result is that some women in later life often find little or no joy in eating.

This is often enough to trigger an eating disorder.

>>> A Widow with Cancer Loses Her Joy in Eating

Researchers tell the story of Mrs. B, an 82-year-old widow who developed an eating disorder after she lost pleasure in food. Mrs. B experienced a series of events that all contributed to her loss of taste for food. First, she was widowed; second, she lost both her son and daughter-in-law; third, she was diagnosed with cervical cancer, which was cured with radiation; and, finally, because of the radiation therapy, she lost control of her bowels. This last indignity embarrassed her to the point that she began to "dread the sight of" certain foods. Then she drastically restricted her diet—to the point that, at 5-foot-2, she weighed 81 pounds. She was so emaciated and stricken with mouth ulcers and cold sores—from the chemotherapy and lack of proper nutrition—that she had to be hospitalized.

Becoming Sick to Reclaim Power

Some older women use eating disorders as a form of protest or as a way to assert themselves. Townsend notes that in many of the cases that she sees in her nursing home consultations, there is an "attention-seeking component" to these late-life eating disorders. They may be a first-time episode or a relapse as a woman in later life attempts to re-create the attention she garnered when she was sick as a younger person.

>>> QD's Hunger Strike

Researchers document the story of an 82-year-old widow named QD. When she learned that her children wanted to put her in a nursing home, she refused to eat for six weeks. The problem worsened as her time came to enter the home. She insisted that she was unable to walk. Paramedics had to take her into the facility by stretcher.

QD had suffered multiple losses. When her husband died, she had moved in with her only son and daughter-in-law. There she grew despondent, homesick for her old friends and neighborhood. When she lost her sister, she stopped driving and gardening, declaring herself too old and frail to engage in such activities. As her emotional stability deteriorated, her son and his wife realized that the problem was beyond their caretaking abilities and chose to move her to the nursing home. This decision completely backfired when QD stopped eating. Her story ends when, after a stint in the psychiatric ward of a local hospital, QD realized that her son and daughter-in-law were not going to let her move back with them. Meanwhile, the hospital staff explained that the nursing home would not take her back until she started eating. Choosing the lesser of two evils, QD accepted small but regular quantities of food and went back to the nursing facility.

Becoming Sick to Reclaim Status

For many women, retirement can be a wonderful opportunity. But for others, it can be a precursor to a late-life eating disorder. In a society that glorifies productivity and vitality, it is logical to predict that leaving a career will open the door to some difficult emotions. For a woman who has stayed at home to raise children, "retirement" is marked by the marriages of her children and their shifting focus to their own families.

In that void, some turn to travel. It is an easy solution to questions about the future: *I'll find meaning in life now by remaining active. I have to see everything before I die.* But if travel becomes an escape from subconscious fears, then that fear may manifest itself as an eating disorder in later life.

In her poem "Why You Travel," Gail Mazur touches upon the fear in a woman who uses travel to try to escape it:

> *You don't want the children to know how afraid*
> *you are. You want to be sure their hold on life*
>
> *is steady, sturdy. Were mothers and fathers*
> *always this anxious, holding the ringing*
>
> *receiver close to the ear; Why don't they answer;*
> *where could they be? There's a conspiracy*
>
> *to protect the young, so they'll be fearless,*
> *it's why you travel—it's a way of trying*
>
> *to let go, of lying. You don't sit*
> *in a stiff chair and worry, you keep moving . . .*
> *Movement can be an expression of fear.*

The fear that Mazur is writing about can involve losing one's identity at the passage from middle age to later life. The fear is particularly exaggerated at this time because this life stage is associated with so much loss and cultural negativity. A woman in this situation may choose instead to keep busy—travel, exercise, be blindly active at all times.

For example, some women use grandparenting as a means of distraction from those fears. Of course, spending time with grandchildren can bring a woman deep fulfillment, as the children remind her of one of her purposes in life. But some women take on the grandma job with a vengeance because they think that is all they have left. In an extreme, some women try to reinvent their status as the matriarch rather than find a new identity that exists apart from her grown children's families.

This tactic has its drawbacks, especially if a grandmother is using her children or grandchildren as an outlet for her own unresolved issues. She will not feel complete no matter what her children and grandchildren do for her. They, in turn, may begin to resent what they perceive to be intrusiveness.

In short, the woman is using her grandchildren as a coping mechanism while not addressing her own conflicting emotions about aging. And if she is a woman who has harbored a latent problem that she has been refusing to confront for most of her life, then the coping mechanisms can obsess her. In the context of eating disorders, exercise, activity, and preoccupation with children can easily become a larger problem.

>>> Nilda's Compulsion to "Organize Her Affairs" Before Death

Nilda, 70, grew up in Brazil, working her way through law school and then landing a job in the federal justice system—all at a time in a country where women did not do those sorts of things. She married, raised four children, and became a forceful leader.

Then, reaching her late sixties, she retired. She was bored at home and felt isolated from other women, all of whom had chosen more traditional paths.

"I could never be one of those old ladies, knitting and gossiping while their husbands are playing," she says. "They are acting as if they are vegetables."

Metaphorically, Nilda acted out this revulsion: she avoided all vegetables, except tomatoes, and she refocused her energies onto her children, whose career and life choices had "disappointed" her. Her grown son, for example, could not find a job. Her daughter is a low-paid activist in a nongovernmental organization. Nilda believed that the responsibility for their lives now was hers.

"Everyone just says, 'Oh, Nilda will do it,'" she says.

And she did.

This is how her eating disorder began. On New Year's Day, she cooked a huge meal for her extended family. Hearing the stories of their current lives, she began to feel sick to her stomach. Her adult children were acting spoiled and helpless, relying too much on her. Unable to eat, she went to bed that night thinking about money from her properties on the beach, her current home, and her investments. She woke up, pushing off the covers with a mission: she had to put her "affairs in order" before she died.

"I want to organize my life so that when death arrives, I am not taken by surprise," she says.

This urgency expressed itself through her body. She described the sensation as an adrenaline rush, a worry about running out of time before she could get everything done. While this sentiment is common in later life, experts such as Townsend point out that anxiety issues can become huge problems in later life. Nilda took her psychological issues to the extreme.

If we ask why and how a woman this late in life becomes sick, the answer is not simple because usually these illnesses do not arise without a history. An eating disorder was not a fluke for Nilda. She recalled that she had always been a "picky eater," and that she rarely allowed herself to feel her emotions throughout her life. Instead, she buried them under a veneer of toughness and activity—and an inability to eat.

Therefore, it was predictable that now, when she was nearing the end of her life, she could not rest, even to eat. After that New Year's Eve dinner, she subsisted for a year and a half on black coffee, buttered toast, and vitamin supplements. Her 5-foot-1 body has dropped to 104 pounds. Her doctor gave her two diagnoses: depression and anorexia nervosa. She is currently taking antidepressants, but she is not convinced that the drugs are working.

What does she want from life?

"When you are at this age, the third age," she says, "you need distraction, a companion, love, and some money."

But distraction does not mean obsession, and it is easy to see how Nilda is getting the two mixed up. She is going to have to make peace with her life, her choices, and her children. She is going to have to face perhaps the greatest obstacle in her life: letting it all go.

COUNTERING LATE-LIFE EATING DISORDERS

Psychotherapy: Reviewing a Life

According to Erikson, a person in later life should be developing a sense of integrity. To Erikson, this means acceptance. Looking back, a well-adjusted woman in later life realizes that she cannot change the past, and that she must make her peace with it. She accepts that the people with whom she interacted and the circumstances that guided her life are part of the texture of her life, for better and worse. She finds dignity in herself and her choices, even when her sense of well-being is threatened by physical, economic, or psychological loss. She can look herself in the mirror each day and say, *I tried to do my best with what I was given; I do not need to beat myself up.*

But a woman like Nilda, as she is today, is unable to sort through all her experiences and integrate them into her sense of self. She, along with the others who bear mental or physical vulnerabilities, is at risk. Without the developmental skills to cope, this kind of woman in late life will begin to despair; she yearns for a life that she did not live.

But as difficult as this phase of life may be, a woman can learn to weather even these losses and emerge as a "wise woman," with a strong sense of who she is. To do this, she has to be willing to do her developmental work. And she can—now, and at any point in her life.

Doctors "used to think that older adults could not really do therapy because of diminished cognitive capacity," Townsend says. "But research has shown this not to be true."

Norris agrees. Based on her private geriatric and nursing home practice, she finds that older adults are in some ways *better* patients.

"They are more receptive because they have years of life experience," she says. "They are at a time in life at which they are reflective, sizing things up."

This sentiment touches upon the extensive work of Robert N. Butler, professor of geriatrics at Mount Sinai and president of the International Longevity Center. In the early 1960s, Butler pioneered a promising concept called "life review." It encourages reminiscing.

During the 1950s, aging experts did not perceive the value of "looking back"; they thought that telling the same story over and over was a sign of senility. But as a young researcher at the National Institute of Health, Butler worked with healthy older adults, who talked endlessly about their lives. He was struck by the importance of it— the energy, the value, and the effort to come to terms with people and events. He has since woven the process into a kind of therapy.

He asked older people to recall unresolved conflicts that may have happened many years before. He found that the reexamination, the mulling over, the writing down or talking to anyone who would listen, helped older people to come to terms with their pasts. This may have involved some reconciliation, say, with a long-estranged relative or friend. Or it may have meant self-forgiveness, an often teary and cathartic experience. However it emerged, the person's age-old conflict spun into a story that had a new significance. A person realized in the repeated storytelling that his or her life had meaning. This lessened anger, depression, and anxiety and so prepared the person for a peaceful death.

According to Butler, "Life reviews are extremely complex, often contradictory, and frequently filled with irony, comedy, and tragedy."

While it is hard to get people with eating disorders to do these life reviews, this approach, under the guidance of a therapist, could be very beneficial. People with eating disorders are running away, avoiding their pasts, or trying to numb themselves to the past sources of pain. Eating disorders retard a person's development and distract them from their inner work. A therapeutic life review might well help an older woman begin to reflect more, not less, and begin to heal.

Sometimes older people remember the past with more clarity than they see the present, and this may offer a lift over one of the greatest hurdles experienced by the current generation of women in later life: they are not comfortable talking about feelings.

So why not ask them to tell a story of their past instead?

They might get to the place depicted in a poem by Louis McKee:

SECOND CHANCE

In my dream I return
to the place I went
wrong, and given this
chance to change
things, I go on
down the way I went
before. Even in sleep
I know there is only one go—
and it went well
the first time. Where
it didn't—well, it will
be good to see her again.

This approach applies to anyone. Even with all her physical ability impaired, a woman can still enjoy a renewed ability to free-associate, to express nostalgia, and cope with the regrets and guilt she passes along the way. This approach may take longer to get to the heart of the matter, but it may work better than bottles of medication, particularly for the purest form of anorexia tardive, which, like traditional anorexia nervosa, does not respond to drugs.

Antidepressants and Other Drugs

Butler's studies are not saying that medication is never effective. As case histories have confirmed, eating disorders in later life represent a panoply of conditions. Anorexia can result secondary to many other ailments, physical or mental. And often these conditions, which do respond to medication, need to be treated along with the eating disorder. The first step is to untangle the multiple illnesses and social factors that may be contributing to an older adult's weight loss.

"When I see somebody is losing weight," Morley says, "I've got to work my way through all of these psychological and medical things that might be going on." To simplify matters, his team has come up with the mnemonic MEALSONWHEELS to describe the varied causes of weight loss in older adults. In the context of eating disorders, M stands for medication effects, where an older person is losing weight because of a prescription drug she is taking for another condition. E stands for emotional problems, especially depression and anxiety. A stands for true anorexia nervosa, a problem that probably began much earlier in life. And so on.

If a woman understands these distinctions, she can become more aware of what kinds of treatment are best for her. For example, if she is suffering from depression and stops eating because of that, then she is a very good candidate for antidepressants such as those from a class called monoamine oxidase inhibitors (MAOIs). These drugs relieve depression by preventing the enzyme monoamine oxidase from breaking down the neurotransmitters norepinephrine, serotonin, and dopamine in the brain.

Right now the medical community is debating whether medication, psychotherapy, or some combination of the two is the best way to treat late-life depression. In a study reported in the *New England Journal of Medicine*, researchers found that antidepressants did better than psychotherapy in helping patients older than 65 to feel better. But the details of the study are also telling. When doctors used Paxil and a monthly psychotherapy session, the combination relieved the worst symptoms of depression. Then, once the patients felt better, drugs alone worked better than therapy alone in maintaining their recovery. The bottom line, say physicians such as Morley and Norris, is that they do not advocate medication alone for older patients, in part because there are often multiple illnesses going on at once—and with isolation, loneliness, and anxiety so prevalent, personal interaction may be paramount to helping a person in late life to cope.

Medication does have its place in treatment of late-life eating problems. For example, geriatric physicians often prescribe an appetite-boosting drug called Megace (megestrol acetate), a synthetic version of the hormone progesterone. It apparently works well to help a woman who has lost her appetite to recover it, at least somewhat. And since 2005, patients have the option of a newer form of the drug, Megace ES, which they can take on an empty stomach, a huge bonus for women who have been fasting.

However, drugs cannot cure deeply established eating disorders. Of course, there is a catch: a person has to want the drug to work, which explains why Megace, first approved by the FDA for marketing in 2001, does not successfully treat younger patients with classic anorexia nervosa. If a woman who has anorexia in later life has a disease with deep roots, ones that go way back to her youth, her odds of full recovery are slim—no matter if the treatment is medication or psychotherapy or a combination of the two. Her habits are simply too entrenched and her body and brain chemistry may have been changed permanently.

"The best you can do is to get her not to be malnourished any-more," Morley says.

Treatment Outside the Box

What can a person do when medication and psychotherapy don't work? Tacie Vergara, who has committed herself to this group of older women with chronic disorders, puts it this way: "If you have to think outside the box, you can always find more creative and innovative ways to work with people."

Sometimes that means helping a family with caretaker fatigue or encouraging members to spend mealtimes with their older rela-tives. This fits in with the idea of getting Meals-on-Wheels workers to sit with older people while they eat, especially when family mem-bers and friends cannot be regular dinner companions.

In working with older clients, Norris has had to find ways to circumvent common communication problems. People in later life coming to psychotherapy are often suffering from hearing prob-lems or cannot speak loudly or clearly, perhaps because of a stroke or other disease. An older patient may also have trouble concen-trating, requiring more help from the therapist to focus on the topic at hand.

At the same time, Norris says her patients love to tell her stories about themselves, as sometimes she is the only one who will listen to them. Rather than trivializing the tangents, Norris often uses them as a springboard to generate behavioral change. She lets her clients ramble.

"One of my challenges in terminating the session," she says, is that "they don't want to stop."

When family members ask what they can do for their ill relative, Norris always responds, "The best gift you can give is your time."

Meanwhile, Townsend, who deals with mental health care on a larger, more community-centered level, says that she has to think about ways *to go to* older adults offering help or education, rather than expecting them to come to her. The population is much less mobile than younger patients and often has complicated problems that need multipronged solutions.

"Simply bringing an older adult to the community mental health clinic for their appointments and medications may not work," she says.

With late-life eating disorders, patients who are ill and the people who care for them are often overwhelmed with the amount of care needed: mental health, medical and social services, as well as needs around housing, nutrition, and aging. Therefore, public health and social programs in states such as New Hampshire are now employing case managers whose job is solely to coordinate all the necessary services.

Another approach, termed a gatekeeper model, involves educators going into communities to train people who have constant contact with older adults—postal workers, Meals-on-Wheels delivery people, and pharmacists, for example—as to what constitutes a possible eating disorder, as well as concurrent depression and anxiety problems.

HOW TO SPOT A PROBLEM IN A PERSON IN LATER LIFE

Weight Loss

Given that a misdiagnosis can be a fatal mistake, Morley has developed a simple tool to help people spot eating disorders quickly in a group of women who, because of lifestyle and other factors, often escape detection. Where does one begin?

"Weight loss, weight loss, *weight loss*," answers Morley.

Based on results from 247 residents in nine long-term-care centers in St. Louis as well as 868 members from the community who were not institutionalized, Morley used a short test that is about 80 percent accurate. He simply circles—or asks an older person to circle—the correct answer to eight questions and tally the score based on the following scale: a =1, b = 2, c = 3, d = 4, e = 5. A score less than or equal to 28 indicates that the person is at risk of losing at least 5 percent of his or her body weight within six months. Here are four of the most indicative questions:

1. My appetite is
    a. very poor
    b. poor
    c. average
    d. good
    e. very good

2. When I eat, I feel full after eating
    b. about a third of the meal
    c. over half a meal
    d. most of the meal
    e. I hardly ever feel full

3. Food tastes
    a. very bad
    b. bad
    c. average
    d. good
    e. very good

4. Normally I eat
    a. less than one meal a day
    b. one meal a day
    c. two meals a day
    d. three meals a day
    e. more than three meals a day

Low scores should serve as a warning to have a candid talk with a doctor or eating disorder expert to help thwart a larger problem.

Unhealthy Exercise

Other indicators of an eating disorder, especially in the current population of young-olds now reaching later life, are exercise habits. In this life stage, the body's physiological changes affect a person's ability to exercise safely. The pumping capacity of the heart declines with age. This causes slower oxygen delivery to the muscles and, therefore, lowers cardiovascular fitness. The arteries, in turn, lose some of their elasticity. Meanwhile, bones are becoming brittle and more prone to fracture. Joints lose flexibility, and it takes the body much longer to recover from muscle strain.

This is not to say that an older person should stop exercising. Quite the opposite. According to researchers at the Mayo Clinic, an older woman should stay active. But a woman in later life should modify her exercise activities. She might switch from jogging to walking, or from aerobic step classes to yoga or Pilates. But if a 70-year-old woman is increasing the intensity of workouts or going from no regimen to "hard-core" in a matter of weeks, she may be signaling that she is in trouble.

In a case like this, it might be helpful to think about what else is going on in the person's life. When a woman is using exercise or a diet to deal with the death of a loved one, or if she bears an excessive interest in her body size or image, then she is at risk for a disorder. It is not wrong for a loss, real or metaphoric, to inspire zeal about working to acquire better health. But workouts have to fall within appropriate age and physical-condition limits. And a woman going through loss, which indeed is stressful, has to treat her psychological self as well as her physical body.

NUMINOSITY IN LATER LIFE

Summing this all up, a woman in later life, now more than ever, is experiencing the devastating impact of invisibility. At any age, a woman wants to be special. She wants to feel beautiful. She wants to feel good, not worried or anxious. Carl Jung would say that to do this, no matter what her life circumstances, she has to achieve numinosity, defined as a transformative process by which a person first comes apart and then is put back together, restored to "wholeness." Numinosity refers to an unusual, heightened state of psychological awareness. It is an "aha" sensation that brings a woman a sense of peace.

At its Latin roots, numinosity loosely translates to "agree with a nod of the head" or to affirm. An older woman has to be affirmed by others in society. She also has to learn how to affirm herself. She has to realize that she is beautiful, with an inner radiance not measured by a scale or cultural standards of beauty.

When a woman of a certain age is suffering from an eating disorder, she has not learned to reject the culture's negative message that those who are beautiful are thin; that those who can discipline themselves not to eat, to exercise more, and to hold in their feelings are to be admired. But with numinosity she can come to accept that she is beautiful, that her life does have meaning—simply because she lived it.

8

Healing

The Ongoing Chapter in an Eating-Disordered Life

But now that I am in love
With a place that doesn't care
How I look and if I am happy,
Happy is how I look and that's all.
My hair will grow grey in any case,
my nails chip and flake,
my waist thicken, and the years
work all their usual changes.

If my face is to be weather beaten as well,
It's little enough lost
For a year among the lakes and vales
Were simply to look out my window
At the high pass
Makes me indifferent to mirrors
And to what my soul may wear
Over its new complexion.

(FLEUR ADCOCK, "WEATHERING")

Healing is akin to wearing a new complexion, becoming indifferent to that which does not nurture. Healing allows the winds of emotion to blow freely. Still, despite all we might know about healing, it is hard not to get knocked down. In that emotional storm, we may cling to our destructive habits, as if they were roots, simply because they are familiar to us.

I once said to a friend, "When I am stressed, I go back to my eating disorder. It makes me feel safe." And my friend said, "Anorexia is a disease, not a safe haven. Let's call it what it is."

An eating disorder *is* a disease. It's a prison. But we can break out by naming what we have: "I have an eating disorder." This sounds so simple but, of course, healing is never this easy. I know this first-hand. Decades after I was diagnosed with anorexia, and years after I stopped fitting the official diagnosis, I still have trouble.

In the course of writing this book, I began a program called cognitive behavioral therapy (CBT). The first step was to keep a log of what I ate, when, and how I felt as the food went into my mouth. This was a telling act. I knew that if I could not keep a food log and make sure to weigh myself each week—but only once a week—or if I felt extreme emotions as I wrote down "1/2 grapefruit" or "2 scoops Ben and Jerry's Pistachio Pistachio ice cream," these were signals that something was amiss. Indeed, something was amiss with me.

I learned that I have managed my eating disorder through avoidance. For example, for years I have refused to set foot on a scale. In fact, I would ask my doctor not to let me know the number. "Just write it down in your charts and let me know if there is a problem," I would tell the physician's assistant.

But here are the signs that I have more work to do: buying a scale and keeping a food log got to me. I remember standing for thirty-five minutes in Bed Bath & Beyond. I could not decide upon the "right scale," and when I finally said, "Stop this, already," and threw one into the cart, my hands were shaking. I had no idea how reluctant I would be to do this.

I realized, too, that, as a habit, I eat almost nothing until dinner. I have done this for ten years, since my divorce. And in researching this book, I also learned that this food habit is not unique; many women with eating disorders, particularly those with either anorexia or bulimia, restrict their food intake by putting off meals. I do it for nearly twenty-four hours, sometimes eating only once a day.

I would have called my habit a "food issue," not an eating disorder.

And I still do since today I do not fit the diagnosis of anorexia nervosa. Yet as I began the next step of the CBT program, eating three meals and two snacks each day, I was terrified. What if I gained weight? Who would I be if I were heavier?

And this exercise, precisely because of its difficulty for me, told me that I certainly am still suffering. And now I have a name for it. Subthreshold disorder.

Naming is the first step in the process.

If what you are doing, what you have, may be a less serious problem on the spectrum of eating disorders and disordered eating, you may ask why I am suggesting that you jump through this hurdle. You may argue, *Isn't this just pathologizing something that is relatively benign? What woman doesn't have a food or body issue?*

Naming is an admission that something is wrong. If you have a "food issue" or a bona fide eating disorder, chances are that it interferes with your life and relationships; therefore, you are not living to your fullest. You, and your habits, are affecting the lives of your partner, children, and friends. Ask them what they think. You may get some shocking answers.

Naming is only the first step toward healing. The next is to reach out for help. Throughout *Lying in Weight,* I have referred to this approach as "gathering support" or "amassing the tools for recovery." For it is upon these tools and supports that we will have to rely when the going gets really tough, that is, when we are staring our beast straight in the face, fear pumping adrenaline into our circulation.

Ultimately, and with support, you are going to have to look inside yourself in order to heal. No one, no program, can do it for you. But looking inside often comes later in the healing process.

And it is a *process.* It takes a lifetime. As you take the steps toward healing, you are, in essence, learning to float, to keep your head above water more easily, rather than thrashing and panicking as the waters get choppy. In the process of healing, you may feel that you are drowning. Relax. Trust that you can learn to float.

This chapter is by no means comprehensive. There are long lists of names and resources out there for you. In fact, the information can be overwhelming. I will help you navigate the initial process. This chapter is meant to simplify your journey and inspire you to continue.

STEP ONE: IDENTIFYING THE PROBLEM

A Minor Problem?
Or a Full-Fledged Eating Disorder?

To heal, you first need to be honest. This is tough because an eating disorder exists on a foundation of denial and deceit. Honesty is a heart-to-heart talk with someone whom you love. If you are a woman in trouble, you can approach your partner or family member and say, *I have been hiding this thing for a long time. Help me. What do you experience when you are with me?*

If you are a partner, sister, friend, or child of a woman who might be ill, you may have been suspecting something for years, biting your tongue. You can sit her down and say to her, *I love you, and therefore I have to tell you what I am seeing.*

If you are not sure how serious the problem is, there are at least three self-tests you can use. The most standard is the Eating Attitudes Test, or EAT-26. It asks for personal information as well as eating and exercise behaviors. The result is a score. Although the test alone cannot say definitively that you have an eating disorder, a high score (above 20) raises a red flag. At this signal, you would do well to make an appointment with a professional who can diagnosis the situation more accurately.

If you do score high, do not despair. This does not automatically mean that you have an eating disorder. For example, you may have an undiagnosed illness, such as depression, which can mimic the symptoms of a true eating disorder. Again, someone versed in eating disorders can give a second, more comprehensive assessment.

If you get to this step, then you can expect to walk away from that appointment with a name. A diagnosis. A beginning.

Another self-test, developed by therapists at Remuda, can help determine whether you overexercise. This is particularly relevant if you are an older woman, turning to exercise as an antidote to aging.

Do You Overexercise?

1. Do you feel guilty if you miss your workout?

2. Do you still exercise if you are sick or hurt?

3. Would you miss going out with friends or spending time with family just to ensure you got your workout in?

4. Do you become emotionally upset if you miss a workout?

5. Do you calculate how much to exercise based on how much you eat?

6. Do you have trouble sitting still because you're not burning calories?

7. If you are unable to exercise one day, do you feel compelled to cut back on what you eat that day?

If you answer yes to one or more of these questions, you may have a problem. It may not be a full-blown eating disorder. Nonetheless, as an older woman, you could be damaging your health.

Another self-test, developed by eating disorders researcher Mary Boggiano, will help you pinpoint a problem with bingeing. The definition of a binge is highly subjective and often hard for even the most seasoned experts to pin down. But Boggiano has surveyed many women and come up with a list of questions. Here is a sampling:

Do You Binge Eat?

During a "binge" have you:

1. Eaten with bad table manners (licking plates or scooping out food with your fingers)?

2. Eaten canned food straight out of the can, frozen food while still frozen, and/or food that was too hot?

3. Eaten food that was soiled or taken from the floor?

4. Thrown food in the trash but later picked it out of the trash and eaten it?

5. Eaten food that you knew may have been spoiled?

6. Eaten food raw that was meant to be cooked (e.g., cookie dough, meat)?

7. Eaten food from other people's plates while you were washing them?

8. Had diarrhea, intestinal bloating, belching, or flatus because of the bingeing?

9. Skipped social or important events in order to stay home and binge?

10. Hidden or saved food until you could be alone to binge it?

11. Manipulated situations or persons so that you could binge?

12. Acted or felt defensive about your food?

13. Taken extraordinary measures to secure binge foods (e.g., late-night food runs, going shop to shop)?

14. Taken drastic measures to resist binges (e.g., drunk liquids to "fill up," eaten nonedible things first, chewed and spat out food)?

15. After binge eating, have you ever punished yourself?

The Definition of a Binge

Bingeing is eating, in a discrete period of time (e.g., within any two-hour period), an amount of food that is definitely larger than most people would eat during a similar period and under similar circumstances. Bingeing is also accompanied by a feeling that one cannot stop eating or control what or how much one is eating. Binge eating episodes are associated with three (or more) of the following:

1. Eating much more rapidly than normal

2. Eating until feeling uncomfortably full

3. Eating large amounts of food when not feeling physically hungry

4. Eating alone because of being embarrassed by how much one is eating

5. Feeling disgusted with oneself, depressed, or very guilty after overeating

Another reference to help you in defining a bingeing problem is psychiatrist Christopher Fairburn's book *Overcoming Binge Eating*.

STEP TWO: REACHING OUT FOR HELP

How to Contact a Professional

If you decide that you want to seek help, the key is to develop a trusting relationship with a health professional. Getting the right person is a highly personal and sometimes very complicated task. There is the style of therapy to consider, as well as the location itself. In this day and age, adequate insurance coverage is also a major factor.

One place to start is by contacting the Academy for Eating Disorders (www.aedweb.org). Also, the National Eating Disorders Association has an information and referral help line (800-931-2237)

and a website with a treatment referrals section (www.national-eatingdisorders.org).

It is important to seek out someone adept in eating disorders and not simply a friend who happens to be a doctor or a religious counselor. The latter can help with healing, most certainly, but eating disorders are extraordinarily complex, and it takes someone aware of and trained in that complexity to guide the healing process.

An eating disorders specialist can usually diagnose a problem as well as rule out some other physical cause for the behaviors. Doctors will also recommend treatment based upon your symptoms.

The most important—and daunting—task is to be truthful; lying about how long your symptoms have gone on and with what severity can handicap treatment. Remember, these diseases have high rates of relapse. Lying only makes the situation worse.

Where Do I Go and What Will It Look Like When I Get There?

Hospitals

The good news is that more often than not health-care practitioners opt for treatments that do not involve hospitalization. Studies show that a hospital, while providing a protective environment, does not allow a patient to apply her discoveries and new attitudes to real-life situations. The downside is that once a patient is back in the real world with all its stresses, she may be more vulnerable to relapses.

However, inpatient treatment is often necessary when:

➤ You have already tried outpatient treatment unsuccessfully.

➤ You have additional medical problems that require immediate medical attention.

   The most common physical consequences of eating disorders include osteoporosis (thinning of the bones), heart problems (especially irregular heart rhythms) due to electrolyte imbalance, kidney problems (resulting from repeated dehydration), and brain abnormalities (enlarged spaces in the brain). Because eating disorders revolve around the gastrointestinal system, complications in this area are also common. They include constipation, diarrhea, reflux, nausea, and heartburn. Hospitalization may be necessary to deal with these medical complications, as well as the eating disorder itself.

➤ You are suicidal or too ill to make use of outpatient treatment.

Often when a woman has an eating disorder, she also has associated mental illnesses. These include obsessive-compulsive disorder, anxiety, depression, social phobias, trauma, and chemical dependencies. These co-morbidities may require additional treatment in a hospital or a clinic.

➤ You are pregnant and unable to curtail your eating disorder symptoms.

The most common problems for a mother-to-be with an eating disorder include gestational diabetes and pre-eclampsia. The unborn baby risks miscarriage, low birth weight, or premature birth. There is a higher rate of cesarean deliveries. For these reasons, pregnant women with a serious and active eating disorder need aggressive day-to-day care.

➤ Your insurance will cover you only if you are admitted to a hospital or treatment center.

Believe it or not, the majority of insurers in the United States do not categorize an eating disorder as a mental illness. Therefore, when seeking medical coverage, a woman may find that her insurer will not pay for regular visits to a therapist. Ironically, the insurer oftentimes will pay if a woman is extremely sick or her eating disorder has associated medical complications. In fact, Lynn Grefe says she knows of cases in which women with anorexia were not emaciated enough to qualify for insurance coverage. The women actually had to lose *more* weight, and then enter the hospital, to get the coverage that they needed.

Eating Disorders Centers

As an alternative to standard hospitalization, there are special centers where you can reside while being treated for an eating disorder. Appendix 2 gives a comprehensive list of residential treatment centers, designed specifically for this medical condition.

Each center has its own personality. For example, Remuda Ranch puts treatment in a Christian-based context, while Mirasol opts for a more alternative approach, including biofeedback therapy, which teaches you how to control the state of your body using electrical impulses coming from your brain. Other centers such as Renfrew have many satellite locations, which might be important if, for example, you have young children and want to be as close to home as possible.

Some older women are reluctant to begin treatment not only because of the stigma attached to it but also because institutional services for their age group are lacking. The top centers are now aware of this problem. They are gearing up their resources to adapt to women of all ages. For example, Renfrew has special group therapy that addresses relationships with partners. Another group deals with issues of aging, while another addresses family and parenting needs. Remuda, Mirasol, and the Mayo Clinic have also begun to understand and cater to the special needs of older women.

The intensity of treatment will vary according to the type and severity of your illness. The top clinics can provide very aggressive treatment. A typical day would include therapy sessions, meetings with nutritionists and physicians, support groups, educational classes, and introductions to structured meals. Issues discussed and debated would center on body image, stress management and coping skills, assertiveness training, art and music therapy, and expressive writing.

In terms of relapse prevention, some treatment facilities offer step-down programs that will help bridge the journey from an institutional to a home environment. For example, Remuda and some of the Renfrew centers now have apartments where you could spend additional time after leaving intensive treatment. This functions as a practice space. Living in an apartment-style setting with other recovering women will provide a chance to try out new meal plans, attitudes, and behaviors. This is one step before reentering your day-to-day life and confronting all the stresses that brought about the illness in the first place.

Nonresidential Treatment

In addition to hospitals and centers, there are intensive eating disorder treatment programs that operate on an outpatient basis. The Cambridge Eating Disorders Center (CEDC) in Massachusetts, for instance, offers a mix of programs at varying levels of intensity, from aggressive day-long therapy programs to simple weekly group therapy.

Seda Ebrahimi, a veteran of eating disorders treatment, started the center to "prevent an eating disorder from becoming a lifestyle." When she worked at McLean Hospital, she treated many chronically ill patients. For these women, recovery was usually followed by a relapse. This has special relevance to older women, who might be the ones deeply concerned about issues of aging.

Ebrahimi launched CEDC in 2003 as an alternative to inpatient and residential treatment. Her idea was to provide treatment for women with eating disorders, but in such a way that allowed them to live in context with the rest of their lives.

CEDC is not the only clinic to offer this type of outpatient treatment, but its smorgasbord of programs is well designed to meet the special needs of older women. For example, you may need to support yourself and your children while you are in treatment. Your employer may not allow you extensive sick leave. With more flexible therapy programs, you could work your day job or take care of children at home and still attend therapy sessions in the evenings. Eating disorders researchers are finding that flexibility is key—not only to lifestyle issues, but also in paralleling the way healing happens in real time.

"Recovery itself is not a straight line," Ebrahimi says. "It is full of bumps and pitfalls."

Ebrahimi notes that it not uncommon for a patient who has overcome her symptoms after intensive treatment to assume that she is fully recovered. She leaves the program with high hopes. But those hopes can be dashed if she resumes her old life, faces the same stresses, and reacts in the same old way. She has to have made some kind of internal change in order for her therapy to work in her day-to-day life.

If a woman chooses or is forced to leave her program prematurely, she will have to begin the process again. And the second, third, or fourth time around can be that much more daunting because, with time and failed attempts, the woman is beginning to believe she is a failure.

This almost happened to Christine, 34. She entered a residential treatment facility to treat her anorexia because she was forced to do so. She was so ill and suicidal that her husband and therapist presented the "choice" of voluntary admission to an inpatient center or commitment to that treatment by the state. She chose the former, but once treatment began, Christine plotted how to make it end as quickly as possible. She went through the motions, gained the weight that she needed, and said "the right words." And then she checked out. She went home to all the life stresses she had left. Within a year she had relapsed into her old habits.

The relapse almost did her in. But that is not the end of her story. *Recovery is not a straight line. It is full of bumps and pitfalls.*

Today, Christine is more ready than ever to go back into treatment. But she has decided that it is better for her to engage in therapy outside of a residential center. She feels that she has more control, and control is a big issue in this disease.

The practical lesson here is that treatment is never one-size-fits-all. Often, a woman has to be willing to try many different approaches until she finds the right one at the right time in her life and disease stage.

Private Therapists

For some, particularly those with less severe problems, one-on-one therapy unaffiliated with an eating disorders center is the best approach. There are hundreds, perhaps thousands, of therapists who deal in private practice with women who have eating disorders. This kind of regular therapy often works well if the patient is either functioning well or has an eating problem at the subclinical level.

In her book *The Body Myth*, psychologist Margo Maine gives a list of questions that anyone can ask a potential therapist when first seeking help. These include:

➤ Are you a specialist in eating and body image problems?

➤ How long have you specialized in this area?

➤ What other problems do you treat?

➤ What are your fees?

➤ What is your treatment approach or philosophy?

For help in finding a private practitioner, contact NEDA, AED, or a nearby treatment center for a recommendation.

STEP THREE: CONSIDERING THE OPTIONS
The Styles and Approaches of Therapy

Just as it is important to consider the bricks and mortar of where, how, and at what intensity treatment takes place, you also need to think about style and approach. There are a number of designs for treatment of eating problems. Four of the most popular are cognitive behavioral therapy (CBT), interpersonal psychotherapy (IPT), drug treatment, and group therapy. These are not the only treatments available, or necessarily the best for a given patient. But these are ones that have supporting evidence for their effectiveness.

For more information about general treatment approaches and styles, see J. Kevin Thompson's *Handbook of Eating Disorders and Obesity* or Carolyn Costin's *The Eating Disorder Sourcebook.*

Cognitive Behavioral Therapy: Changing Actions First

When asked what treatments they recommend for an eating disorder, experts more often than not refer to cognitive behavioral therapy (CBT).

CBT is based on a model created by Aaron T. Beck to treat depression. Therapy hinges on a premise: when you face a certain situation, whether it is a screaming baby or a shouting husband, how you feel and what you do is mediated by your perceptions and thought patterns.

In short, your thinking motivates your actions; your actions then feed back to change your thinking patterns.

Thus, CBT asserts that if you get sick, both your *behaviors* and your *thoughts* are probably sick; therefore, your eating disorder operates on several behavioral and cognitive levels.

Level 1 represents the surface thoughts and behaviors that are easy to see: *I binged at four P.M. today; I feel guilty. Tomorrow, I will begin to diet again.*

Level 2 includes automatic thoughts that lie just beneath the surface of a particular situation: *I am mad at my husband for staying late at work. Therefore, I am going to punish him (and myself) by bingeing and purging.*

Level 3 gets to the core that transcends any thought or behavior in the moment. *I deserve punishment because I am not a worthwhile person.*

The ultimate goal of CBT is to get to these core doctrines and help massage them into less rigid, more forgiving truths. CBT attempts to treat an eating disorder by tackling all levels of the disease, starting with level 1. Here is how it works:

The first stage of CBT treatment focuses on behaviors and offers education. If you participate in CBT, you will begin by self-monitoring, through a food log and weekly weigh-ins. You will be planning your meals and strategizing how to reduce your damaging behaviors.

Once you get a handle on these outward behaviors, you will enter the second stage, with its more "cognitive" focus. You will be thinking about why you believe that you need to diet or binge eat. You will gradually be replacing the patterns of dieting and bingeing with problem-solving skills. You will be learning how to deal with life stresses or intolerable emotions through better thought patterns and strategies.

In the third and final stage, you will be able to plan for the future in order to avoid a return to the unhealthy habits.

The research done so far suggests that CBT works best for people with bulimia. Fairburn, who tailored CBT for people with eating disorders, claims that it worked to reduce binge eating symptoms in 90 percent of his patients with bulimia. Further, he showed that his patients maintained their recovery, both one and six years after treatment.

Others experimenting with CBT also quote success, but more modestly. For example, researchers report that only half of their patients remained symptom-free at the end of treatment. They also noted that CBT "is not a panacea." Some pointed out CBT's limitations, including problems with getting the therapy to remain effective in the long term.

If you have an eating disorder other than bulimia, you may not respond as well to CBT. For example, studies show that women with binge eating disorder quickly relapse back into bingeing and that anorexia is extraordinarily resistant to treatment.

But therapists are not giving up. They are now modifying CBT in the hopes of making it a more universal treatment. For example, researchers have concluded that a missing piece to CBT involves women using their eating disorders as narcotics, attempts to self-regulate an unwieldy emotional world. *You took away my eating habits. What will I have left when I get upset?*

To deal with that, therapists are now trying to combine CBT with other techniques, such as motivational therapies that have been used successfully in the treatment of drug and alcohol addictions. The main idea is to come up with better ways for women to manage the negative feelings the eating disorder has been masking and to help women rekindle feelings of personal power. Early studies with these integrative approaches are showing promise.

Overall, CBT is a good choice for first-level treatment, both because it has experimental data to validate it and because it gets to the psychology behind the damaging behaviors of an eating disorder. Since it does not work for a substantial number of women, however, other therapies are also worth exploring.

Focal/Interpersonal Psychotherapy: Changing Motivations First

While CBT moves from symptoms to core issues, interpersonal psychotherapy (IPT) works from the core first. The premise of IPT is that you are using your eating disorder to cope with some deep psychological issue, probably something from your past. Thus, IPT will begin with your personal history.

IPT all but avoids mention of symptoms. It acknowledges that an eating disorder is its own beast, deserving of attention. But IPT asserts that the eating disorder is chameleon-like, changing with circumstances and time. For example, if you purged by vomiting when you were younger, you may now purge through overexercise instead. The eating disorder has changed its appearance but not its purpose, which is to manage negative feelings.

Rather than going after the behaviors of vomiting or overexercising, IPT starts with what's behind those behaviors. It unfolds in three basic stages:

The first is the *discovery period*. Researchers have found that three-fourths of individuals diagnosed with anorexia or bulimia reported that they had experienced significant life-changing stress within a year before the onset of the illness. *Lying in Weight* has extensively detailed what these triggers might be, life stage by life stage.

While your stressor may not "cause" your eating disorder, it probably plays a huge role in sparking and feeding your problem. Thus, in the first stage you would work with a therapist to pinpoint the origins of your illness and the current situations that are fueling it. Once brought to light, they become the focus of therapy.

For older women in particular, some focal areas might include grief, life transitions, identity changes, and role disputes in relationships. For example, if you are a woman in mid- to late life, you may have been devastated by the death of a loved one. The goal of therapy might be to face the loss and then find new outlets and interests to balance your life again.

If you recently divorced or remarried, you may be having trouble adapting to your new role as a single woman or second wife. IPT may focus on helping you work through the fears of taking on a new identity.

If you and your partner are experiencing trouble, you may have mismatched expectations of each other. For example, Tracy enjoyed working but ultimately felt overburdened by the demands of raising her two boys as well. Tracy's husband expected her to take on a completely domestic role. She found herself miserable and searching for an outlet. She went back to her old habits, born from bulimia; she dieted and obsessed about her weight.

IPT might help Tracy. Instead of focusing on her body as the source of her problem, she and her husband might work in therapy to pinpoint where their differences lie. The couple could then work toward better communication about their respective needs and expectations and thereby problem-solve and renegotiate their roles.

Once you discover your areas of stress, you progress to the second stage of IPT, which recants week-to-week progress. You would start reviewing your progress during each subsequent therapy session. You may recant the issues bothering you at the moment. Your therapist, meanwhile, would gradually step back and let you take charge of your own healing. Ultimately, you would learn how to problem-solve on your own so that in the final stage, you and your therapist deal mainly with closure.

As with CBT, IPT has been most successful for women with bulimia. IPT therapists are working to find ways to modify the therapy for women with anorexia and binge eating disorder, hoping to make it a more universal form of treatment.

Published reports conclude that CBT and IPT have the same overall success rates, but IPT requires more time to start working. This makes sense: it takes time to discover the issues at the core of an eating disorder. However, IPT might be preferable to CBT if there is a single, obvious issue behind the eating disorder—a history of sexual abuse, for example. And IPT's effects can be lasting, making it a good choice of treatment for bulimia, particularly if you tried CBT and found that therapy lacking.

Medication: Changing Biology First

Eating disorders have an addictive component to them. Even if you have an eating disorder and want to heal, your body may be so changed by your behaviors that it cannot easily stop its familiar habits. You may crave the behaviors that make you sick.

How can you overcome a hurdle that is as much biological as psychological? One answer is medication. The psychiatric community is now engaged in a great debate about whether or not addiction, and mental illness in general, can be treated like purely physical illnesses such as diabetes.

Historically, doctors have used antipsychotic drugs on patients with anorexia nervosa. But the drugs did not work well, and as a result, medications for eating disorders fell out of vogue for at least two decades. But in 1982, psychiatrists thought there could be a breakthrough.

James Hudson and Harrison Pope published a paper showing the benefits of the antidepressant Prozac in treating women with bulimia. Although other studies have disputed the value of Prozac, it did offer hope to a desperate group of women.

Do drugs work to treat eating disorders? It depends. Right now the best results are coming from selective serotonin reuptake inhibitors (SSRIs) in the fluoxetine (Prozac) family. Based on an analysis of more than twenty clinical studies, the Food and Drug Administration (FDA) has approved Prozac to treat bulimia nervosa. To date, it is the only FDA-approved drug for this condition.

For some women, like Ruth, 45, the drug helps reduce binge eating. "The Prozac had an immediate effect on me," she recalls. "By the third day I had taken it, it was just like this realization that something was different."

Her experience fits with those of many other women with bulimia, who have reported that after taking Prozac, they have experienced a 50 to 60 percent reduction in their binge eating and vomiting. Women also described better moods and less concern about their weight and shape.

But there is a caveat. Although patients are showing improvement in symptoms, the percentage of women who are actually symptom-free is low. At the same time, relapse occurs frequently. According to Chris Fairburn, the effects of antidepressants are often short-term, sometimes lasting only a matter of weeks.

Ruth's experience shows us one reason why. When she was actively symptomatic, she was exhausted between binge-purge episodes. She frequently slept for long periods of time, up to fourteen hours. "I slept so that I wouldn't have to think about food," she notes.

But after the Prozac took effect, she binged less frequently and her sleep binges also began to wane. As she spent more time awake, she began thinking about food and purging more often. That caused her symptoms to pick up again. So the drugs alone were inadequate.

Another downside: antidepressants carry side effects, including weight loss or gain. Studies show that a class of antidepressants called tricyclics can prompt weight gain, while Prozac, in general, promotes weight loss. Any weight change is critical to eating disorders recovery. Weight fluctuations can impact long-term recovery in a negative way.

For example, Mary, who suffered from bulimia, found that she lost weight when taking Prozac. At first, she was thrilled. But then her weight began dropping too low.

"People were telling me that I was too thin," she says. "Then I realized that the game was up."

She eventually started gaining the weight back, but that process was extraordinarily difficult, made more so because she kept comparing her body to its earlier shape, when she was thinner.

In other case studies, women who take Prozac often reduce their bingeing but simultaneously increase their dieting. This gets to another limitation of antidepressants used without psychotherapy: they can stop bingeing and purging, but they do not bring about recovery. True healing means psychological relief from deeper fears: *I am afraid of getting fat, even if I eat "normally."* And that degree of healing cannot come from simply popping a pill.

"There is a lot of depth that is missing in eating disorders treatment," says Joanna Poppink. "Yes, the behavior can change, but then we have the relapse business."

For this reason, and due to the fact that women with anorexia nervosa experience almost no benefit from taking drugs, therapists are stepping back from their initial enthusiasm for medications for eating disorders.

This is not to say that the medication book is closed. Treatment of binge eating disorder is very much on the frontier. Published reports show some promise in small studies of drugs such as topiramate (Topamax)—traditionally used to treat epilepsy—and others such as fluvoxamine and sibutramine. These appear both to reduce binge eating and cause weight loss in obese patients with binge eating disorder. Still other drugs, such as desipramine, imipramine, and d-fenfluramine, have reduced binge eating but not affected weight loss. But if coupled with other forms of weight-loss interventions, these and other medications such as rimonabant, an experimental weight-loss drug, might help patients in recovery.

One last hope comes from a hormone called leptin, now being tested to help treat infertility problems in women with histories of anorexia. Leptin also showed initial promise in helping overweight patients to maintain weight loss after dieting for up to a year. The hormone may be the link between diabetes and obesity: leptin helps to control the balance of a person's blood sugar.

The *Handbook of Eating Disorders and Obesity* has a comprehensive chapter on the subject of drugs and eating disorders. In general, psychologists and psychiatrists agree that drugs may help, particularly if the eating disorder is bulimia. But drugs cannot be a substitute for psychological therapy.

Group Therapy: Changing Support Structures First

If you are an older woman suffering from an eating problem, you are probably dealing with troubled relationships—partners, children, or coworkers who increase your stress load and worsen your symptoms. Group therapy can be an outlet to vent about these troubles as well as a safe space in which to share long-kept secrets.

In general, group therapy for eating disorders involves education, interpersonal psychotherapy, cognitive behavioral therapy, or a mixture of all three. CBT and IPT have been described above. The first of the approaches, education, might be more formal. At the University of Toronto specialists used a lecture format to help a group understand what an eating disorder actually is. Group members may generate new information by talking about personal stories, failures, and successes.

Thus, if you are a woman who has a more severe problem, your personal therapist might recommend group therapy as an add-on to individual therapy. If you are ill and cannot afford the costs of individual therapy, a group offers a more affordable venue. If you have binge eating disorder, or are simply an older woman who is still extraordinarily ashamed of your problem, group therapy might seem like an easier place to begin. You could spend sessions quietly listening while drumming up the courage to speak. Finally, if you have a subclinical disorder and need only a touch of support, a group might be ideal for you.

If you want to try group therapy, you would do well to look at the group's composition. Some groups are homogenous, including only people with the same disorder—all women with anorexia, for example. Other groups are mixed—women with anorexia and women with bulimia.

Group composition can be important. For example, if you have anorexia nervosa and your potential group is mixed, you may not be able to relate to someone with binge eating disorder. Another consideration is age. The Cambridge Eating Disorders Center organizes groups based on members' age, decade by decade. Renfrew organizes groups by topic of discussion: family issues, relationships, or aging, for example.

St. Paul's Hospital in Vancouver employs yet another commonality: parenting. Dietician Kim Williams started a playgroup for new moms with eating disorders. The group was an offshoot of an eating disorders program that St. Paul's runs for pregnant women. Williams and her colleagues realized that the postpartum period was one of the most difficult times for women with histories of eating disorders. Why not allow the new mothers to share their struggles and gain support during this trying time?

But not every group runs perfectly. Williams's experience shows just how crucial it is that an eating disorders group falls under the guidance of a leader with experience. As the mothers in the St. Paul's group came together with their infants and toddlers in tow, the new moms quickly gravitated toward discussion of what they were feeding their children. *Maddy won't eat anything except chicken nuggets. Austin is a chowhound; I am worried that he is going to get fat.*

"I had to limit it," Williams says. "I had to remind them continually, 'This is a time for us to talk about what is going on with you. And you need to talk to someone else about what is going on with your child.'"

After that, the discussions moved to relationships, communication, in-laws, and how they were coping. And because of these ground rules, the women found support in the experiences of others.

As a general rule, if you are considering group therapy, you should check out the structure, style of therapy, kind of people in the group, group focus, and the credentials and experience of the facilitator.

Marital and Family Therapy:
Changing Relationships First

While group therapy can serve as an adjunct to individual therapy, so can marital or family therapy. Family dynamics have long been a part of the treatment strategy for eating disorders. But traditionally, this has been about young women with issues of individuation and separation from their families of origin.

Researchers now extend the eating disorder treatment to the family—the daughter, the wife, the mother, the stepmother, the grandmother. Family therapy can mean husband and wife coming in for couples counseling. Family therapy can also mean mother and daughter, both dealing with their own eating disorders. Researchers point out that one of the best reasons for which an older woman might choose family therapy is remarriage.

"We are talking about women who may have been married ten or twenty years," says Edward Cumella. "They have raised their children with one man."

If this is the case in your situation, the second time around, you may find yourself in a strange, complicated realm.

In traditional family therapy, the old philosophy was that if a girl is sick, it is her family that is sick. While this precipitated a great deal of unhealthy mother-blaming, now researchers view the family as the "container," the "holding environment," of a woman's mental health. While family dynamics may not be the cause of a woman's problem, they are nonetheless going to feed and fuel it.

If you are a woman with a problem and decide to engage in family therapy, perhaps to treat an eating disorder rising up after a second marriage, a family therapist is likely going to be working with your husband, your ex-husband, even your new husband's ex-wife. If all these people can bring their experiences and perceptions to the table, it can help move therapy along. Family therapy does not exist to lay blame, but a family therapist is going to work to help you disengage from your previous family and establish a new bond in your new family, even working with children and stepchildren to examine their role in the family's dysfunction.

Another version of family therapy is couples therapy. If you and your partner are having trouble, that tension can instigate your eating-disordered behaviors. Couples counseling may offer you and your partner a fresh perspective. This therapy is not meant to be a substitute for individual healing work, but rather, an adjunct that brings to light previously hidden facets of the illness.

The ideal, says Joanna Poppink, is that you have your own individual therapist, your partner has his, and then the two of you have a couples therapist, who is different. As you and your partner start healing, your recovery is likely to upset the foundation of your relationship. Therapy will address ways that can help both partners heal.

Yet another situation warranting family therapy is if you have experienced an eating disorder and then your child begins to struggle with one as well. Even if you are in recovery, your daughter may only now begin to realize the impact of your former behaviors. She may feel angry and rebellious, sickening herself, and demanding to know, *Where were you when I needed you, Mom?* In truth, you may not remember, having been consumed by the rituals of your eating disorder.

"This is where you get big clashes," Poppink says. "Tremendous anger and tears. Because of memory blanks."

Poppink says that even if you are a mother who has healed from her own problem, the pain that you will face when you recognize your part in your child's illness will be overwhelming. If you are in this situation, it would be wise for you and your daughter to engage in family therapy. There can be a positive outcome. Poppink says that if a mother in this situation can tolerate the anguish of recognition, then tremendous catharsis can occur for all who are involved.

Twelve-Step Programs: Changing Addiction First

Some women, particularly those who binge, have found relief in programs such as Overeaters Anonymous (OA). The treatment philosophy is that you are sick because you are hooked. For this reason, twelve-step programs, which have effectively treated many addictions, look attractive to women with eating disorders. On the surface, binge eating does have addictive qualities. People who binge eat are like people who drink because they

> ➤ Experience cravings to engage in the behavior

> ➤ Feel a loss of control over their behavior

> ➤ Are preoccupied with thoughts about the behavior

> ➤ Might use the behavior to defuse tension

> ➤ Deny the severity of their behavior

> ➤ Attempt to keep their behavior secret

> ➤ Persist in the behavior despite adverse effects

> ➤ Often make repeated unsuccessful attempts to stop.

Mary Boggiano's work adds a biological factor to that list: binge eating might be influencing the same brain centers as alcoholism, though the extent and specific neurological pathways are not yet fully understood. Nonetheless, the potential connection between eating disorders and addiction suggests that a program meant to treat alcoholism might successfully treat binge eating.

Indeed, OA worked to stop the symptoms of Marianne, who suffered for years from bulimia. Twelve years after her first meeting, Marianne still swears by OA and practices "abstinence" from trigger foods, including those that contain sugar.

But Fairburn cautions that alcohol is not the same thing as food; you can abstain from alcohol but you cannot survive without eating. Thus, while twelve-step programs encourage abstinence, eating disorders treatment has to do the opposite—allow you to eat, but in a different way.

Another difference between alcoholism and binge eating treatments involves relapse. With alcoholism, simply taking a drink, because of what it can lead to, is considered a relapse. Twelve-step programs also emphasize that "going back to the bottle," even to take a sip, defines a relapse.

With eating disorders there cannot be "abstinence"; that, in eating disorder terms, is severe anorexia nervosa. Therefore, if you are a woman with an eating disorder, you have a harder task than alcoholics because you must learn how to coexist with food. Understand that a relapse is almost expected. "You just try to minimize them," says James Hudson at McLean Hospital. "You don't get all caught up in the catastrophe of having them."

The last consideration has to do with a prevalent thinking often seen in eating disorders. Fairburn terms this thinking "all or nothing." He notes that a woman who typically binges wants it *all*, but between binges she probably feels so guilty that she eats *nothing*. Twelve-step programs can actually encourage this faulty thinking by pushing more for abstinence (nothing), which will in turn prompt more bingeing (all).

Treatment for eating disorders, then, should involve working toward a middle ground, not abstinence. This is not to say that twelve-step programs are irrelevant. But if you are a woman with a bingeing problem, you should be aware of the differences among alcoholism, substance abuse, and binge eating.

STEP FOUR: CONSIDERING ALTERNATIVES

As good as CBT, IPT, and other gold-standard therapies are, they do not work for everyone—at least in the time frame normally used for measuring success rates. In one study, Stuart Agras and colleagues at Stanford University in California estimated that only a third of women with eating disorders were eating disorder–free one year after standard treatment. Those statistics indicate that something in these treatments is missing.

"With some people, you can do talk therapy until they are blue in the face," says Jeanne Rust at Mirasol. "They are not gonna get better."

But instead of asking, What's wrong with the person? Rust says that it is better to ask, Why can't we reach them?

The quest is on to find new ways of reaching out. But before describing some cutting-edge approaches, a piece of advice: do not consider treatment a failure if the first attempt was not a success. Eating disorders require a long period of recovery. They are stubborn. And it may take a long time and many creative attempts to tame them.

The Internet: Breaking New Ground

An alternative to more traditional therapies is the Internet, where many with eating disorders already seek information. Indeed, a Pew Foundation report documented that 62 percent of all Internet users and nearly three-fourths of women seek health information on the Internet. And despite skepticism about the accuracy of the information, 70 percent of users reported that the information they received influenced their decisions.

Treatment pioneers are seizing this opportunity. They are offering online help with everything from self-assessment tests to information, advice, and emotional support. Internet-based interventions have their advantages over traditional therapy: compared to conventional therapies, the Internet is cheaper, or even free if you log on at a public library. It can open doors for treatment if a therapist is unaffordable. Also, if insurance offers only a minimum of coverage, the Internet can provide a stopgap treatment source when coverage runs out.

If you are a woman homebound by child care or infirmities, as in later life, transportation can be an issue. The Internet does not require a trip in a car to a therapist's office. Additionally, the Internet provides flexibility: you can get help at the time that you most need it. Even in the middle of the night.

Another advantage of the Internet, and the one that women with eating disorders cite most, is its perceived anonymity and privacy. Eating disorders breed shame and secrecy. If you are a woman with a problem and are avoiding institutional help because of a high-powered job or fear that your spouse or coworkers will learn about your struggles before you are ready to tell them, you may like the idea of an online alias.

Will the Internet work to treat or manage your eating disorder?

Yes, but only to a degree and only in some cases. It is important to note that, to date, no Internet-directed treatment for eating disorders has ever been effectively tested in women with full-blown eating disorders. Studies conducted thus far have involved only women with subthreshold symptoms or those who are merely at risk for developing an eating disorder.

The phrase "at risk" in the context of adult women includes one or more of the following situations:

➤ You recently left a treatment facility for an eating disorder.

➤ You have "eating issues," but have not progressed to diagnosable status.

➤ You have a history of an eating disorder and are now facing a particularly stressful period of your life, i.e., pregnancy or the death of a loved one.

The Internet can be helpful in one of two general ways: getting information and communicating with others. One example is the EAT-26 test, which is now available online. If the score is high, some websites will provide a list of eating disorder treatment specialists. Other sites offer information for further diagnosis.

The Internet also works amazingly well in the arena of education. A Google search can provide information about the latest findings on eating disorders, as well as resources to learn about healthier nutrition, exercise, and tips to manage damaging attitudes, thoughts, and emotions.

The downside is that some of this information is inaccurate and, in some cases, actually harmful. In one study of an eating disorders support group online, researchers analyzed three hundred bulletin board messages: 12 percent were inaccurate. Also, much of the "education" is purposefully or inadvertently *pro*–eating disorder. For example, many websites discuss how to diet or exercise "better," meaning more intensely. Meanwhile, more than four hundred websites in the "pro-anorexia" and "pro-bulimia" vein have users with eating disorders discussing the nuts and bolts of their illnesses. This is not education. So be careful: check out the source. If you are unsure of its credibility, check with a reputable organization such as NEDA, the largest national organization that deals with eating disorders.

If you are searching for more engagement, there are many chat rooms, bulletin boards, and other interactive sites. Chat rooms give real-time feedback, usually from others who are in similar situations. Bulletin boards are less spontaneous, but they offer the advantage of flexibility in timing and convenience.

When you first log on, you might be overwhelmed by the plethora of sites dealing with eating disorders. The key to wading through them is to identify who is running them. For example, the website something-fishy.org is run by Amy and Tony Medina. They began their website in 1995, as Amy was recovering from anorexia. The site is still very popular today because it is very comprehensive and works "in the trenches." Users come from countless backgrounds, in all stages of recovery. There are special rooms for partners and loved ones as well as bulletins broken down by type of eating problem. That diversity and the energy of the users make the website work.

Another kind of eating disorders website is one that is moderated by a therapist. Psychologist Joanna Poppink, for example, provides educational and inspirational materials as well as an online bulletin board.

Before every message gets posted, Poppink reviews it, filtering out the spam and content. For example, one woman had an eating disorder and her boyfriend posted a message about her. The woman asked to have the message removed for fear that her mother would see it. Poppink immediately did so.

But she, or any therapist facilitating a website, cannot control everything. For example, visitors swap e-mail addresses and communicate offsite. In addition, Poppink cannot offer treatment online and she cannot respond to a visitor's psychological crisis. There are also ethical considerations, such as the fact that Poppink can neither guarantee visitors total anonymity and confidentiality, nor ascertain whether people who register on her site are who they say they are. So if you choose this avenue for help, you should be aware of the risks.

While offering many advantages, the Internet should not be used as a substitute for standard treatment if that is available. The Internet and related technologies, as they stand today, should be viewed more as supplements to one's knowledge base about the disorders.

As to the impact of the Internet, it is profound. Internet applications now being tried include therapists who communicate with patients between sessions, perhaps offering support, monitoring, or prescription refills; and real-time, moderated discussion groups, which are more on a par with group therapy. In yet another approach, some women with eating disorders are actually creating their own websites and blogs that serve to express their own recovery.

Future applications could include tools such as Web-based body image journals, and tools to monitor events that trigger dissatisfaction. Perhaps someone will come up with graphic "avatars" that simulate what a woman might look like at a different, healthier size.

For a more detailed discussion of Internet-based interventions, consult "Internet-Based Treatment Strategies" by Andrew Winzelberg and colleagues in the *Handbook of Eating Disorders and Obesity*.

"We do not view Internet or other advances in communication technologies as a panacea for the treatment of eating disorders," the authors write, "but rather, as a useful tool to aid in the identification and treatment of these disorders."

Meditation: Balancing Emotions

One of the hallmarks of eating disorders is intense emotion. One way to cope with it is through meditation. And there are many forms of it. For example, a technique called transcendental meditation (TM) seeks to quiet ordinary thinking patterns, often through the use of a mantra repeated over and over. "Mindfulness" meditation will teach you how to guide your attention to your inner sensations, using breathing, body sensation, and movement. Breathing techniques can help calm you and restore mental balance between thoughts and feelings.

While not the cure, these meditative approaches do have evidence—randomized, and controlled clinical trials—backing up their effectiveness. For example, in one study of 202 people, 55 and older, researchers found that TM decreased death rates by a quarter, and mindfulness meditation, while not quite as potent, nonetheless significantly reduced death rates from heart problems and cancer. Other studies have shown meditation's success in extending longevity. Psychologists Jean Kristeller and Ruth Quillan-Wolever, speaking at the Academy of Eating Disorders annual meeting in 2004, discussed the promise of mindfulness meditation as a treatment specifically for eating disorders. And women with bulimia who participated in a six-week clinical trial of guided imagery reduced their bingeing and vomiting, felt better able to comfort themselves, and improved their feelings about their bodies and eating.

To explore how this works in more detail, psychiatrist Thawatchai Krisanaprakornkit, who runs the Meditation Therapy Clinic at Khon Kaen University in Thailand, offers an eight-step program. It helped ease the anxiety, moods, and symptoms of distress in patients suffering from depression and anxiety. In fact, patients who practiced tended to sleep better and reported better relationships with their families. While depression and anxiety disorders are not eating disorders, they share some similar symptoms with the former.

"In eating disorders, fear and dread are the phenomena of the mind at the moment," Krisanaprakornkit notes. "If the patients can be better aware, they can manage better. They can regulate better."

Meditation is not for everyone, as evidenced by high dropout rates in the clinical studies that have been published. However, because it is rarely harmful, why not try? The only caution is that meditation should not be used instead of other treatments, especially when an eating disorder is severe.

"We urge meditation to be used with group support, guided imagery, physical exercise," says James Gordon, chairman of the 2002 White House Commission on Complementary and Alternative Medicine Policy in a press release published by the Cochrane Collaboration in Washington, D.C. "It's too much of a burden on meditation to use it on its own."

Yoga, Pilates, and Related Disciplines: Aligning Body and Mind

Eating disorders are all about body preoccupation. To change that, you should not necessarily *avoid* thinking about the body. Rather, healing might be learning how to focus on your body, but in a healthy way. Yoga, Pilates, and related disciplines promote acceptance of the body the way it is, rather than sculpting or beating it into some ideal.

In general, Pilates is a form of exercise meant to realign and strengthen the body as well as balance it with inner sensations. There are many forms of Pilates. The original Pilates is truest to its creator, Joseph Pilates, but contemporary adaptations have also emerged, adding advances in physical therapy, spinal research, and biomechanics.

Similarly, there are many basic approaches to yoga, some highly meditative, others more outwardly physical. Yoga schools such as raja yoga, trika yoga, and kundalini yoga fit into the more meditative branches. Techniques such as pranyama work with breathing and attention to inner sensations. Practices such as iyengar and ashtanga yoga synchronize the breath with a series of progressive postures. Because your body is stretched to its physical limits or sweating out toxins, it calls for focused attention on postures and breathing.

These techniques open paths to healing: reconnecting your thoughts to your body in a healthy way after years, perhaps decades, of self-abuse.

"Yoga is, for some women, the only time when they and their bodies are allies," says Linda Sparrowe, a longtime iyengar yoga instructor and someone who has suffered from an eating disorder. "They can say to themselves, 'With my eyes closed, on my own mat, where there are no mirrors, I can be safe and good at something that is not dependent on how I look or what people think of me.'"

At the same time, yoga or Pilates can more gently substitute for the intense aerobic workouts that may be dangerous to you as you age.

But there is at least one disadvantage to yoga and Pilates: often instructors ask participants to avoid eating—or eat lightly—for an hour or two before a session. If that means *I can starve myself before class and then take several classes back-to-back, not eating for most of the day,* this defeats the purpose of these healing tools. As with everything else, yoga and Pilates should be practiced with care and moderation.

Biofeedback: Gaining Awareness and Control

Just as yoga, Pilates, or related disciplines position the body to affect your mental state, so does another experimental approach, called biofeedback training. Started in the late 1970s, the technique began with a question: Can humans exert control over involuntary body processes, including brain wave patterns?

Working first with epilepsy and attention-deficit disorder patients, investigators learned that individuals could in some cases be taught to control normally involuntary processes, such as heart rate, blood pressure, and muscle tension.

Now biofeedback is being applied to eating disorders. The basic idea is that if you are a woman with an eating disorder, you may have significant cognitive deficits, including problems with memory, thinking clearly, and other brain-related issues. These problems might be depicted by changes in one or more of four known types of brain waves.

According to clinical psychologist Peter Smith, who in conjunction with Mirasol in Tucson, Arizona, is studying biofeedback in women with eating disorders, these sorts of faulty patterns show up the most in women who are severely underweight. One application of biofeedback might be to identify those with the most "faulty" brain patterns, indicating the most resistance to treatment. "If you have compromised brain function," Smith says, "you could be sitting in rehab but not absorbing anything."

If you were to test as one of these highly resistant types, therapists would know not to launch into a demanding treatment because at this point you would simply not be able to process it mentally. Gradually, as you gained back weight and commensurate cognitive function, biofeedback therapists could teach you how to transform your brain waves into healthier patterns.

You would begin this therapy with an electroencephalogram (EEG), which is a recording of brain electrical activity measured by electrodes placed on the scalp. You would then be asked to wear an "electrode cap" and sit down in front of a computer screen, where you would play a game, much like Tetras on a Game Boy, except that the game screen would display your own brain waves as a series of bars. You would watch the bars, and try to alter your thoughts to create waves appropriate for the required task. When you succeeded, you would hear a sound change. In this way, you would learn to control something about yourself, something other than food.

STEP FIVE: MOVING DEEPER

Shifting Perspective

Now that we have explored therapies, which help by bringing in outside assistance, it is important to shift inward—where, ultimately, healing has to take place. "Deeper healing" means that something internal and fundamental has to change. Perhaps we can begin by changing how we think about eating disorders.

With the publication of DSM-IV, much of mental illness treatment has gravitated toward labeling clusters of behaviors as diseases—anorexia, bulimia, binge eating disorder, EDNOS, and so on—and viewing the behaviors themselves as symptoms. This is what psychologist Melanie Katzman referred to as the "medicalization" of eating disorders.

The first question in healing is, Do my behaviors, my vulnerability, qualify as an eating disorder? But the next one has to be, Does fitting the criteria really matter?

While naming the eating disorder is an important first step in healing, because it removes denial, staying with the names and etching them into our psyches brands us with eating problems and supports our being ill.

Look at the semantics: we say "symptoms" when we mean "behaviors." We say "disease" when we mean "psychological coping tool." As a society, we see eating disorders as self-inflicted "diseases" with hurtful "symptoms," such as those young girls develop when drowning in a world of fashion magazines and dieting tips.

Based on my symptoms, I have a disease dubbed "atypical" or "subclinical" anorexia nervosa. If I stay focused on that and if I react in the way that the language in the DSM-IV leads me to react, I begin to envision myself as sick. True or not, where does that get me? I walk away with my head down, hair spilling over to cover my face. I see myself as "anorexic." And in the worst case, the "disease" progresses until it becomes my identity. *I am an anorexic.*

How do we heal from this? I argue that we cannot. We can only stop the "symptoms."

But if we continue to see ourselves and others with eating disorders as anorexics, bulimics, and binge eaters, then we all see ourselves as "diseased."

I suggest that we shift perspective. For example, there is a component to anorexia that is actually positive. I am an overachiever, bursting with ambition. I accomplish. If I did not harbor this innate drive, how else could I have driven myself to 89 pounds?

Now, as I heal, after I have admitted that I have a problem and done a great deal of work to stop the symptoms, I want to change the name of my "disease." What if I could see myself as "powerful" and "gifted" instead of sick, and my "behaviors" as clever devices that protected me psychically when I was faced with intolerable circumstances?

By viewing anorexia as a perversion of a powerful personality, I can heal myself by channeling my gifts into something healthy. This affords me something positive to work with—instead of a personality flaw that I cannot ever change.

I think Jeanne Rust at Mirasol has got it right. She says, "We have been doing the same thing with CBT since the early 1980s and it is not working for everyone. We need to begin to look for other ways."

Her way is to start working on the positive instead of the negative. "Then recovery is going to be so much faster because women are going to fall in love with life again," she says.

Similarly, Rob Brezsny, in his book *Pronoia Is the Antidote for Paranoia*, has started the ball rolling. Instead of viewing the world through a prism of paranoia, seeing everyone as out to get him, Brezsny chooses pronoia instead, which argues that the world is dead set on bestowing him with blessings. Start there. Shift the perspective.

The psychological community can do the same. Brezsny actually pokes fun at DSM-IV and its propensity to pathologize human behavior. What isn't an illness these days? Listed in the DSM, for example, are caffeine-induced sleep disorder and nightmare disorder.

Brezsny is not arguing that the DSM-IV needs to be eliminated. Rather, it may have swung too far in the direction of sickness. Too much sickness precipitates too much passive "treatment." *You are sick and so I will give you this.* None of *this* belongs to the patient, who may feel helpless as therapists spoon-feed her therapy.

I assert that healing in the realm of eating disorders demands a change of attitude in the direction of personal power. Rather than seeing myself as sick, I can see myself as blessed. I have been endowed with a certain nature. It is good. The goal of healing is not to erase myself; rather, it is to find the strength, gather the remnants of self-esteem, and put them together in a picture of hope.

And how do I begin to find this hope? I offer you my own story of inside-out healing that is working for me today: writing this book.

As any author knows, to write is a daunting task. My editor tells me that she has witnessed many authors who shelve their dream projects, even after the contract has been signed.

I now understand why.

I began this book with an idea. An idea is not enough. I also had to write a proposal, find an agent, contract with a publisher, and create a manuscript. I had never done this before, and I really had no idea where to begin.

But there was the idea, gnawing at me. To sabotage it, I came up with a long list of reasons why I could not write this book: I am a single mother. How could I manage my daughter's life and my own enterprise? How could I pay my bills if I took time away from free-lancing? Worse, what memories would I dig up? What issues would emerge that I had long since put to bed?

And as the list got longer, one theme began to emerge as the real reason why I did not write: fear.

You see, I knew that I had an eating disorder as a teenager. Past tense. And I was afraid of what I would find—afraid that I could relapse. Did that proclivity ever go away? Because I knew that a part of the eating disorder never does.

I have to admit that the fear was nearly paralyzing. So I did what I always do when the emotions are overwhelming: I researched the topic. I went to libraries and read books. I talked to people about agents and proposals. I talked to eating disorders experts. I talked to many women. And the motivation came. In story after story, the women said the same thing to me: the eating issue lingers in some way and there is little to nothing out there for us older women to draw from for support.

With this, I realized that there was nothing left for me to do except write.

But I could not. I could not begin.

Except that I could. One January evening, I set the alarm for 5 A.M. When National Public Radio blasted out—and after I hit the snooze button many times—I got out of bed. I made tea. Indian tea. I had never done this before. This small action was something new. It was a beginning. I started with something I could do easily: brewing Indian tea, from scratch.

I remember the smells of cardamom, cloves, coriander, and ginger. I remember the bubbles of milk almost giggling in the pan. And with those spices, I imagined exotic places. I thought of India and China. I imagined some Sri Lankan woman, maybe one who was starving, plucking green tea leaves, steaming, drying, and rolling them. Before long, a circle of women were in my kitchen, as my tea was seeping, urging me on.

I looked outside. I saw a lone streetlight, and my neighbor's Christmas lights, still up in early January. They were blinking, winking at me. And the moon. Oh, the moon, almost full.

I was somewhere else. I was in a magical place.

I began to write. I wrote for three hours that day. And three more the next. And in two weeks more, I had a proposal. Later, I had a chapter. And much, much later, I had this book to offer as a contribution to that circle of women.

I am not saying it was consistently easy. There were mornings that the negative "voices" I so dreaded did come. They told me a now familiar story, that in order to succeed, I would have to starve; I would have to be thinner to be better.

And some days the voices would be so loud that I would have to take time out, sit with my cats, and recite the litany of what happens when I do not eat: I tax my relationships; people who love me wonder why I deprive myself, and why I come across as cranky and icy. I lose my periods and, therefore, increase my risk of spending later life in a wheelchair from osteoporosis. Worst of all to me, I model an eating disorder for my daughter, who, now at age 10, needs a role model more than ever.

And sometimes with the self-talk I won the arguments. Each day that I did was one more day of healing.

This, for me, is what it means to *want* to get better.

And you?

Creative Endeavor: Expressing the Self

As in my case, one very common theme of healing is self-expression. Among the nearly four dozen women I have interviewed for this book, those who have reached bottom and then somehow found their way back up have usually embraced some kind of creative endeavor. This is an internal rather than an external approach to healing.

It could be that as a woman begins to heal, she finds her voice again and is willing to let it be heard in a myriad of ways. But, equally possible, a woman might actually animate her own healing process by embarking upon some project or artistic exploration.

For example, Laura, who suffered from anorexia as a teenager and relapsed after her father's death, turned to painting. An artist and museum educator by profession, Laura harnessed these artistic skills to support her resilience and recovery. Her watercolors and prints became her voice. She used them to help others. In fact, the images she made during her recovery have been reproduced not only in artistic exhibits but also in journals of health and humanities. This story of recovery shows how healing is synchronous in nature; it not only helped Laura to recover her own sense of being on solid ground but also others whom she touched.

Jenny Lauren, the child model and ballerina who suffered from anorexia and bulimia, took up painting as well. Then, after a difficult time while in the hospital for depression, she began writing her memoir, *Homesick,* telling her story in all its horrific detail. The experience of writing about her disorder helped to curtail her symptoms.

"Just knowing I was going to share this story, knowing that I had something important to do and to explain it, gave me sort of a project," she says. "Any project helped me get out of the eating disorder. The writing became a new addiction, but at least, you know, a positive one."

Indeed, reaching out in any form can help heal as well as act as an outward sign of progress. Because eating disorders tend to be very egocentric disorders, it is probably forcing you to be preoccupied with your pain and your body. You may have totally lost sight of your creative potential. But it is there.

In fact, "an eating disorder, at its core, is a creative act," says Poppink.

That is because you probably came up with an eating disorder as a means to survive extraordinary psychological pain.

Healing, according to Poppink, "involves gently and slowly cutting down on the eating-disordered behaviors." But when those do come down, something else has to take their place.

Why not try something else, equally creative? By virtue of your previous behaviors, you already know you can.

You do not have to paint your pain or make picture frames to hold the "new image of you." Indeed, one woman told me how she abhorred making picture frames during the art therapy segment of her inpatient treatment. But you may benefit from some other means of communication.

As noted above, the Internet can be very useful as a tool of not only communication but also self-expression. Sarah Mason, who suffered from bulimia, put together her own website with poetry, inspirational passages, and stories of sickness and healing. She also formed a larger support group called Payson Road, which helps those in recovery. Mary Pat, who suffered from EDNOS, wrote a book, *Reflecting Grace,* about spirituality and healing. Grace Over-bake, who suffered from anorexia, produced and directed a play about eating disorders called *Schoolgirl Figure.*

Other ways of communicating include talks and speaking engagements. Carrie, who became Mrs. Ohio in 2004, used her crown as a platform to increase attention to eating disorders. She told her story to university co-eds who were also struggling with disorders. She spoke at luncheons with donors who might fund research and public awareness endeavors.

Similarly, Gail, who suffered from bulimia, launched the F.R.E.E.D Foundation. She and her husband have raised more than $200,000 to help women who cannot pay for treatment, to change insurance regulations, and to promote eating disorders awareness programs. These are just examples. Your expression can be modest at first—making a daily journal entry, for instance.

Find something that you can do, that you like to do, something apart from food. If you find yourself even brainstorming the possibilities, realize that you are on your way. Self-expression is both a tool and a sign of healing.

Spirituality: Another Path

For many women with eating problems, healing has a spiritual component. This may fall under the rubric of a formal religion. For example, Cindy, who suffered from EDNOS, found great comfort in the Christian framework of Remuda Ranch. She had all but given up her religious roots when her eating disorder emerged during her early twenties.

She found great comfort in "giving her problem over" to a higher power. Her faith has kept her together decades after her own recovery, even when her daughter was diagnosed with anorexia nervosa. She recalls the time when her daughter "crashed and burned," ending up in the hospital and suffering from complications of her illness.

"My heart was pounding in my chest for days," Cindy recalls.

"But I could sit down, feel it pounding, mentally picture her in a bad place, start to cry, and think, 'But I am not in charge here. God loves her more than I do.'"

True, trust in God did not take Cindy's anxiety away. "But it meant that I could rest," she says, "knowing that I did not have to do anything at that moment other than trust God."

Others have found that the religion of their childhood was part of their problem. Tracy all but gave up her strict Protestant upbringing. But then, after suffering from alcoholism and bulimia, and going through AA, she felt a spiritual void. She began to accept the "higher power" idea that AA preaches. Long after her symptoms of bulimia subsided, she joined a Unity Church that she read about on the Internet. Today, she is seeing a counselor there. He offers psychotherapy, but it has a more spiritually focused perspective, which bodes well for Tracy, who is not comfortable with CBT or other formal therapies.

Spirituality does not have to mean "God." It can be any approach involving a search for something larger in one's life, a search for meaning. In order to begin this search, you need a *contextual* understanding of your behaviors. This book has provided a general one, based on the issues at each phase of life. But you are going to have your own context, be it your relationships, racial or ethnic heritage, class struggles, economic definition—all such elements.

Putting it all in context can help you reveal the meaning attributed to the eating disorder: *It is my friend. It is my fallback. It is my weapon.*

Starting with the right vocabulary, which you can learn by working with a therapist or a book like this one, you can find the words for telling your story. You can then construct your own narrative as it captures your struggles and focuses on your healing. This is what it means to recover your voice. And once you have it back, you will start to realize the larger meaning in your life.

To illustrate this concept of spirituality, Tracy tells the story of her first experience with recovery. In one of the worst phases of her bulimia, she was in Hawaii, staying with her sister. Living 35 miles from Honolulu, she had to take a bus to reach her job, and so she had to be at the stop by 4:30 each morning. One morning, Tracy found herself eating butterscotch Tasty Cake and drinking a Diet Coke. She looked up at the sky and felt it.

"All of a sudden I got it," she said. "I felt universal love. I realized love is everything and it is in me and around me."

And with that, Tracy changed her behaviors. Not dramatically at first—but from that point on, she never returned to the intense pain and worry that had been permeating her whole life.

Recovery often hinges on those "aha" moments that come with the realization that you are not alone with your pain. The recovery stories that I hear are less about therapy sessions and meal plans— although these factor in—and more about a moment, that moment when suddenly, inexplicably, something has changed. Some call it a miracle. Others say it is like feeling a deep sense of self. It is this spiritual aspect of healing, while hard to define or prescribe, that seems to be experienced by every woman who has made her way into recovery.

Feminist Healing: Countering Cultural Forces That Create Eating Disorders

Looking at the basis of an eating disorder from the feminist viewpoint, culture and society have long projected their sick politics and sick conflicts onto women's bodies. They are templates, dry-erase boards that get marked up by a sick culture. "Sick" in this context means practices and attitudes that are riddled with gender inequity, homophobia, oppression against women, abuse, invalidation, and dislocation.

Psychologist Melanie Katzman noted that patients being treated for eating disorders reported that "being understood" was one of the most important linchpins for recovery to occur. In others words, women begin to heal when they begin to be heard.

In the parlance of pop culture, eating disorders occur when a woman "loses her voice," "is silenced," or "is not seen." Disorders, then, arise from feelings of powerlessness. They can happen for many reasons. And they need to be addressed.

For example, Paola in Brazil took up vomiting to cope with the pressures of straddling two disparate worlds: the old Brazilian culture, as embodied by her mother, and the new São Paulo culture, where women could be attorneys. Paola understood the impossibility of satisfying the conflicting or competing expectations of both worlds. She coped by bingeing and purging: a symbolic gesture for ingesting the new culture, feeling guilty, and purging it back out in appeasement to the old culture.

This is one example of the larger social and cultural forces that shape eating disorders. There are more. The saints of old tell stories of self-deprivation, couched as asceticism to mortify their bodies. Today, self-denigration, starvation, and self-abuse go hand in hand once a girl becomes aware that her opportunities for outside recognition and advancement are slim. She buys into the directive to be submissive, but only superficially. Inside, through her eating rituals, she is cultivating her personal power.

This means that eating disorders go far beyond fat phobia, and therefore, healing has to go beyond that as well. When you are working with a therapist, you may wish to explore ways to help redress the larger cultural and social causes of these problems. At first, this might take the form of group therapy. The idea is that if you are in an oppressive situation, you may have grown so used to it that you will have a hard time even imagining living in an open atmosphere. If you are moving to a new home, taking on a new role such as "mother," or transitioning in any significant way, you are likely experiencing feelings of disconnection and isolation. As a counter, you might need to surround yourself with others who are in a similar set of circumstances, a new culture.

Finding or founding a group, either inside or outside of therapy, creates a safe space to explore how to live in a new shape, with a new identity, and new rules for living.

Advocacy: Tackling the Bigger Picture

Another solution, particularly for women in more advanced stages of healing, is advocacy. It is the projecting of personal power outward rather than inward. There are many issues to choose from. Engaging in these causes, and helping others, can inspire healing.

Holding Insurance Providers Accountable

Many women with eating problems who are trying to get outside help often encounter a major hurdle: cost. Just when you finally get up enough courage to attempt recovery, you may find that it is prohibitively expensive. While this is a tragic consequence of the U.S. health system, organizations such as NEDA are working hard for change.

Insurers, in general, tend to be unsupportive of eating disorders. Right now, thirty-five states have laws enacting mental health parity. This means that insurance companies must cover treatment for mental illness as readily as physical illness. The catch, however, is that only twelve states—California, Connecticut, Delaware, Maine, Maryland, Minnesota, New York, North Dakota, Rhode Island, Vermont, Washington, and West Virginia—include eating disorders in their list of mental illnesses. Also, the treatment covered often falls short of what is needed. For example, if you have anorexia nervosa, binge-purge subtype, and residential treatment is recommended for sixty days, your insurance benefits may cover only ten days.

Lynn Grefe at NEDA tells stories of women having to charge treatment costs to their credit cards, maxing out on their credit, depleting their savings, and taking second mortgages. Some women who are denied treatment and become even sicker may find that they do get coverage, but only because they have developed a heart murmur or other physical complication.

While it may be extraordinarily difficult to get insurance reimbursement for necessary treatment, "fight with your insurance carrier," Grefe says. "Be willing to document everything and keep records."

NEDA's website gives a list of steps to take in this battle. They include (1) having the evaluating physician or specialist write a letter documenting the level of care needed; (2) appealing to the medical director of the insurance company if you are denied; (3) taking up the issues with your employer, who might be able to negotiate with the insurer; and, as always, (4) appeal the denied coverage, hiring a lawyer to help if necessary.

Gail and her husband, Rob, found themselves in this situation when Gail needed inpatient treatment for long-term bulimia. The treatment center wanted payment up front. Gail suddenly needed to come up with $40,000. She and her husband took out a second mortgage.

"If it had cost a million bucks, I would have raised it somehow," Rob says.

Later, he had to fight the matter with their insurer, who gave him a hard time. After six months of aggressive effort, he was able to get back a large portion of that money. But not without extensive phone calls, letter writing, and information gathering.

It may be impossible for you to fight an insurer when you are also fighting an illness. Still, keep the records and at least begin the process. You may be able to revisit it later. For a more comprehensive list of steps to take, go to NEDA's website, www.nationaleating-disorders.org, and look under "Survival Kit." In addition, the Family and Friends Action Council shares stories of families' struggles to get help and coverage.

Upping the Ante for Research and Public Awareness

As with insurance, funding is also scarce for eating disorders awareness and research, particularly for women who are older. The National Institute of Mental Health in 2005 appropriated only $21 million to study eating disorders, even though they affect 15 to 20 million people, including those with binge eating disorder and

EDNOS. Meanwhile, officials earmarked $650 million for research into Alzheimer's, which afflicts only 4.5 million.

"I'm not saying that we shouldn't fund Alzheimer's," Grefe at NEDA notes. "But when you look at how many it is affecting, there is an enormous disparity." And because eating disorders, when left untreated, cost so much more in dollars as well as emotional pain, it would be better to get many more people into treatment that much earlier.

While NEDA is working for change state by state, the Eating Disorders Coalition for Research, Policy and Action (EDC), the lobbying arm of NEDA, is working at the federal level. Headquartered on Pennsylvania Avenue in Washington, D.C., this group of nonprofit organizations, treatment centers, and other businesses wants legislators and policy makers to recognize eating disorders as a public health priority. By educating members of Congress, surveying past federal agency efforts, raising the visibility of eating disorders, and general advocacy, the group hopes to increase federal support and resources for eating disorders.

You might want to join EDC's Family and Friends Action Council, which has lobby days, in which you can be part of a group contacting federal officials about the need for funding research and treatment. Your own story will add to those of others, documenting personally how tragic eating disorders can be. Some members have actually testified before Congress to help push for change.

If this is too intimidating, you might want to work more at your local level; there are many grassroots efforts that you can join. For example, Lifelines Foundation promotes education, awareness, and prevention of eating disorders throughout Texas.

If your religious activities provide a path of comfort to you, you may want to address eating disorders within your faith community. For example, one woman told her story in a newsletter put out by the National Association for Women in Catholic Higher Education.

Another avenue is through organizations associated with your ethnicity. Eating disorders are now showing up in minority groups such as African Americans and Native Americans, where such disorders have been historically underreported. Since many minority groups in the United States and many women in developing countries are also in lower socioeconomic classes, these groups are markedly underserved by research, prevention, and treatment strategies.

Mothers with histories of eating disorders, or those who are worried about their daughters, might get involved in school-based programs such as Full of Ourselves. Developed by a Harvard researcher and an acclaimed curriculum designer, this program addresses critical issues of body preoccupation and reduces the risk for disordered eating in girls in grades 3 to 8.

In short, find your niche and step up.

One other alternative, if you want to take up other issues not directly related to the eating disorders themselves: there are many groups that work for economic parity, maternity leave, protection from violence and abuse, and appreciation of parenting, as opposed to money making. These are a few of the many opportunities for involvement as you recover. The key is to project your voice to the larger world rather than inward toward your body, where the energy can do such massive damage. Healing is about reclaiming your personal power.

STEP SIX: SHEDDING DEAD LEAVES

I am certain you can heal. That is because I am certain that you have your own dream, lying on the back shelf of your mind. I ask you one question: When are you going to let yourself start toward that dream? Of course, I know the answer: When you are ready.

I also know that no one can make you ready, not your therapist, your partner, your friends, or your children. Therapy is a tool, an outside-in approach, nothing more. Healing, on the other hand, is inside out, a mystery that needs patience, persistence, and nurturing to unfold.

In thinking about this, it is useful to imagine ourselves as different as species of trees. Some of us are like gingkoes, which shed their leaves at the first sign of cold. Others are more like pin oaks, which wait as long as possible, clinging to their brittle foliage. But one fine day, maybe the shortest day of the year, even the most stubborn tree will be ready to let go.

Maybe today's healing is reading this chapter. Later, another leaf will fall. If we lose enough leaves, we may feel barren for a while. But if we stay rooted in our selves, even as we lose the bad habits that we think we are saving us, then spring, and the new leaf buds that it brings, will arrive.

Helpful Organizations

Academy for Eating Disorders
   (AED)
www.aedweb.org
(874) 498-4274
60 Revere Drive, Suite
   500
Northbrook, IL 60062

Council on Size and Weight
   Discrimination, Inc.
www.cswd.org
(845) 679-1209
PO Box 305
Mount Marion, NY 12456

Eating Disorders Anonymous
   (EDA)
www.eatingdisordersanonymous.
   org
Check website for local address
   and phone number

Eating Disorders Coalition for
   Research, Policy, and Action
www.eatingdisorderscoalition.org
(202) 543-9570
611 Pennsylvania Avenue SE,
   Suite 423
Washington, D.C. 20003-4303

Eating Disorders Information
   Network
www.edin-ga.org
(404) 816-3346
2964 Peachtree Road NW,
   Suite 324
Atlanta, GA 30305

Eating Disorder Referral and
   Information Center
www.edreferral.com
(858) 792-7463
2923 Sandy Pointe, Suite 6
Del Mar, CA 92014

International Association
   of Eating Disorders
   Professionals
www.iaedp.com
(800) 800-8126
PO Box 1295
Pekin, IL 61555-1295

Massachusetts Eating Disorders
   Association (MEDA)
www.medainc.org
(617) 558-1881; (866) 343-MEDA
92 Pearl Street
Newton, MA 02458

National Association of Anorexia
   Nervosa and Associated
   Disorders (ANAD)
www.anad.org
(847) 831-3438
PO Box 7
Highland Park, IL 60035

National Eating Disorders
   Association (NEDA)
www.nationaleatingdisorders.org
(800) 931-2237
603 Stewart Street, Suite 803
Seattle, WA 98101

National Eating Disorders
   Screening Program (NEDSP)
www.mentalhealthscreening.org/
   college/eating.aspx
(781) 239-0071
1 Washington Street,
   Suite 304
Wellesley Hills, MA 02481

Overeaters Anonymous
   Headquarters (OA)
www.oa.org
(505) 891-2664
Check website for local address
   and phone number

The Elisa Project
www.theelisaproject.org
(214) 369-5222
8100 Lomo Alto,
   Suite 262
Dallas, TX 75225

We Insist on Natural Shapes
   (WINS)
www.winsnews.org
(800) 600-9467
PO Box 19938
Sacramento, CA 95819

Directory of Treatment Facilities

Alexian Brothers Behavioral
   Health Hospital
www.alexian.org
(847) 882-1600
1650 Moon Lake Boulevard
Hoffman Estates, IL 60194

The Bella Vita
www.thebellavita.com
(626) 304-0800
200 South Los Robles Avenue,
   Suite 540
Pasadena, CA 91101

at Los Angeles:
766 Colorado Boulevard
Los Angeles, CA 90041
(323) 255-0400

at BHC Alhambra:
4619 North Rosemead Boulevard
Rosemead, CA 91770
(626) 286-1191

Belmont Behavioral Health
www.estein.edu/facilities/
   belmont/index.html
(215) 877-2000
4200 Monument Road
Philadelphia, PA 19131

Cambridge Eating Disorder
   Center (CEDC)
info@CEDCmail.com
(617) 547-2255
www.eatingdisordercenter.org
3 Bow Street
Cambridge, MA 02138

Canopy Cove
info@canopycove.com
(800) 236-7524
2300 Killearn Center
    Boulevard
Tallahassee, FL 32309

Casa Palmera
info@casapalmera.com
(888) 481-4481
14750 El Camino Real
Del Mar, CA 92014

Castlewood
info@castlewoodtc.com
(888) 822-8938
800 Holland Road
St. Louis, MO 63021

Center for Change
info@centerforchange.com
(801) 224-8255
1790 North State Street
Orem, UT 84057

Center for Discovery
eatingdisorders@
    centerfordiscovery.com
(562) 882-1265
9844 Pangborn Avenue
Downey, CA 90240

Center for Eating Disorders at
    Sheppard Pratt
info@sheppardpratt.org
(410) 938-5252
6501 North Charles Street
Baltimore, MD 21285

Center for Hope of the Sierras
info@centerforhopeofthesierras.
    com
(877) 828-4949
1453 Pass Drive
Reno, NV 89511

Children's Hospital of Denver
webmaster@tchden.org
(800) 624-6553
1056 East 19th Avenue
Denver, CO 80218

Denver Health
(877) 228-8348
777 Bannock Street
Denver, CO 80204-4507

Eating Disorders Center of
    Denver
info@edcdenver.com
(866) 771-0861
950 South Cherry Street,
    Suite 1010
Denver, CO 80246

Eating Disorders Institute
(701) 234-2000
PO Box M.C.
Fargo, ND 58122

Fairwinds Treatment
    Center
fairwinds@fairwindstreatment.
    com
(800) 226-0301
1569 South Fort Harrison
Clearwater, FL 33756

Harmony Grove
Lauriedaily@yahoo.com
(800) 990-8052
3656 Torrey View Court
San Diego, CA 92130

Laureate Psychiatric
    Clinic
webadministrator@saintfrancis.
    com
(918) 491-5600
6655 South Yale Avenue
Tulsa, OK 74136

Laurel Hill Inn
lhi@laurelhillinn.com
(781) 396-1116
PO Box 368
Medford, MA 02155-0004

Loma Linda University
    Behavioral Medicine Center
cmcgrath@ahs.llumc.edu
(909) 558-9200
1710 Barton Road
Redlands, CA 92373

Lotus House
info@lotusgroup.biz
(317) 774-8080
11950 Fishers Crossing Drive
Fishers, IN 46038

McCallum Place
info@mccallumplace.com
(800) 828-8158
100 South Brentwood, Suite 350
Clayton, MO 63105

McLean Hospital/Harvard
    Medical School
info@mclean.harvard.edu
(800) 333-0338
115 Mill Street
Belmont, MA 02478

Menninger
www.menningerclinic.com
(800) 351-9058
2801 Gessner Drive
PO Box 809045
Houston, TX 77280-9045

Mirasol
jrust@mirasol.net
(888) 520-1700
7650 East Broadway,
    Suite 303
Tucson, AZ 85710-3773

Monte Nido
mntc@montenido.com
(310) 457-9958
27162 Sea Vista Drive
Malibu, CA, 90265

Montecatini
monte@tns.net
(760) 436-8930
2524 La Costa Avenue
La Costa, CA 92009

Oceanaire
info@oceanaireinc.com
(310) 377-3200
30175 Avenida Tranquila
Rancho Palos Verdes, CA
    90275

Penn State
www.hmc.psu.edu/
    eatingdisorders/
(717) 531-2099
905 West Governor Road,
    Suite 250
Hershey, PA 17033

Presbyterian Hospital of Dallas
www.texashealth.org/hospitals
(214) 345-6789
8200 Walnut Hill Lane
Dallas, TX 75231-4402

Puente de Vida
info@puentedevida.com
(877) 995-4337
PO Box 86020
San Diego, CA 92138

Rader Programs
rader@raderprograms.com
(800) 841-1515
2130 North Ventura Road
Oxnard, CA 93036

Rebecca's House
www.rebeccashouse.org
(800) 711-2062
23861 El Toro Road, Suite 700
Lake Forest, CA 92630

Remuda Ranch
info@remudaranch.com
(800) 445-1900
1 East Apache Street
Wickenburg, AZ 85390

Renfrew Center
foundation@renfrew.org
(877) 367-3383
475 Spring Lane
Philadelphia, PA 19128

Ridgeview Institute
www.ridgeviewinstitute.com
(800) 329-9775
3995 South Cobb Drive
Smyrna, GA 30080

River Centre Clinic
info@river-centre.org
(419) 885-8800
5465 Main Street
Sylvania, OH 43560

River Oaks Hospital
Kim.Epperson@uhsinc.com
(800) 366-1740
1525 River Oaks Road West
New Orleans, LA 70123

Rogers Memorial Hospital
www.rogershospital.org
(800) 767-4411
11101 West Lincoln Avenue
Milwaukee, WI 53227

Rosewood Ranch
info@rosewoodranch.com
(800) 845-2211
36075 South Rincon Road
Wickenburg, AZ 85390

Santé Center for Healing
www.santecenter.com
(800) 258-4250
PO Box 448
Argyle, TX 76226

Shades of Hope
info@shadesofhope.com
(800) 588-4673
PO Box 639
Buffalo Gap, TX 79508

Sierra Tucson
Outreach@SierraTucson.com
(800) 842-4487
39580 South Lago del Oro
    Parkway
Tucson, AZ 85739

The Ranch
info@recoveryranch.com
(800) 849-5969
PO Box 38
Nunnelly, TN 37137

University Medical Center
    at Princeton
www.princetonhcs.org/
    page2646.aspx
(609) 497-4490
253 Witherspoon Street
Princeton, NJ 08540

Walden Behavioral Care
info@waldenbehavioralcare.com;
www.waldenbehavioralcare.com
(781) 647-6700
9 Hope Avenue,
Suite 500
Waltham, MA 02453-2711

Western Psychiatric Institute
    and Clinic
http://wpic.upmc.com/
(412) 624-2100
3811 O'Hara Street
Pittsburgh, PA 15213-2593

Westwind
westwindedrc@mts.net
(888) 353-3372
458 14th Street
Brandon, MB R7A 4T3
Canada

Women's Center
info@pinegrove-treatment.com
(888) 574-4673
2255 Broadway Drive
PO Box 16389
Hattiesburg, MS 39404

The Clinical Definitions of Eating Disorders

ANOREXIA NERVOSA

A. Refusal to maintain body weight at or above a minimally normal weight for age and height (e.g., weight loss leading to maintenance of body weight less than 85 percent of that expected; or failure to make expected weight gain during period of growth, leading to body weight less than 85 percent expected).

B. Intense fear of gaining weight or becoming fat, even though underweight.

C. Disturbance in the way in which one's body weight or shape is experienced, undue influence of body weight or shape on self-evaluation, or denial of the seriousness of the current low body weight.

D. In postmenarcheal females, amenorrhea, i.e., the absence of at least three consecutive menstrual cycles. (A woman is considered to have amenorrhea if her periods occur only following hormone administration, e.g., estrogen, administration.)

SPECIFY TYPE:

Restricting type: During the current episode of anorexia nervosa, the person has not regularly engaged in binge eating or purging behavior (i.e., self-induced vomiting or the misuse of laxatives, diuretics, or enemas).

Binge eating/purging type: During the current episode of anorexia nervosa, the person has regularly engaged in binge eating or purging behavior (i.e., self-induced vomiting or the misuse of laxatives, diuretics, or enemas).

BULIMIA NERVOSA

A. Recurrent episodes of binge eating. An episode of binge eating is characterized by both of the following:

1. Eating, in a discrete period of time (e.g., within any two-hour period), an amount of food that is definitely larger than most people would eat during a similar period of time and under similar circumstances.

2. A sense of lack of control over eating during the episode (e.g., a feeling that one cannot stop eating or control what or how much one is eating).

B. Recurrent inappropriate compensatory behavior in order to prevent weight gain, such as self-induced vomiting; misuse of laxatives, diuretics, enemas, or other medications; fasting; or excessive exercise.

C. The binge eating and inappropriate compensatory behaviors both occur, on average, at least twice a week for three months.

D. Self-evaluation is unduly influenced by body shape and weight.

E. The disturbance does not occur exclusively during episodes of anorexia nervosa.

SPECIFY TYPE:

Purging type: During the current episode of bulimia nervosa, the person has regularly engaged in self-induced vomiting or the misuse of laxatives, diuretics, or enemas.

Nonpurging type: During the current episode of bulimia nervosa, the person has used other inappropriate compensatory behaviors, such as fasting or excessive exercise, but has not regularly engaged in self-induced vomiting or the misuse of laxatives, diuretics, or enemas.

BINGE EATING DISORDER

A. Recurrent episodes of binge eating. An episode of binge eating is characterized by both of the following:

   1. Eating, in a discrete period of time (e.g., within any two-hour period), an amount of food that is definitely larger than most people would eat during a similar period of time and under similar circumstances.

   2. A sense of lack of control over eating during the episode (e.g., a feeling that one cannot stop eating or control what or how much one is eating).

B. The binge eating episodes are associated with three (or more) of the following:

   ➤ Eating much more rapidly than normal

   ➤ Eating until feeling uncomfortably full

   ➤ Eating large amounts of food when not feeling physically hungry

   ➤ Eating alone because of being embarrassed by how much one is eating

   ➤ Feeling disgusted with oneself, depressed, or very guilty after overeating

C. Marked distress regarding binge eating is present.

D. The binge eating occurs, on average, at least two days a week for six months.

NOTE: The method of determining frequency differs from that used for bulimia nervosa. Future research should also address whether the preferred method of setting a frequency threshold is counting the number of days on which binges occur or counting the number of episodes of binge eating.

E. The binge eating is not associated with the regular use of inappropriate compensatory behaviors (e.g., purging, fasting, excessive exercise) and does not occur exclusively during the course of anorexia nervosa or bulimia nervosa.

Source: American Psychiatric Association, *Diagnostic and Statistical Manual of Mental Disorders*, 4th ed. (Washington, D.C.: APA, 1994).

Introduction | CONFIDENCES AND LIES

Page

xv 8 million women with eating disorders: Anorexia Nervosa and Related Eating Disorders (ANRED), Academy of Eating Disorders (AED), and American Academy of Child and Adolescent Psychiatry (AACAP). See the ANRED website, specifically http://www.anred.com/stats.html, and the AED website, specifically http://www.aedweb.org/eating_disorders/prevalence.cfm.

xvi 10 million with anorexia or bulimia: Lynn Grefe, National Eating Disorders Association, interview with the author, July 15, 2004. See the ANRED website, specifically http://www.anred.com/stats.html, and the American Academy of Child and Adolescent Psychiatry website, specifically http://www.aacap.org/publications/factsfam/eating.htm.

xx will eventually die: Anorexia Nervosa and Related Eating Disorders (ANRED). See ANRED website as cited above.

xxi African American, Native American, Latino: Denise Brodey, "Blacks Join the Eating-Disorder Mainstream," *New York Times*, September 20, 2005; for a review of literature, see M. Crago, C. M. Shisslak, and L. S. Estes, "Eating Disturbances Among American Minority Groups: A Review," *International Journal of Eating Disorders* 19: 239–248, 1996.

xxi economic success and celebrity: A. E. Becker, "Television, Disordered Eating, and Young Women in Fiji: Negotiating Body Image and Identity During Rapid Social Change," *Culture, Medicine and Psychiatry* 4: 533–559, 2004.

1 | CHRONICITY

Page:

2 reports track the outcomes: P. F. Sullivan, "Course and Outcome of Anorexia and Bulimia Nervosa," in C. Fairburn and K. Brownell, eds., *Eating Disorders and Obesity: A Comprehensive Handbook*, 2d ed. (New York: Guilford, 2002), pp. 226–232; D. B. Herzog et al., "Recovery and Relapse in Anorexia and Bulimia Nervosa: A 7.5-Year Follow-up Study," *Journal of the American Academy of Child and Adolescent Psychiatry* 38: 829–837, 1999; P. Keel et al., "Long-Term Outcome of Bulimia Nervosa," *Archives of General Psychiatry* 56: 63–69, 1999; E. D. Eckert et al., "Ten-Year Follow-up of Anorexia Nervosa: Clinical Course and Outcome," *Psychological Medicine* 25: 143–156, 1995; H. C. Steinhausen, C. Rauss-Mason, and R. Seidel, "Follow-up Studies of Anorexia Nervosa: A Review of Four Decades of Outcome Research," *Psychological Medicine* 21: 447–454; M. Strober, R. Freeman, and W. Morrell, "The Long-Term Course of Severe Anorexia Nervosa in Adolescents: Survival Analysis of Recovery, Relapse, and Outcome Predictors over 10–15 years in a Prospective Study," *International Journal of Eating Disorders* 22: 339–360, 1992; S. Collings and M. King, "Ten-Year Follow-up of 50 Patients with Bulimia Nervosa," *British Journal of Psychiatry* 164: 80–87, 1994; M. M. Fichter and N. Quadflieg, "Six-Year Course of Bulimia Nervosa," *International Journal of Eating Disorders* 22: 361–384, 1997; S. Zipfel et al., "Long-Term Prognosis in Anorexia Nervosa: Lessons from a 21-Year Follow-up Study," *Lancet* 355: 721–722, 2000; D. Reas et al., "Prognostic Value of Duration of Illness and Early Intervention in Bulimia Nervosa: A Systemic Review of the Outcome Literature," *International Journal of Eating Disorders* 30: 1–10, 2001.

2 according to criteria: *American Psychiatric Association, Diagnostic and Statistical Manual of Mental Disord*ers: *DSM-IV* (Washington, D.C.: American Psychiatric Association, 1994).

5 body dysmorphic disorder: Margo Maine and Joe Kelly, *The Body Myth: Adult Women and the Pressure to Be Perfect* (Hoboken, NJ: John Wiley & Sons, Inc., 2005), 79–109.

5 *most* eating disorders: Binge eating disorder (BED) traditionally has been classified as EDNOS. Some researchers still do not count it as its own disorder. C. G. Fairburn et al, "The Natural Course of Bulimia Nervosa and Binge Eating Disorder in Young Women," *Archives of General Psychiatry* 57: 659–665, 2000.

6 a diagnostic manual: PDM Task Force, *Psychodynamic Diagnostic Manual* (Silver Spring, MD: Alliance of Psychoanalytic Organizations, 2006).

6 one of fourteen personality types: B. Carey, "For Therapy, a New Guide with a Touch of Personality," *New York Times,* January 24, 2006.

6 at least three personality types: D. L. Franko, "Diagnosis and Classification of Eating Disorders," in J. Kevin Thompson, ed., *Handbook of Eating Disorders and Obesity* (Hoboken, NJ: John Wiley & Sons, Inc., 2005), 65–66.

6 acts compulsively and has poor coping strategies: Women with this personality type tend to fare the worst at recovering.

9 Jamie-Lynn describes: Mike Falcon, "Jamie-Lynn 'Gets Wise' to Eating Disorder," *USA Today,* November 25, 2002.

10 based on unconditional love: http://www.amazon.com/exec/obidos/tg/detail/-/0375750185. This is a claim made in Peggy Claude-Pierre's book *The Secret Language of Eating Disorders* (New York: Vintage, 1997), page 131 in particular.

10 raise money for treatment: "Curing Eating Disorders," *New York Times,* December 6, 1992, p. V15.

10 Semantics also cause trouble: F. Feretti, "Eating Disorders: New Treatments," *New York Times,* September 2, 1985, p. 22.

13 Herzog's team found: D. B. Herzog et al., "Recovery and Relapse in Anorexia and Bulimia Nervosa: A 7.5-Year Follow-up Study," *Journal of the American Academy of Child and Adolescent Psychiatry* 38: 829–837, 1999.

14 Recovery did not always stick: A separate study of 173 patients with bulimia reported more than half had relapsed within three years of treatment. A relapse was defined as bingeing and purging for at least four weeks after having stopped for at least four weeks. P. Keel et al., "Long-Term Outcome of Bulimia Nervosa," *Archives of General Psychiatry* 56: 63–69, 1999.

15 she may be lying: Patients with eating disorders are notorious for secrecy. "They lie to doctors all the time," says psychologist Tacie Vergara, who treats older woman at Renfrew Center, an eating disorders treatment facility, headquartered in Philadelphia, Pennsylvania. In fact, in a description of one style of treatment, researchers went so far as to include a special section entitled "Deception in Treatment." K. Pike et al., "Cognitive-Behavioral Therapy in the Treatments of Anorexia Nervosa, Bulimia Nervosa, and Binge Eating Disorder," in J. Kevin Thompson, ed., *Handbook of Eating Disorders and Obesity* (Hoboken, NJ: John Wiley & Sons, Inc., 2004), 151–152.

15 not a particularly fabulous definition: Keel went so far as to check the accuracy of self-reporting by phone. When she was collecting data from a cluster of women with bulimia, women who had entered an eating disorders clinic at the University of Minnesota, she found a discrep-

ancy. Almost a third of the women admitted in face-to-face interviews that they were still engaging in bulimic behaviors. But on questionnaires, that fraction was larger; more women *wrote* that they were not symptom-free than *said* so in a personal interview. "That directly speaks to the issue of these women not being comfortable acknowledging the extent of their illness," Keel says. And that clearly is a problem when coming up with estimates such as the rule of third.

16 recovery rates for adults: http://www.remudaranch.com/eating_disorders/education.asp; http://www.renfrew.org/treatment-outcomes.asp. Jeanne Rust, director and founder of Mirasol in Tucson, Arizona. Interview with the author, March 17, 2005.

17 relapse rates vary: M. P. Olmsted, A. S. Kaplan, and W. Rockert, "Rate and Prediction of Relapse in Bulimia Nervosa," *American Journal of Psychiatry* 151: 738–743, 1994; J. Carter et al., "Relapse in Anorexia Nervosa: A Survival Analysis," *Psychological Medicine* 34: 671–679, 2004.

19 What does the term "recovered" really mean?:   A. Field et al., "Distinguishing Recovery from Remission in a Cohort of Bulimic Women: How Should Asymptomatic Periods Be Described?" *Journal of Clinical Epidemiology* 50: 1339–1345, 1997.

21 telltale behaviors do stop: E. D. Eckert et al., "Ten-Year Follow-up of Anorexia Nervosa: Clinical Course and Outcome," *Psychological Medicine* 25: 143–156, 1995.

2 | ADOLESCENCE

Page

25 power in a time of seeming powerlessness: Melanie A. Katzman and Sing Lee, "Beyond Body Image: The Integration of Feminist and Transcultural Theories in the Understanding of Self Starvation," *International Journal of Eating Disorders* 22: 385–394, 1997.

26 flow chart: C. Fairburn, *Overcoming Binge Eating* (New York: Guilford Press, 1995), 58.

27 Minnesota Semistarvation Experiment: A. Keys et al., *The Biology of Human Starvation* (Minneapolis: University of Minnesota Press, 1950).

28 theories of what should happen during adolescence: One of the pioneers in describing psychological development is Eric Erikson. While his theories, particularly for women, have since fallen upon controversy, his main contribution still is that development happens through a sequence of steps. Erikson further stressed the importance of the independent and autonomous self as the pinnacle of development. While this chapter references those ideas, it is not espousing all of Erikson's

thinking. Indeed, in his classic, *Identity and the Life Cycle,* Erikson supposed that until a girl finds a partner, her sense of identity remains
incomplete. But psychologists such as Carol Gilligan in her feminist
classic, *In a Different Voice,* and Jean Baker Miller, who trailblazed
women's psychology, asserted that women do not develop in isolation.
Rather, they develop in connection to others, and the connections are at
least as important as what and whom they connect. (See C. Robb's *The
Relational Revolution in Psychology,* Farrar, Straus & Giroux, 2006).

NOTE: It is not the goal of this book to determine who is more correct,
Erikson or Gilligan. In fact, both psychologists have their critics. (R.
Barnett and C. Rivers, *Same Difference: How Gender Myths Are Hurting Our Relationships, Our Children, and Our Jobs* [New York: Basic
Books, 2004]; A. M. Paul "This Changes Everything," *New York Times
Book Review,* March 12, 2006.) In this chapter, the development of girls
is presented from a more individualist perspective, with the idea that
an eating disorder blunts the qualities that Erikson celebrates: autonomy and independence. The more relational development that Gilligan
salutes is addressed in this chapter when describing the "social self" and
"cultural self," and also in the next three chapters, which deal with partnership, pregnancy, and parenting, involving some of the most intimate
interrelationships of a woman's life.

29 *Homesick*, a graphic self-portrait: Jenny Lauren, *Homesick: A Memoir
of Family, Food and Finding Hope* (New York: Atria Books, 2004), 8–31.
31 overall development of a child: E. H. Erikson, *Identity and the Life
Cycle* (New York, London: W. W. Norton and Company, 1980), 49–107.
35 as a group of interacting mini-selves: Mary Pipher, *Reviving Ophelia:
Saving the Selves of Adolescent Girls* (New York: Ballantine Books, 1994),
45–73.
37 and take up the burden of self-criticism: Ibid., 57.
37 $9.4 billion plastic surgery business: The American Society of Aesthetic
Plastic Surgeons, "Cosmetic Plastic Surgery Research: Statistics and
Trends for 2001, 2002, 2003." http://www.cosmeticsurgerystatistics.com/
statistics.html.
37 a mere thirteen minutes: S. L. Turner, H. Hamilton, M. Jacobs et al.,
"The Influence of Fashion Magazines on the Body Image Satisfaction of
College Women: An Exploratory Analysis," *Adolescence* 32 (Fall): 603–
614, 1997.
37 Miss America Pageant contestant: D. M. Garner et al., "Cultural Expectations of Thinness in Women," *Psychological Reports* 47: 483–491, 1980.
37 contestants weighed 15 percent below: C. V. Wiseman et al., "Cultural

Expectations of Thinness in Women: An Update," *International Journal of Eating Disorders* 11: 85–89, 1992.

37 runway models: Eric Wilson, "When Is Thin Too Thin?," *New York Times,* September 21, 2006.

38 elementary school students: M. E. Collins, "Body Figure Perceptions and Preferences Among Preadolescent Children," *International Journal of Eating Disorders* 10: 199–208, 1992.

38 10-year-olds are afraid of being fat: E. Koff and H. Rierdan, "Perceptions of Weight and Attitudes Toward Eating in Early Adolescent Girls," *Journal of Adolescent Health* 12: 307–312, 1991.

38 underweight girls think they are overweight: L. Mellin et al., "A Longitudinal Study of the Dietary Practices of Black and White Girls 9 and 10 Years Old at Enrollment: The NHLBI Growth and Health Study," *Journal of Adolescent Health* 20: 27–37, 1991.

38 body dissatisfaction has gone global:

Africa—D. Legrange et al., "The Meaning of 'Self-Starvation' in Impoverished Black Adolescents in South Africa," *Culture, Medicine and Psychiatry* 28: 439–461, 2004. M. Frith, "Zulu Women Follow Western Trend for Eating Disorders" *Independent,* April 16, 2004.

Australia—K. Rolland, D. Farnill, and R. A. Griffiths, "Children's Perceptions of Their Current and Ideal Body Sizes and Body Mass Index," *Perceptual and Motor Skills* 82: 651–656, 1996; K. Rolland, D. Farnill, and R. A. Griffiths, "Body Figure Perceptions and Eating Attitudes Among Australian Schoolchildren Aged 8 to 12 Years, *International Journal of Eating Disorders* 21, 273-278.

Brazil—A. P. Pinheiro, E. Regina, and J. Giuliani, "Body Dissatisfaction in 8-to-11-year-old Brazilian Schoolchildren: Prevalence and Associated Factors." *Rev Saude Publica* 40(3): 489–496, June 2006.

China—C. Davis and M. Z. Katzman, "Perfection as Acculturation: Psychological Correlates of Eating Problems in Chinese Male and Female Students Living in the United States," *International Journal of Eating Disorders* 25 (1999): 65–70; Yangfeng Wu, "Overweight and Obesity in China: The Once Lean Giant Has an Obesity Problem That Is Growing Rapidly," *British Journal of Medicine* 333: 362–363, 2006.

Croatia—J. Markovic, A. Votavaraic, and S. Nikolic, "Study of Eating Attitudes and Body Image Perception in the Preadolescent Age," *Collegium Anthropologicum* 22: 221–232.

Fiji—A. E. Becker et al., "Eating Behaviours and Attitudes Following Prolonged Exposure to Television Among Ethnic Fijian Adolescent Girls," *British Journal of Psychology* 180: 480–482; A. E. Becker, "Television,

Disordered Eating, and Young Women in Fiji: Negotiating Body Image and Identity During Rapid Social Change," *Culture, Medicine and Psychiatry* 4: 533–559.

Ghana—BBC Online, "Anorexia Found in Rural Africa," July 5, 2000, http://news.bbc.co.uk/1/hi/health/818725.stm.

Great Britain—A. J. Hill, E. Draper, and J. Stack, "A Weight on Children's Minds: Body Shape Dissatisfaction at 9 Years Old," *International Journal of Obesity* 18: 383–389, 1994.

Israel—A. Sasson, C. Lewin, and D. Roth, "Dieting Behavior and Eating Attitudes in Israeli Children," *International Journal of Eating Disorders* 17: 67–72, 1995.

Japan—H. Ontahara, T. Ohzeki, K. Hanaki, H. Motozumi, and K. Shiraki, "Abnormal Perception of Body Weight Is Not Solely Observed in Pubertal Girls: Incorrect Body Image in Children and Its Relationship to Body Weight," *Acta Psychiatrica Scandinava* 87: 218–222, 1993; T. Nadaoka et al., "An Epidemiological Study of Eating Disorders in a Northern Area of Japan," *Acata Psychiatrica Scandinavia* 93: 305–310, 1996.

Mexico—G. G. Perezmire, "Body Image Disturbances in a Mexican Sample of Preadolescent Students," *Revista Mexicana de Psicologia* 14: 31–40, 1997.

Sweden—B. Edlund, K. Halvarsson, and P. Sjoden, "Eating Behaviors, and Attitudes to Eating, Dieting and Body Image in 7-Year-Old Swedish Girls," *European Eating Disorders Review* 4: 40–53, 1996.

38 ages 6 to 12 have been on at least one diet: *Teen Magazine* (Fall 2003).

38 eventually progress to unhealthy, compulsive dieting: Anorexia Nervosa and Related Eating Disorders website. Viewed online at http://www.anred.com/welcome.html.

39 creating a brain map of the teenage emotional self: Abigail Baird and Jane C. Viner, "Frenemies: Using Cognition to Mediate the Effects of Relational Aggression," Cognitive Neuroscience Society Conference, March 2005, New York.

40 learn how to sit with painful feelings: Charlotte Kasl, *If the Buddha Got Stuck: Handbook for Change on a Spiritual Path* (New York: Penguin Books, 2005), 30–34.

43 differently to boys and girls: American Association of University Women Educational Foundation, *How Schools Shortchange Girls,* Washington D.C., 1992. Viewed online at http://www.aauw.org/research/hssg.pdf. Amy Huang, Ashley Ring, Teresa Torres et al., *Tech Savvy: Educating Girls in the New Computer Age*, American Association of University Women Educational Foundation, Washington, D.C., 2000. Viewed

online at http://www-cse.stanford.edu/classes/cs201/projects/gender-gap-in-education/page6.htm

43 as their male counterparts: U.S. Department of Labor, Bureau of Labor Statistics, *Women in the Labor Force: A Databook*, Washington, D.C., 2005, pp. 50–56. Viewed online at http://www.bls.gov/cps/wlf-databook2005.htm.

47 had been sexually harassed: Diana Jean Schemo, "1 in 4 College Students Surveyed Cite Unwanted Sexual Contact," *New York Times*, January 25, 2006.

47 physically hurt by a date: Jay G. Silverman, Anita Raj, and Karen Clements, "Dating Violence and Associated Sexual Risk and Pregnancy Among Adolescent Girls in the United States," *Pediatrics* 114: e220–e225, 2004.

48 next to headlines about weight loss: *Marie Claire*, August 2005 cover; *Self*, July 2005 cover.

49 girls who had been abused: Jay G. Silverman et al., "Dating Violence Against Adolescent Girls and Associated Substance Use, Unhealthy Weight Control, Sexual Risk Behavior, Pregnancy and Suicidality," *Journal of the American Medical Association* 286: 572–579, 2001.

51 at a gut level: Erikson, 1980, pp. 49–107.

51 religious doctrine: Jill Burcum, "The Struggle with 'Ana,'" *Star Tribune*, May 1, 2005.

51 Pro-ana . . . pro-mia: Mim Udovitch, "A Secret Society of the Starving," *New York Times Magazine*, September 8, 2002.

51 more than four hundred: Anna M. Bardone-Cone and Kamila M. Cass, "Investigating the Impact of Pro-Anorexia Websites: A Pilot Study," *European Eating Disorders* 14: 156–262, 2006.

52 self-abusing saints: Rudolph Bell, *Holy Anorexia* (Chicago: University of Chicago Press, 1985).

52 no such higher ideal: Jennifer Egan, "Power Suffering," *New York Times Magazine*, May 16, 1999.

52 Too much help from parents: Erikson, 1980, pp. 49–107.

57 teenage girls in Nadroga, Fiji: Anne Becker, Rebecca A. Burwell, Stephan E. Gilman et al., "Eating Behaviors and Attitudes Following Prolonged Exposure to Television Among Ethnic Fijian Adolescent Girls," *British Journal of Psychiatry* 180: 509–514, 2002.

58 generation of women still deeply confused: Kim Chernin, *The Hungry Self* (New York: Times Books, 1985), 17.

59 being authentic and being loved: Alice Miller, *The Drama of the Gifted Child* (New York: Basic Books, 1981).

3 | YOUNG ADULTHOOD

Page

62 It is only after a reasonable sense of identity: Erikson, 1980, p. 101.

66 Finnish researchers found: "Sexual Function and Attitudes Among Women with Eating Disorders," *Eating Disorders Review* 15: 6, 2004.

66 fewer women with anorexia tend to marry: David M. Garner and Paul E. Garfinkle, eds., *Anorexia Nervosa: A Multidimensional Perspective* (New York: Brunner/Mazel, 1982).

67 more negative attitudes toward sexuality: "Sexual Function and Attitudes Among Women with Eating Disorders," op. cit.

68 three groups of couples: Stephan Van den Broucke, Walter Vandereycken, and Jan Norre, *Eating Disorders and Marital Relationships* (London and New York: Routledge, 1997), 40–85.

70 theory of attachment: J. Bowly, *Attachment and Loss, Vol. 1: Attachment* (New York: Basic Books and London: Hogarth Press, 1969).

70 alienation from their fathers: Joeanne Gutzwiller, J. M. Oliver, and Barry M. Katz, "Eating Dysfunctions in College Women: The Roles of Depression and Attachment to Fathers," *Journal of the American College Health* 52: 27–32, 2003.

71 her father's absence: Victoria Secunda, *Women and Their Fathers: The Sexual and Romantic Impact of the First Man in Your Life* (New York: Delacorte Press, 1992), 140–141.

75 fit the men into three categories: Peter Dally, "Anorexia Tardive: Late Onset Marital Anorexia Nervosa," *Journal of Psychosomatic Research* 18: 423–428, 1984.

79 Psychological abuse by a husband: Linda Berg-Cross, "Intimate Relationships, Psychological Abuse and Health Problems," *The Register Report*: 20–27, Spring 2005.

79 partners of bulimic women . . . had psychiatric disorders: J. H. Lacey, "Homogamy: The Relationships and Sexual Partners of Normal-Weight Bulimic Women," *British Journal of Psychiatry* 161: 638–642, 1992.

80 twenty-one men: Van den Broucke et al., 1997, pp. 40–85.

81 tell their partners up front: Blake Woodside, M.Sc., M.D. University of Toronto, interview with the author, March 7, 2005.

84 when a full-blown illness first emerged: Dally, 1984, pp. 423–428.

86 connection between substance abuse and eating disorders: National Center on Addiction and Substance Abuse, *Food for Thought: Substance Abuse and Eating Disorders* (New York: Columbia University, December 2003).

88 *after* marrying: Debora Bussolotti, Fernando Fernandez-Aranda, Raquel

Solano et al, "Marital Status and Eating Disorders: An Analysis of Its Relevance," *Journal of Psychosomatic Research* 53: 1139–1145, 2002.

88 turn out to be sicker: Van den Broucke et al., 1997.

95 to suffer from depressive disorders: B. Wittmund, H. U. Wilms, and M. C. Angermeyer, "Depressive Disorders in Spouses of Mentally Ill Patients," *Social Psychiatry and Psychiatric Epidemiology* 37: 177–182, 2002; Michael Crowe, "Couples and Mental Illness," *Sexual and Relationship Therapy* 19: 308–318, 2004.

4 | PREGNANCY

Page

98 distinct developmental phase in a woman's life: Joan Offerman-Zuckerberg, *Critical Psychophysical Passages in the Life of a Woman: A Psychodynamic Perspective* (New York: Plenum Press, 1988),1–2; Grete L. Bibring, Thomas F. Dwyer, Dorothy S. Huntington et al., "A Study of the Psychological Processes in Pregnancy and of the Earliest Mother-Child Relationship," *Psychoanalytic Study of the Child* 16: 9–72, 1961; Melanie A. Katzmann, "When Reproductive and Productive Worlds Meet: Collision or Growth," in *Feminist Perspectives on Eating Disorders* (New York: Guilford Press, 1994),132–135.

99 strikes against her efforts: Dottie C. James, "Eating Disorders, Fertility and Pregnancy: Relationships and Complications," *Journal of Perinatal and Neonatal Nursing* 15: 36–48, 2001.

100 structuring her life around rules: Debra L. Franko and Emily B. Spurrell, "Detection and Management of Eating Disorders During Pregnancy," *Obstetrics and Gynecology* 95: 942–946, 2000.

102 ban in Madrid, Spain: Harold Heckle, "Madrid Fashion Show Bans 5 Thin Models," *Washington Post*, September 16, 2006.

102 associate fertility with fleshiness: O. Wayne Wooley, ". . . And Man Created 'Woman': Representations of Women's Bodies in Western Culture," in *Feminist Perspectives on Eating Disorders* (New York and London: Guilford Press, 1994), 17–52.

102 painter Fons Van Woerkom: Wooley, p. 20.

102 mothers' limited academic or career opportunities: Deborah Perlick and Brett Silverstein, "Faces of Female Discontent: Depression, Disordered Eating, and Changing Gender Roles," in *Feminist Perspectives on Eating Disorders*, 82–83.

105 women with bulimia often lose their periods: Suzanne Abraham, "Sexuality and Reproduction in Bulimia Nervosa Patients Over 10 Years," *Journal of Psychosomatic Research* 44: 491–502, 1998; John Farnill

Morgan, J. Hubert Lacey, and Philip M. Sedgwick, "Impact of Pregnancy on Bulimia Nervosa," *British Journal of Psychiatry* 174: 135–140, 1999.

105 overactive sex drives: Donna Stewart, "Reproductive Functions in Eating Disorders," *Annals of Medicine* 24: 287–291, 1992.

105 246 women in the study sample: Mark A. Blais, Anne E. Becker, Rebecca A. Burwell et al., "Pregnancy: Outcome and Impact on Symptomatology in a Cohort of Eating-Disordered Women," *International Journal of Eating Disorders* 27:140–149, 2000.

106 most of the pregnancies are unplanned: Suja Srikameswaran, St. Paul's Hospital, Vancouver, B.C., interview with the author, November 23, 2004.

106 links between bulimia, irregular periods, and an overzealous sex drive: Morgan et al., 1999, pp. 135–140.

107 higher rates of miscarriage: James E. Mitchell, Harold C. Seim, Debbie Glotter et al., "A Retrospective Study of Pregnancy in Bulimia Nervosa," *International Journal of Eating Disorders* 10: 209–214, 1991; M. Brinch, T. Isager, and K. Tolstrup, "Anorexia Nervosa and Motherhood: Reproduction Pattern and Mothering Behavior of 50 Women," *Acta Psychiatrica Scandinavica* 77: 611–617, 1988; Cynthia M. Bulik, Patrick F. Sullivan, Jennifer L. Fear et al., "Fertility and Reproduction in Women with Anorexia Nervosa: A Controlled Study," *Journal of Clinical Psychiatry* 60: 130–135, 1999.

107 who do not miscarry: Blais et al., 2000, pp. 140–149.

108 earlier menstruation: J. K. Lake, C. Power, and T. J. Cole, "Women's Reproductive Health: The Role of Body Mass Index in Early and Adult Life," *International Journal of Obesity and Related Metabolic Disorders* 21: 432–438, 1997.

108 PCOS   the   cause: http://www.havingbabies.com/infertility-weight. html; David A. Ehrmann, "Polycystic Ovary Syndrome," *New England Journal of Medicine* 352: 1223–1236, 2005.

109 3,586 Australian women: J. X. Wang, M. Davies, and R. J. Norman, "Body Mass and Probability of Pregnancy During Assisted Reproduction Treatment: Retrospective Study," *British Medical Journal* 321: 1320–1321, 2000.

110 adult female athletes: Steven J. Anderson, Bernard A. Griesemer, Miriam Johnson et al., "American Academy of Pediatrics Committee on Sports Medicine and Fitness: Medical Concerns of the Female Athlete," *Pediatrics* 106: 610–613, 2000.

110 survey of female athletes: K. L. Kubas and P. S. Hinton, "Psychosocial Correlates of Disordered Eating in Female Collegiate Athletes:

Validation of the ATHLETE Questionnaire," *Journal of American College Health*: 149–162, November 1, 2005.

110 subclinical disorders: Stewart, 1992, pp. 287–291.

111 keeping this group in check: Ibid.

111 simply reaching a normal weight: Ibid.

112 1.2 million women: Centers for Disease Control and Prevention, "Assisted Reproductive Technology (ART) Report," Atlanta, Georgia, 2002. Viewed online at http://www.cdc.gov/ART/index.htm.

112 66 women who visited a fertility clinic: Stewart, 1992, pp. 287–291.

112 the criteria for an eating disorder: Suzanne Abraham, Michael Mira, and Derek Llewellyn-Jones, "Should Ovulation Be Induced in Women Recovering from an Eating Disorder or Who Are Compulsive Exercisers?" *Fertility and Sterility* 52: 566–568, 1990.

112 Micali found: Nadia Micali, King's College, London, U.K., interview with the author, November 9, 2005.

113 18 to 43 percent: Centers for Disease Control and Prevention, "Assisted Reproductive Technology (ART) Report: 2003 Fertility Clinic Report by State: National Summary," Atlanta, Georgia, 2003. Viewed online at http://apps.nccd.cdc.gov/ART2003/national03.asp.

115 will fulfill them personally: Raymond Lemberg and Jeanne Phillips, "The Impact of Pregnancy on Anorexia and Bulimia Nervosa," *International Journal of Eating Disorders* 8: 285–295, 1989; J. F. Morgan, J. H. Lacey, and P. M. Sedgewick, "Impact of Pregnancy on Bulimia Nervosa," *British Journal of Psychiatry* 174: 135–140, 1999.

115 unconditional love: Leanne Domash, "Motivations for Motherhood and the Nature of the Self-Object Tie," in *Critical Psychophysical Passages in the Life of a Woman: A Psychodynamic Perspective* (New York: Plenum Press, 1988).

116 get over their eating disorder: Lemberg and Phillips, 1989, pp. 285–295.

117 are chilling: Franko and Spurrell, 2000, pp. 942–946; Debra Franko, Mark A. Blais, Anne E. Becker et al., "Pregnancy Complications and Neonatal Outcomes in Women with Eating Disorders," *American Journal of Psychiatry* 158: 1461–1466, 2001.

118 born with birth defects or die: Ibid.; Mitchell et al., 1991, pp. 209–214; Brinch et al., 1988, pp. 611–617.

118 underweight pregnant rats: M. H. Vickers, B. H. Breier, D. McCarthy et al., "Sedentary Behavior During Postnatal Life Is Determined by the Prenatal Environment and Exacerbated Postnatal Hypercaloric Nutrition," *American Journal of Physiology-Regulatory, Integrative and Comparative Physiology* 285: 271–273, 2003.

118 hyperemesis gravidarum: Stewart, 1992, pp. 287–291.

118 most doctors do not know: Franko and Spurrell, 2000, pp. 942–946.

119 tend to miscarry more often: Mitchell et al., 1991, pp. 209–214; Franko et al., 2001, pp. 1461–1466.

119 suffer multiple miscarriages: Nadia Micali, King's College, London, U.K., interview with the author, November 9, 2005.

121 cultures worshipped goddesses: Wooley, 1994, pp. 17–52.

121 actress Kate Hudson: Rebecca Traister, "Pregnancy Porn," Salon.com, July 31, 2004. Viewed online at http://www.salon.com/mwt/feature/2004/07/31/pregnancy_porn/.

121 pregnant CIA operative: Jodi Kantor, "Pregnancy Won't Stop 'Alias' Star from Being Adventurous, Even Sexy" New York Times, October 6, 2005.

122 this obsession: Laurie Abraham, "The Perfect Little Bump," New York magazine, September 27, 2004, pp. 21–25.

124 relinquish their unhealthy behaviors: Morgan et al., 1999, pp. 135–140.

125 do relatively well: Franko et al., 2001, pp. 1461–1466; Cecilia Ekeus, L. Lindberg, and A. Hjern, "Birth Outcomes and Pregnancy Complications in Women with a History of Anorexia Nervosa," An International Journal of Obstetrics and Gynecology 113: 925, 2006.

126 cesarean sections more often: J. Hubert Lacey and G. Smith, "Bulimia Nervosa: The Impact on Mother and Baby," British Journal of Psychiatry 150: 777–781, 1987; Bulik et al., 1999, pp. 130–135.

128 within nine months: Franko et al., 2001, pp. 1461–1466.

128 worse symptoms after pregnancy: Lacey and Smith, 1987, pp. 777–781; Morgan et al., 1999, pp. 135–140.

128 unrealistic expectations: Wendy Jenkin and Marika Tiggemann, "Psychological Effects of Weight Retained After Pregnancy," Women and Health 25: 89–98, 1997.

129 six months after giving birth: L. Walker, "Weight-Related Distress in the Early Months After Childbirth," Western Journal of Nursing Research 20: 30–44, 1998.

129 these unrealistic models: Suzanne Abraham, Alan Taylor, and Janet Conti, "Postnatal Depression, Eating, Exercise, and Vomiting Before and During Pregnancy," International Journal of Eating Disorders 29:482–487, 2001; Franko et al., 2001, pp. 1461–1466.

129 taking antidepressants: Lee S. Cohen, Lori L. Altshuler, Bernard L. Harlow et al., "Relapse of Major Depression During Pregnancy in Women Who Maintain or Discontinue Antidepressant Treatment," Journal of the American Medical Association 295: 499–507, 2006.

129 persistent pulmonary hypertension: Christina D. Chambers, Sonia Hernandez-Diaz, Linda J. Van Marter et al., "Selective Serotonin-Reuptake Inhibitors and Risk of Persistent Pulmonary Hypertension of the Newborn," *New England Journal of Medicine* 354: 2188–2190, 2006.

131 Emme Aronson: Emme Aronson, interview with the author, September 14, 2004. Viewed online at http://www.safesearching.com/officia-lemme/allaboutemme/bio.shtml.

133 obstetricians and fertility experts: Franko and Spurrell, 2000, pp. 942–946.

135 Abandonment is often a huge issue: Naomi Berne, "Psychology of Childbirth," in *Critical Psychophysical Passages in the Life of a Woman: A Psychodynamic Perspective* (New York: Plenum Press, 1988), 123–131.

5 | PARENTING YEARS

Page

138 child's connection to food: Chernin, 1985, pp. 99–105.

138 soothed by candy: Susan L. Johnson and Leann L. Birch, "Parents' and Children's Adiposity and Eating Style," *Pediatrics* 94: 653–661, 1994.

139 mothers who diet excessively: Kathleen M. Pike and Judith Rodin, "Mothers, Daughters and Disordered Eating," *Journal of Abnormal Psychology* 100: 198–204, 1991; "Restrictive Feeding Can Make Children Overeat," *Eating Disorders Review* 7, January/February 2003.

139 relatives of women with anorexia: Lisa R. Lilenfeld, Walter H. Key, Catherine G. Greeno et al., "A Controlled Family Study of Anorexia Nervosa and Bulimia Nervosa," *Archives of General Psychiatry* 55: 603–610, 1998; Michael Strober, Roberta Freeman, Caryln Lampert et al., "Controlled Family Study of Anorexia Nervosa and Bulimia Nervosa: Evidence of Shared Liability and Transmissions of Partial Syndromes," *American Journal of Psychiatry* 157: 393–401, 2000.

139 Binge eating disorder: James I. Hudson, Justine K. Lalonde, Judith M. Berry et al., "Binge Eating Disorder as a Distinct Familial Phenotype in Obese Individuals," *Archives of General Psychiatry* 63: 313–319, 2006.

139 predisposing a child: Cynthia M. Bulik, Patrick F. Sullivan, Federica Tozzi et al., "Prevalence, Heritability, and Prospective Risk Factors for Anorexia Nervosa," *Archives of General Psychiatry* 63: 305–312, 2006.

141 Public health practitioners: Roni Rabin, "Breast-Feed or Else," *New York Times*, June 13, 2006.

141 less than women without such disorders: Rebecca J. Park, Rob Senior, and Alan Stein, "The Offspring of Mothers with Eating Disorders," *European Child and Adolescent Psychiatry* 12: 110–119, 2003; Elizabeth Waugh and Cynthia M. Bulik, "Offspring of Women with Eating Disorders," *International Journal of Eating Disorders* 25: 123–133, 1999.

141 highest concerns about weight and shape: Waugh and Bulik, 1999, pp. 123–133.

144 500 extra kilocalories: Karen S. Wosje and Heidi J. Kalkwarf, "Lactation, Weaning, and Calcium Supplementation: Effects on Body Composition in Postpartum Women," *American Journal of Clinical Nutrition* 80: 423–429, 2004.

145 grow up to be obese adults: Rabin, 2006.

145 mothers obsessed about fatness: Christopher G. Owen, Richard M. Martin, Peter H. Whincup et al., "The Effect of Breastfeeding on Mean Body Mass Index Throughout Life: A Quantitative Review of Published and Unpublished Observational Evidence," *American Journal of Clinical Nutrition* 82: 1298–1307, 2005.

145 failed to thrive: P. J. Cooper and C. F. Fairburn, "The Depressive Symptoms of Bulimia Nervosa," *British Journal of Psychiatry*, 148: 268–274, 1986; A. Stein, L. Murray, P. Cooper et al., "Infant Growth in the Context of Maternal Eating Disorders and Maternal Depression: A Comparative Study," *Psychological Medicine* 26: 569–574, 1996; Alan Stein, Helen Woolley, Sandra D. Cooper et al., "An Observational Study of Mothers with Eating Disorders and Their Infants," *Journal of Child Psychology and Psychiatry* 35: 733–748, 1994.

145 Danish mothers: M. Brinch, T. Isager, and K. Tolstrup, "Anorexia Nervosa and Motherhood: Reproduction Pattern and Mothering Behavior of 50 Women," *Acta Psychiatrica Scandinavica* 77: 611–617, 1988.

145 who ration food: G. F. M. Russell, J. Treasure, and I. Eisler, "Mothers with Anorexia Nervosa Who Underfeed Their Children: Their Recognition and Management," *Psychological Medicine* 9: 429–448, 1998.

146 March of Dimes: Viewed online at http://www.marchofdimes.com/professionals/681_1153.asp.

146 hyperkinetic disorder: K. M. Linnet, K. Wiskborg, E. Agorbo et al., "Gestational Age, Birth Weight, and the Risk of Hyperkinetic Disorder," *Archives of Disease in Childhood* 91: 655–660, 2006. Viewed online at http://press.psprings.co.uk/adc/june/ac88872.pdf.

146 infantile anorexia: Irene Chatoor, Jody Ganiban, Robert Hirsch et al., "Maternal Characteristic and Toddle Temperament in Infantile Anorxia," *Journal of the American Academy of Child and Adolescent Psychiatry* 39: 743, 2000.

146 below the fifth percentile: Alice Lawrence, "Feeding Disorders of Infants and Toddlers: Infantile Anorexia," *The Child Avocate*, 2003. Viewed online at http://www.childadvocate.net/infantile_anorexia.htm.

146 back to parents: Nancy C. Winters, "Feeding Problems in Infancy and Early Childhood," *Primary Psychiatry* 10: 30–34, 2003.

147 were more insecure: "Eating Disorders, Mother's Insecurity and Child Temperament Can Lead to Infantile Anorexia," *Health and Medicine Week*, August 19, 2000, pp. 15–16.

147 trust versus mistrust: Erikson, 1980, pp. 49–107.

147 children adopted into American families: Alison B. Wismer Fries, Toni E. Ziegler, Joseph R. Kurlan et al., "Early Experience in Humans Is Associated with Changes in Neuropeptides Critical for Regulating Social Behavior," *Proceedings of the National Academy of Sciences* 102: 17237–17240, 2005.

148 suckle differently: Stewart Agras, Lawrence Hammer, and Fiona McNicholas, "A Prospective Study of the Influence of Eating-Disordered Mothers on Their Children," *International Journal of Eating Disorders* 25: 253–262, 1999.

149 do not fail to thrive: Waugh and Bulik, 1999, pp. 123–133; Cecilia Ekeus, L. Lindberg, and A. Hjern, "Birth Outcomes and Pregnancy Complications in Women with a History of Anorexia Nervosa," *An International Journal of Obstetrics and Gynecology* 113: 925, 2006.

150 blogs written by parents: David Hochman, "Mommy and Me: A Generation of New Parents Are Telling Tales from the Crib in Blogs That Revel in Self-Absorption," *New York Times,* January 30, 2005.

150 TV shows: Ginia Bellafante, "Children, Apples of Parents' Eyes, Face Arrows on TV," *New York Times,* November 19, 2005.

152 throughout the first year postpartum: Raymond Lemberg and Jeanne Phillips, "The Impact of Pregnancy on Anorexia Nervosa and Bulimia," *International Journal of Eating Disorders* 8: 285–295, 1989.

152 their eating issues again: Priti Patel, Rebecca Wheatcroft, Rebecca J. Park, and Alan Stein, "The Children of Mothers with Eating Disorders," *Clinical Child and Family Psychology Review* 5: 1–19, 2002.

154 than children of healthy mothers: Cooper and Fairburn, 1986, pp. 268–274.

154 below the fifteenth percentile: Stein et al., 1994, pp. 733–748.

154 "dawdling" during mealtimes: Agras et al., 1999, pp. 253–262; Sami Timimi and Paul Robinson, "Disturbances in Children of Patients with Eating Disorders," *European Eating Disorders Review* 4 (1996): 183–188, 1996.

155 tended to score higher: J. B. McCann, A. Stein, C. G. Fairburn et. al.,
    "Eating Habits and Attitudes of Mothers and Children with Non-Organic
    Failure to Thrive," *Archives of Disease in Childhood* 70: 234–236, 1994.

155 reported him as greedy: Timimi and Robinson, 1996, pp. 183–188.

155 should be venturing out: Erikson, 1980, pp. 67–77.

156 children in the study overate: Eric Stice, W. Stewart Agras, and Law-
    rence D. Hammer, "Risk Factors for the Emergence of Childhood Eating
    Disturbances: A Five-Year Prospective Study," *International Journal of
    Eating Disorders* 25: 375–387, 1999.

158 videotaped the mothers: Stein et al., 1994, pp. 733–748.

159 tends to emerge: D. Blake Woodside, Lorie F. Shekter-Wolfson, J. S.
    Brandes, and J. B. Lackstrom, *Eating Disorders in Marriage: The Couple
    in Focus* (New York: Brunner/Mazel, 1993).

160 overdependent relationship with her daughter: Ute Franzen and
    Monika Gerlinghoff, "Parenting by Parents with Eating Disorders: Ex-
    periences with a Mother-Child Group," *Eating Disorders* 5: 5–14, 1997.

161 learned to comfort their mothers: Ibid.

161 take over household chores: Waugh and Bulik, 1999, pp. 123–133;
    D. Blake Woodside and Lorie F. Schekter-Wolfson, "Parenting by Pa-
    tients with Anorexia Nervosa and Bulimia Nervosa," *International Jour-
    nal of Eating Disorders* 9: 303–309, 1990.

161 were so preoccupied with vomiting: J. H. Lacey and G. Smith, "Bulimia
    Nervosa: The Impact of Pregnancy on Mother and Baby," *British Journal
    of Psychiatry* 150: 777–781, 1987.

161 physically abused her son: Franzen and Gerlinghoff, 1997, pp. 5–14.

163 one in six U.S. children: Cynthia L. Ogden, Margaret D. Carroll,
    Lester R. Curtin et al., "Prevalence of Overweight and Obesity in the
    United States, 1999–2004," *Journal of the American Medical Associa-
    tion* 295: 1549–1555, 2006.

163 the normal weight range: Alison E. Field, Nancy R. Cook, and Matthew
    W. Gillman, "Weight Status in Childhood as a Predictor for Becoming
    Overweight or Hypertensive in Early Adulthood," *Obesity Research* 13:
    163–169, 2005.

163 national campaigns to prevent childhood obesity: Eric Stice, Heather
    Shaw, and C. Nathan Marti, "A Meta-Analytic Review of Obesity Pre-
    vention Programs for Children and Adolescents: The Skinny on Inter-
    ventions That Work," *Psychological Bulletin* 132: 667–691, 2006.

164 survey of 1,300 organizations: "Shaping America's Youth Initiative,"
    presented at the Institute of Food Health Technologists' 2004 annual
    meeting, Portland, Oregon.

165 they are simply ignoring: "Parents: Is Your Child Obese (Think Care-fully)," *New York Times,* May 23, 2006; Harriet Brown, "Well-Intentioned Food Police May Create Havoc with Children's Diets," *New York Times,* May 20, 2006.

165 high-calorie fast foods: Dan Mitchell, "Supersize Comeback for Fast Food," *New York Times,* November 12, 2005.

165 overweight but not obese: Gina Kolata, "Still Counting on Calorie Counting," *New York Times,* April 29, 2005.

165 supersize themselves: Timothy Egan, "With Potbellies Back In, Buffet Pots Are Humming," *New York Times,* May 3, 2005.

165 change children's growth charts: Betsy McKay, "When Is a Baby Too Fat?," *Wall Street Journal,* May 18, 2006.

165 pharmaceutical industry: Ray Moynihan, "Obesity Task Force Linked to WHO Takes Millions from Drug Firms," *British Medical Journal* 332: 1412, 2006.

166 tofu and greens for lunch: Gina Kolata, "Thinning the Milk Does Not Mean Thinning the Child," *New York Times,* February 12, 2006; Melanie Warner, "Industry Urged to Offer More Nutritious Foods for Children," *New York Times,* May 3, 2006; Marian Burros, "Bill Strikes at Low-Nutrition Foods in Schools," *New York Times,* April 6, 2006; Alice Waters, "Eating for Credit," *New York Times,* February 24, 2006; Mireya Navarro, "Playtime at the Health Club," *New York Times,* January 22, 2006.

166 Mother's Day: Woodside and Schekter, 1990, 303–309.

167 they thought about their shape and weight: Linda Smolak, Michael P. Levine, and Florence Schermer, "Parental Input and Weight Concerns Among Elementary School Children," *International Journal of Eating Disorders* 25: 263–271, 1999.

167 critical comments: Alison E. Field, S. B. Austin, Ruth Striegel-Moore et al., "Weight Concerns and Weight Controls: Behaviors of Adolescents and Their Mothers," *Archives of Pediatric and Adolescent Medicine* 159: 1121–1126, 2005.

167 heaviest students: A. J. Hill, E. Draper, and J. Stack, "A Weight on Children's Minds: Body Shape Dissatisfactions at 9 Years Old," *International Journal of Obesity* 18: 383–389, 1994.

168 children in grades 3 to 6:   Michael J. Maloney, Julie McGuire, Stephen R. Daniels et al., "Dieting Behavior and Eating Attitudes in Children," *Pediatrics* 84: 482–489, 1989.

168 develop full or partial eating disorders: C. Barr Taylor, Tamara Sharpe, Catherine Shisslak et al., "Factors Associated with Weight Concerns in

Adolescent Girls," *International Journal of Eating Disorders* 24: 31–42, 1998.

169 by the age of 7:   Leann Birch, Jennifer Orelt Fisher, and Kirsten Krahn-stoever Davison, "Learning to Overeat: Maternal Use of Restrictive Feeding Practices Promotes Girls' Eating in the Absence of Hunger," *American Journal of Clinical Nutrition* 78: 215–220, 2003.

169 mothers who dieted the most: Andrew J. Hill, Claire Weaver, and John E. Blundell, "Dieting Concerns of 10-Year-Old Girls and Their Mothers," *British Journal of Clinical Psychology* 29: 346–348, 1994.

171 weight was important: A. E. Field, S. B. Austin, R. Streigel-Moore et. al., "Weight Concerns and Weight Control Behaviors of Adolescents and Their Mothers," *Archives of Pediatric and Adolescent Medicine* 159: 1121–1126, 2005.

171 amounts of fat that mothers and daughters ate: Cassandra Stanton, Elizabeth Fries, and Steven J. Danish, "Racial and Gender Differences in the Diets of Rural Youth and Their Mothers," *American Journal of Health* 27: 336–347, 2003.

176 1,200 pairs of female twins: K. L. Klump, M. McGue, and W. G. Iacono, "Differential Heritability of Eating Attitudes and Behaviors in Prepubertal Versus Pubertal Twins," *International Journal of Eating Disorders* 33: 287–292, 2003.

177 gene that encodes an estrogen receptor: K. Rosenkrantz, A. Hinney, A. Zieglar et al., "Systematic Mutation Screening of the Estrogen Receptor Beta Gene in Probands of Different Weight Extremes: Identification of Several Genetic Variants," *Journal of Clinical Endocrinology and Metabolism* 83: 4524–4527, 1998.

178 testosterone exposure in the womb: K. L. Klump, K. L. Gobrogge, P. S. Perkins et al., "Preliminary Evidence That Gonadal Hormones Organize and Activate Disordered Eating," *Psychological Medicine* 36: 539–546, 2006.

183 cutting back on sugar and fat: W. A. Walker and Courtney Humphries, *Eat, Play, and Be Healthy: A Harvard Medical School Guide to Healthy Eating for Kids* (McGraw-Hill: New York, 2005).

183 Institute of Medicine: Committee on Prevention of Obesity in Children and Youth, *Preventing Childhood Obesity: Health in the Balance* (Washington, D.C.: The National Academies Press, 2005). Viewed online at http://fermat.nap.edu/catalog/11015.html.

183 a variety of foods: Diane Neumark-Sztainer, *"I'm, Like, SO Fat!" Helping Your Teen Make Healthy Choices About Eating and Exercising in a Weight-Obsessed World* (New York: Guilford Press, 2005).

184 eat together most nights: Elsie M. Taveras, Sheryl L. Rifas-Shiman, Catherine S. Berkey et al., "Family Dinner and Adolescent Overweight," *Obesity Research* 13: 900–906, 2005.

184 create a positive atmosphere: Neumark-Sztainer, 2005.

184 rather than weight loss: Eric Stice, Katherine Presnell, and Heather Shaw, "Psychological and Behavioral Risk Factors for Obesity Onset in Adolescent Girls: A Prospective Study," *Journal of Consulting and Clinical Psychology* 73: 195–202, 2005; L. L. Birch, S. L. Johnson, and G. Andresen et al., "The Variability of Young Children's Energy Balance Intake," *New England Journal of Medicine* 324: 232–235, 1991.

184 videotapes of themselves: Stein et al., 1994.

184 focus less on weight gain or weight loss: Neumark-Sztainer, 2005.

184 more important than their weight and shape: Caroline J. Cederquist, *Helping Your Overweight Child: A Family Guide* (Naples, FL: Advance Medical Press, 2002).

6 | MIDLIFE

Page

189 have begun keeping statistices: Edward Cumella, interview with the author, March 18, 2005; Cynthia M. Bulik and Nadine Taylor, *Runaway Eating: The 8-Point Plan to Conquer Adult Food and Weight Obsessions* (Emmaus, PA: Rodale, 2005).

190 Recent books about bulimia: Ginia Bellafonte, "When Midlife Seems Just an Empty Plate," *New York Times,* March 9, 2003; Bonnie Rothman Morris, "Older Women, Too, Struggle with a Dangerous Secret," *New York Times,* July 6, 2004; Sabrina Rubin Erdely, "The Scary New Way Stress Is Affecting Women," *Redbook,* March 2004, p. 114.

190 trying to juggle multiple roles: Eduardo Porter, "Stretched to the Limit, Women Stall March to Workplace," *New York Times,* March 2, 2006.

190 *Get a face-lift*:   Eryn Brown, "Sometimes, Nips and Tucks Can Be Career Moves," *New York Times,* February 12, 2006.

190 culture casts a body-projection imperative: Debra Waterhouse, *Like Mother, Like Daughter* (New York: Hyperion, 1997), xvi; Bulik and Taylor, 2005, pp. 29–41.

190 engage in pathologic weight control: Susan C. Wooley et al., "Feeling Fat in a Thin Society," *Glamour* magazine, February 1984, p. 198.

191 Women with binge eating disorder: American Psychiatric Association,

Diagnostic and Statistic Manual of Mental Health Disorders: DSM-IV (Washington, D.C.: APA, 1994).

191 researchers surveyed the attitudes: Diane M. Lewis and Fary M. Cachelin, "Body Image, Body Dissatisfaction, and Eating Attitudes in Midlife and Elderly Women," *Eating Disorders* 9: 29–39, 2001.

191 main reason that people are overweight: Paul Taylor, Cary Funk, and Peyton Craighill, "Americans See Weight Problems Everywhere but in the Mirror," *Pew Research Center: A Social Trends Report*, Washington, D.C., April 11, 2006, pp. 1, 8–9. Viewed online at http://pewresearch.org/assets/social/pdf/Obesity.pdf.

192 binge eating disorder afflicts: Debra L. Franko, Stephen A. Wonderlich, Deborah Little et al., "Diagnosis and Classification of Eating Disorders," in Thompson, ed., 2005, p. 72.

192 anatomy of the binge: José Carlos Appolinario, interview with the author, February 28, 2005.

194 to become generative: Erikson, 1980, pp. 103–104.

194 is a mile marker: Bernice Neugarten, *The Meanings of Age* (Chicago: University of Chicago Press, 1995).

195 the eating disorder germinates: Bulik and Taylor, 2005, p. 41.

196 levels of body dissatisfaction: Marika Tiggemann and Jessica E. Lynch, "Body Image Across the Lifespan in Adult Women: The Role of Self-Objectification," *Developmental Psychology* 37: 243–253, 2001; Marika Tiggemann, "Body Image Across the Adult Life Span: Stability and Change," *Body Image* 1: 29–41, 2004.

197 get ahead in the workplace: Brown, 2006.

197 cosmetic surgery in 2005: Cosmetic Surgery National Data Bank, American Society for Aesthetic Plastic Surgery, New York, NY, 2005, pp. 7, 10. Viewed online at http://www.surgery.org/download/2005stats.pdf.

197 with weight-loss side effects: Katherine Zerbe, "Eating Disorders at Middle Age, Part 1 and 2," *Eating Disorders Review* 15: 2–3, 2004.

206 often die: Patrick Sullivan, "Course and Outcome of Anorexia and Bulimia Nervosa," in Chris Fairburn and Kelly Brownell, eds., *Eating Disorders and Obesity: A Comprehensive Handbook,* 2nd ed. (New York: Guilford Press, 2002), 226–32.

206 the story of his mother: Daniel Becker, *This Mean Disease: Growing Up in the Shadow of My Mother's Anorexia Nervosa* (Carlsbad, CA: Gürze Books, 2005).

206 within that group: Sullivan, 2002, p. 227.

206 the majority, partially recover: Ibid., p. 228.

207 cross over into bulimia: Ibid., p. 227.

207 70 percent have been able: Ibid.

208 two reasons why binge eating: Fairburn, 1995, pp. 80–99.

208 rats can learn to binge eat: Mary M. Hagan, Paula C. Chandler, Pamela K. Wauford et al., "The Role of Palatable Food and Hunger as Trigger Factors in an Animal Model of Stress Induced Binge Eating," *International Journal of Eating Disorders* 34: 183–197, 2003.

210 binge eating is addictive: Mary M. Boggiano, Paula C. Chandler, Jason B. Viana et al., "Combined Dieting and Stress Evoke Exaggerated Responses to Opioids in Binge-Eating Rats," *Behavioral Neuroscience* 119: 1207–1214, 2005.

210 gastrointestinal problems, heart attacks: Claire Pomeroy, "Assessment of Medical Status and Physical Factors," in Thompson, ed., 2004, pp. 81–111.

211 sports-related injuries: Consumer Product Safety Commission, *Baby Boomer Sports Injuries,* Gaithersburg, MD, April 2000. Viewed online at http://www.cpsc.gov/library/boomer.pdf.

211 poorer brain function: Janine Giese-Davis, C. Barr Taylor, and Ruth O'Hara, "Stress, the HPA, and Health in Aging," research presented at the Society of Behavioral Medicine Annual Meeting and Scientific Sessions in San Francisco, CA, March 24, 2006.

211 1.5 million osteoporotic fractures: Clifford J. Rosen, "Postmenopausal Osteoporosis," *New England Journal of Medicine* 353: 595–603, 2005.

212 after their first period: M. T. Munoz and J. Argente, "Anorexia Nervosa in Female Adolescents: Endocrine and Bone Mineral Density Disturbances," *European Journal of Endocrinology* 147: 275–286, 2003.

212 lowest bone mineral density: " Ibid.

212 twenty-one years after recovery: B. M. Biller, V. Saxe, D. B. Herzog et al., "Mechanisms of Osteoporosis in Adult and Adolescent Women with Anorexia Nervosa," *Journal of Clinical Endocrinology and Metabolism* 68: 548–554, 1989.

212 36,000 middle-aged women: Rebecca D. Jackson, Andrea Z. LaCroix, Margery Gass et al., "Calcium Plus Vitamin D Supplementation and the Risk of Fractures," *New England Journal of Medicine* 354: 669–683, 2006.

213 diagnosis is osteoporosis: Rosen, 2005.

213 hormone called leptin: Corrine K. Welt, Jean L. Chan, John Bullen et al., "Recombinant Human Leptin in Women with Hypothalamic Amenorrhea," *New England Journal of Medicine* 351: 987–997, 2004.

214 Americans are now suffering from diabetes: American Diabetes Association. Viewed online at http://www.diabetes.org/about-diabetes.jsp.

214 Brazilian researchers: Marcelo Papelbaum, José Carlos Appolinario, Rodrigo de Olivera et al., "Prevalence of Eating Disorders and Psychiatric Comorbidity in a Clinical Sample of Type II Diabetes Mellitus Patients," *Revista Brasileira de Psiquiatria* 27: 135–138, 2005.

214 plagued by an eating disorder: Scott Crow, David Kendall, Barbara Praus et al., "Binge Eating and Other Psychopathology in Patients with Type II Diabetes Mellitus: A Randomized Trial," *International Journal of Eating Disorders* 30: 222–226, 2001.

214 rebel against the strict dietary restrictions: Susan Z. Yanovski, "Diagnosis and Prevention of Eating Disorders in Obesity," in B. Guy-Grand et al., eds., *Progress in Obesity Research* (London: John Libbey, 1999), 229–236.

214 gain more fat: Judith Rodin, Lisa Silberstein, and Ruth Streigel-Moore, "Women and Weight: A Normative Discontent," *Nebraska Symposium on Motivation*, 1984, p. 283.

215 has to be a second priority: James Hudson, interview with the author, September 10, 13, and 27, 2004.

216 assess the risk for type 2 diabetes: Pomeroy, 2004, p. 94.

216 changes at menopause: University of Michigan Disease Center, *About Depression*, Ann Arbor, MI. Viewed online at http://www.med.umich.edu/depression/menopause.htm.

217 after twenty cycles of dieting: Mary Boggiano, interview with the author, June 16, 21, 2004.

217 of women with eating disorders: Walter Kaye, Michael Strober, and David Jimerson, "The Neurobiology of Eating Disorders," in D. S. Chamey and E. J. Nestler, eds., *The Neurobiology of Mental Illness* (New York: Oxford Press, 2004): 112–128.

217 lose their ability to respond: Ursula F. Bailer et al., "Altered Brain Serotonin 5-HT_{1A} Receptor Binding After Recovery from Anorexia Nervosa Measured by Positron Emission Tomography and [Carbonyl^{11}C]WAY-100635," *Archives of General Psychiatry* 62: 1032–1041, 2005; Walter Kaye, Kelly Gendall, and Michael Strober, "Serotonin Neuronal Function and Selective Serotonin Reuptake Inhibitor Treatment in Anorexia and Bulimia Nervosa," *Biological Psychiatry* 44: 825–838, 1998; Walter Kaye, interview with the author, June 29, 2004.

218 tight lid on dieting: Bulik, 2005, p. 85.

220 a study team at University College: H. H. Ehrsson, T. Kito, N. Sadato et al. "Neural Substrate of Body Size: Illusory Feeling of Shrinking of the Waist," *Public Library of Science Biology* 12: e412, 2005.

7 | LATE LIFE

Page

225 does not make sense: Paul Cosford and Elaine Arnold, "Eating Disorders in Later Life: A Review," *International Journal of Geriatric Psychiatry* 7: 491–498, 1992.

227 rheumatoid arthritis, cancer, heart failure: Margaret-Mary Wilson,
David R. Thomas, Lawrence Z. Rubenstein et al., "Appetite Assessment:
Simple Appetite Questionnaire Predicts Weight Loss in Community-
Dwelling Adults and Nursing Home Residents," *American Journal of
Clinical Nutrition* 82: 1071–1081, 2005; American Psychiatric Asso-
ciation, *Diagnostic and Statistic Manual of Mental Disorders: DSM-IV*
(Washington, D.C.: American Psychiatric Association, 1994).

227 biggest decline in nearly seventy years: Arialdi M. Miniño, Melonie
Heron, and Betty L. Smith, "Deaths: Preliminary Data for 2004," *National Vital Statistics Reports*, National Center for Health Statistics,
Hyattsville, MD, 2006. Viewed online at http://www.cdc.gov/nchs/prod-
ucts/pubs/pubd/hestats/prelimdeaths04/preliminarydeaths04.htm.

227 noninstitutionalized U.S. adults: National Center for Health Statistics, *Health United States 2005 with Chartbook on Trends in the Health
of Americans*, Hyattsville, MD, 2005, p. 52.

228 depression is the most common diagnosed cause: John E. Morely, "Anorexia, Sarcopenia and Aging," *Nutrition* 17: 660–663, 2001.

229 in a medical journal: Researchers wrote about two women, 64 and 61
years old, who went on with misdiagnosed eating disorders for 9 and
12 years, respectively. Both women were very worried about becoming
fat. One dealt with her anxiety by dieting and abusing laxatives. The
other nibbled, secreting chewed and unchewed food in her handbag.
Both women suffered from depression. After circling through specialists' offices, accumulating thick medical files and bottles of prescription antidepressants, after aggressive refeeding and close supervision at
home, the two finally landed in an eating disorders clinic, one at five-
foot-five and 74 pounds, the other five-foot-nine, 83 pounds. By then it
was too late; despite intensive treatment, both women died of starvation. Peter Hall and Rick Driscoll, "Anorexia in the Elderly: An Annota-
tion," *International Journal of Eating Disorders* 14: 497–499, 1993.

229 it afflicts 10 percent: National Institute of Diabetes, Digestive and
Kidney Diseases, *NIH Publication* #4, Bethesda, MD, August 2004.
Viewed online at http://www.digestive.niddk.nih.gov/ddiseases/pubs/
diverticulosis/.

229 Greatest Generation: William Strauss and Neil Howe, *Generations:*

The History of America's Future, 1584–2069 (William Morrow & Co.: New York, 1991).

231 even 50 years later: Cosford and Arnold, 1992, pp. 491–498.

232 story about her grandmother: Abby Ellin, "The Measure of a Woman," *New York Times Magazine,* June 19, 2005, p. 70.

233 Mrs. K.:   Sian Cocker, "Onset of Bulimia Nervosa in a 64-Year-Old Woman," *International Journal of Eating Disorders* 16: 89–91, 1994.

234 can shorten a person's life: D. H. Sullivan, J. E. Morley, L. E. Johnson et al., "The GAIN (Geriatric Anorexia Nutrition) Registry: The Impact of Appetite and Weight on Mortality in a Long-Term Care Population," *Journal of Nutrition, Health and Aging* 6: 275–281, 2002.

234 sense of taste and smell: Margaret-Mary G. Wilson and John E. Morely, "Invited Review: Aging and Energy Balance," *Journal of Applied Physiology* 95: 1728–1736, 2003.

234 doubles the chances of dying: D. H. Sullivan et al., 2002, pp. 275–281.

235 associated with longer life: Katherine M. Flegal, Barry I. Graubard, David Williamson et al., "Excess Deaths Associated with Underweight, Overweight and Obesity," *Journal of the American Medical Association* 293: 1861–1867, 2005; Kenneth F. Adams, Arthur Schatzkin, and Tamara B. Harris, "Overweight, Obesity, and Mortality in a Large Prospect Cohort of Persons 50 to 71 Years Old," *New England Journal of Medicine* 355: 763–778, 2006.

236 convergence of factors: Gail Sheehy, *New Passages* (New York: Random House, 1995), 345–368, 294–429.

238 extremely low-cal diets: Alice Dembner, "A Recipe for Longer Life," *New York Times,* August 17, 2004.

238 young mice: R. Weindruch, R. L. Walford, S. Fligiel et al., "The Retardation of Aging in Mice by Dietary Restriction: Longevity, Cancer, Immunity and Lifetime Energy Intake," *The Journal of Nutrition* 116: 641–654, 1984.

238 eating as little as 890 calories: Leonie K. Heilbronn, Lilian de Jonge, Madlyn I. Frisard, et al., "Effect of 6-Month Calorie Restriction on Biomarkers of Longevity, Metabolic Adaptation, and Oxidative Stress in Overweight Individuals: A Randomized Controlled Trial," *Journal of the American Medical Association* 295: 1539–1548, 2006.

239 did not protect the older mice: Linda L. Bellush, Aimee M. Wright, Jon P. Walker et al., "Caloric Restriction and Spatial Learning in Old Mice," *Physiology and Behavior* 60: 541–547, 1996.

239 late-life eating disorders: Cosford and Arnold, 1992, pp. 491–498.

240 Martha's story: Rosalie Hill, Christopher Haslett, and Shailesh Kumar, "Anorexia Nervosa in an Elderly Woman," *Australian and New Zealand Journal of Psychiatry* 35: 246–248, 2001.

242 Meals-on-Wheels study: Y. Suda, C. E. Marske J. H. Flaherty et al., "Examining the Effects of Intervention to Nutritional Problems of the Elderly Living in an Inner City Area," *Journal of Nutrition Health and Aging* 5: 118–123, 2001.

242 when he or she eats alone: John DeCastro, "Eating Behavior: Lessons from the Real World of Humans," *Ingestive Behavior and Obesity* 16: 800–813, 2000.

242 served family-style at the table: Ibid.

243 story of Mrs. B: David M. Clarke, Mark L. Wahlqvist, Con R. Rassias et al., "Psychological Factors in the Nutritional Disorders of the Elderly: Part of the Spectrum of Eating Disorders," *International Journal of Eating Disorders* 25: 345–348, 1999.

244 named QD: Anita Duggal and Robert M. Lawrence, "Aspects of Food Refusal in the Elderly: The 'Hunger Strike'" *International Journal of Eating Disorders* 30: 213–216, 2001.

245 In her poem: Gail Mazur, "Why You Travel," in *Zeppo's First Wife: New and Selected Poems* (Chicago: University of Chicago Press, 2005). Viewed online at http://writersalmanac.publicradio.org/programs/2005/10/17/index.html.

248 sense of integrity: Erikson, 1980, pp. 49–107.

249 mental or physical vulnerabilities: L. K. George Hsu, "Outcome of Anorexia Nervosa: A Review of the Literature (1954–1978)," *Archives of General Psychiatry* 37: 1041–1046, 1980; D. M. Schwartz and M. G. Thompson, "Do Anorectics Get Well? Current Research and Future Needs," *American Journal of Psychiatry* 138: 319–323, 1981; R. H. Ratnasuriya, I. Eisler, G. I. Szmukler, and G. F. Russell, "Anorexia Nervosa: Outcome and Prognostic Factors After 20 Years," *British Journal of Psychiatry* 158: 495–502, 1991.

249 life review: (http://www.ilcusa.org/, http://www.hospicefoundation.org/teleconference/2002/butler.asp); Myrna I. Lewis and Robert Butler, "Life-Review Therapy: Putting Memories to Work in Individual and Group Psychotherapy," *Geriatrics* November: 165–173, 1974; Robert N. Butler, "The Life Review: An Interpretation of Reminiscence in the Aged," *Psychiatry* 26: 65–76, 1963.

250 poem by Louis McKee: Louis McKee, "Second Chance," in *Near Occasions of Sin* (Philadelphia, PA: Cynic Press, 2006). Viewed online at http://writersalmanac.publicradio.org.

251 MEALSONWHEELS: John E Morley and Andrew Jay Silver, "Nutritional Issues in Nursing Home Care," *Annals of Internal Medicine* 123: 850–859, 1995; with additional information from C. M. Reife, "Involuntary Weight Loss," *Medical Clinics of North America* 79: 299–313, 1995.

251 monoamine oxidase inhibitors: John Morley, interview with the author, May 10, 2006.

252 antidepressants did better :   C. F. Reynolds III, M. A. Dew, B. G. Pollock et al., "Maintenance Treatment of Major Depression in Old Age," *New England Journal of Medicine* 354: 1130–1138, 2006.

252 megestrol acetate: Margaret-Mary G. Wilson et al., 2005, pp. 1071–1081.

254 a short test: Ibid.

256 the pumping capacity of the heart: "Aging and Exercise: Modifying Your Routine as You Get Older," *Mayo Clinic Women's HealthSource,* March 2005.

257 achieve numinosity: Michael W. Clark, "SRS 6981: C. G. Jung and Numinosity," August 22, 1994. Viewed online at: http://earthpages. tripod.com/JungNuminosity.html.

8 | HEALING

Page

258 "Weathering":   Fleur Adcock, "Weathering," in *Poems, 1960–2000* (Northumberland, U.K.: Bloodaxe Books, 2000).

261 EAT-26:   David M. Garner, M. Olmstead, M. Bohr, and Paul E. Garfinkle, "The Eating Attitudes Test: Psychometric Features and Clinical Correlates," *Psychological Medicine* 12: 871–878, 1982.

262 whether you overexercise: Courtesy of Edward Cumella, Director of Research, Education, and Quality, Remuda Treatment Centers, March 22, 2005.

262 Another self-test: M. M. Hagan, R. H. Whitworth, and D. E. Moss, "Semistarvation-Associated Eating Behaviors Among College Binge Eaters: A Preliminary Description and Assessment Scale," *Behavioral Medicine* 25: 125–133, 1999.

264 Binge eating episodes: American Psychiatric Association, *Diagnostic and Statistic Manual of Mental Disorders: DSM-IV* (Washington, D.C.: American Psychiatric Association, 1994).

264 defining a bingeing problem: Fairburn: 1995, pp. 3–20; Christopher G. Fairburn, Zafra Cooper, and Roz Shafran, "Cognitive Behavior

Therapy for Eating Disorders: A Transdiagnostic Theory and Treatment," *Behavior Research and Therapy* 41: 509–528, 2003.

265 do not involve hospitalization: Fairburn, 1995, pp. 113–114.

266 constipation, diarrhea, reflux: National Eating Disorders Association, "Eating Disorders Info," viewed online at http://www.nationaleatingdisorders.org; Claire Pomeroy, "Assessment of Medical Status and Physical Factors," in *Handbook of Eating Disorders and Obesity* (Hoboken, NJ: John Wiley & Sons, 2004), 81–111.

267 typical day: *Eating Disorders Resource Catalogue* (Carlsbad, CA: Gürze Books, 2006). Viewed online at www.gurze.com.

268 Cambridge Eating Disorders Center: Viewed online at http://www. cedc-inc.com/.

270 ask a potential therapist: Maine and Kelly, 2005, pp. 200–201.

270 contact NEDA, AED: National Eating Disorders Association web page, viewed online at http://www.nationaleatingdisorders.org; Academy of Eating Disorders web page, viewed online at www.aedweb.org.

271 for more information: Thompson, ed., 2004; Carolyn Costin, *The Eating Disorder Sourcebook* (Los Angeles: Lowell House, 1999).

271 CBT is based on: Aaron T. Beck, *Cognitive Therapy and Emotional Disorders* (New York: International Universities Press, 1976).

272 CBT's limitations: Kathleen M. Pike, Michael J. Devlin, and Katharine L. Loeb, "Cognitive-Behavioral Therapy in the Treatment of Anorexia Nervosa, Bulimia Nervosa, and Binge Eating Disorder," in Thompson, ed., 2004, p. 139.

272 may not respond: Jeremy Holmes, Roger Neighbor, Nicholas Tarrier et al., "All You Need Is Cognitive Behavioral Therapy? (Education and Debate)," *British Medical Journal* 324: (2002): 288–294, 2002.

272 anorexia is extraordinarily resistant: Virginia V. W. McIntosh, Jennifer Jordan, Francis A. Carter et al., "Three Psychotherapies for Anorexia Nervosa: A Randomized, Controlled Trial," *American Journal of Psychiatry* 162 (2005): 741–747, 2005.

273 combine CBT: Agency for Healthcare Research and Quality, "Management of Eating Disorders," *Evidence Report/Technology Assessment* 135, Rockville, MD, April 2006.

273 your personal history: Carol B. Peterson, Stephen A. Wonderlich, James E. Mitchell et al., "Integrative Cognitive Therapy for Bulimia Nervosa," 2004, pp. 245–262.

273 IPT all but avoids: Alix Spiegel, "More and More, Favored Psychotherapy Lets Bygones Be Bygones," *News York Times*, February 14, 2006.

274 significant life-changing stress: U. Schmidt, J. Tiller, M. Blanchard

et al., "Is There a Specific Trauma Precipitating Anorexia Nervosa," *Psychological Medicine* 27: 523–530, 1997.

275 IPT has been most successful: Stacey Tantleff-Dunn, Jessica Gokee-LaRose, and Rachel D. Peterson, "Interpersonal Therapy for the Treatment of Anorexia Nervosa, Bulimia Nervosa and Binge Eating Disorder," in Thompson, ed., 2004, pp. 163–185.

275 engaged in a great debate: James Hudson, McLean Hospital, Belmont, MA, interview with the author, September 10, 13, and 27, 2004.

276 the Food and Drug Administration: Martina de Zwaan, James L. Roerig, and James E. Mitchell, "Pharmacological Treatment of Anorexia Nervosa, Bulimia Nervosa and Binge Eating Disorder," 2004, pp. 186–217.

276 50 to 60 percent reduction: Fairburn, 1995, p. 115; de Zwaan et al., 2004, pp. 195–198.

276 symptom-free: Fairburn, 1995, p. 116.

276 antidepressants are often short-term: Ibid., pp. 114–116.

276 a class of antidepressants called tricyclics: de Zwaan et al., 2004, p. 198; Prozac, in general, promotes weight loss: Ibid., pp. 186–217.

277 experience almost no benefit: B. Timothy Walsh, Allan S. Kaplan, Attia, Evelyn et al., "Fluoxetime After Weight Restoration in Anorexia Nervosa," *Journal of the American Medical Association* 295: 2605–2612, 2006.

277 drugs such as topiramate: Susan L. McElroy, Lesley M. Arnold, Nathan A. Shapira et al., "Topiramate in the Treatment of Binge Eating Disorder Associated with Obesity: A Randomized, Placebo-Controlled Trial," *American Journal of Psychiatry* 160: 255–261, 2003; T. A. Wadden, R. I. Berkowitz, L. G. Womble, et al., "Randomized Trial of Lifestyle Modification and Pharmacotherapy for Obesity," *New England Journal of Medicine* 353: 2111–2120, 2005.

277 rimonabant: In a study of 1,036 nondiabetic obese patients, an experimental drug called rimonabant prompted an average weight loss of 15 pounds in a year and a reduction in risk factors for diabetes and heart disease. But none of the patients in this study had diabetes, even though they were obese. F. Xavier Pi-Sunyer, Louis J. Aronne, Hassan M. Heshmati et al., "Effect of Rimonabant, a Cannainoid-1 Receptor Blocker, on Weight and Cardiometabolic Risk Factors in Overweight or Obese Patients," *Journal of the American Medical Association* 295: 761–775, 2006.

277 leptin: C. K. Welt, J. L. Chan, J. Bullen et al., "Recombinant Human Leptin in Women with Hypothalamic Amenorrhea," *New England Journal of Medicine* 351: 987–997, 2004.

278 maintain weight loss: Michael Rosenbaum, Rochelle Goldsmith, Daniel Bloomfield et al., "Low-Dose Leptin Reverses Skeletal Muscle, Autonomic, and Neuroendocrine Adaptations to Maintenance of Reduced Weight," *Journal of Clinical Investigation* 115: 3579–3586, 2005.

278 partners, children, or coworkers: Costin, 1999, pp. 169–190.

278 might be more formal: Fairburn, 1995, p. 122

278 University of Toronto: Jan Lackstrom, D. Blake Woodside, and Gina Dimitropoulos, "Couples Therapy in the Area of Eating Disorders, Research and Practice," presented at the American Academy of Eating Disorders 2004 Conference, Orlando, Florida, April 29, 2004.

279 Other groups are mixed: Costin, 1999, pp. 155–167.

280 Family dynamics: Deborah M. Michel and Susan G. Willard, "Family Treatment of Eating Disorders," *Primary Psychiatry* 10: 59–61, 2003.

281 not meant to be a substitute: Jim Schettler, family therapist at Remuda Ranch, interview with the author, June 27, 2005.

282 The treatment philosophy: Maine and Kelly, 2005, pp. 204–206.

282 binge eating does have addictive qualities: Fairburn, 1995, pp. 108–111.

284 were eating disorder–free: W. Stewart Agras, Elise M. Rossiter, Bruce Arnow et al., "One-Year Follow-up of Psychosocial and Pharmacologic Treatments for Bulimia Nervosa," *Journal of Clinical Psychiatry* 55: 179–183, 1994; W. Stewart Agras, Christy F. Telch, Bruce Arnow, et al., "One-Year Follow-up of Cognitive Behavioral Therapy for Obese Individuals with Binge Eating Disorder," *Journal of Consulting and Clinical Psychiatry* 65: 343–347, 1997.

284 women seek health information: S. Fox and L. Rainie, "Vital Decisions: How Internet Users Decide What Information to Trust When They or Their Loved Ones Are Sick," Pew Internet and American Life Project, Washington, D.C., May 22, 2002, pp. 4 and 6. Viewed online at www.pewinternet.org/PDF/r/190/report_display.asp.

285 no Internet-directed treatment: Andrew J. Winzelberg, Kristine H. Luce et al., "Internet-Based Treatment Strategies," in Thompson, ed., 2004, pp. 279–296.

285 now available online: Viewed online at http://www.ace-network.com/eatdis/EATtest.htm.

285 information for further diagnosis: Viewed online at http://edreferral.com/assessment.htm.

286 learn about healthier nutrition: Viewed online at http://www.poppink.com.

286 three hundred bulletin board messages: Andrew J. Winzelberg, "The Analysis of an Electronic Support Group for Individuals with Eating Disorders," *Computers in Human Behavior* 13: 393–407, 1997.

286 more than four hundred websites: Mim Udovitch, "The Way We Live Now: 9-8-02: Phenomenon; A Secret Society of the Starving," *New York Times*, September 8, 2002.

286 Amy and Tony Medina: Viewed online at www.something-fishy.org.

286 Another kind of eating disorders website: Viewed online at http://www.poppink.com.

287 Internet applications now being tried: Martin Grunwald and Juliane C. Busse, "Online Consulting Service for Eating Disorders—Analysis and Perspectives," *Computers in Human Behavior* 19: 469–477, 2003.

287 Internet-based interventions: Winzelberg, et al., 2004, 279–296.

288 Mindfulness: C. N. Alexander, E. J. Langer, R. I. Newman et al., "Transcendental Meditation, Mindfulness, and Longevity, an Experimental Study with the Elderly," *Journal Personality and Social Psychology* 57: 950–964, 1998.

288 meditation as a treatment: J. Kristeller and R. Quillian-Wolever, "The Use of Mindfulness Meditation Techniques in Treatment of Binge Eating Disorder," presented at the Academy of Eating Disorders 2004 Conference, Orlando, Florida, April 29, 2004.

288 six-week clinical trial: M. J. Esplen, P. E. Garfinkle, M. Olmsted et al., "A Randomized Controlled Trial of Guided Imagery in Bulimia Nervosa," *Psychological Medicine* 28: 1347–1357, 1998.

288 It helped ease: Thawatchai Krisanaprakornkit, interview with the author, February 8, 2006. Questions can be addressed to drthawatchai@yahoo.com.

289 We urge meditation: Dr. James Gordon quoted in "Meditation," viewed online at http://www.newswise.com/articles/views/517584/.

289 Pilates is a form of exercise: Viewed online at http://www.allaboutpilates.com/welcome.htm.

290 iyengar and ashtanga: Viewed online at http://www.bksiyengar.com and http://www.ashtanga.com.

291 biofeedback is being applied: N. Pop-Jordanova, "Psychological Characteristics and Biofeedback Mitigation in Preadolescents with Eating Disorders," *Pediatrics International* 42: 76–81, 2000; University of Maryland Medical Center's Center for Integrative Medicine, viewed online at http://www.umm.edu/altmed/ConsModalities/Biofeedbackcm.html.

291 You would begin this therapy: See www.eegspectrum.com; the International Society of Neuronal Regulation, viewed online at http://www.isnr.org/; Jim Robbins, *A Symphony in the Brain: The Evolution of the New Brain Wave Biofeedback* (New York: Grove-Atlantic, 2000).

292 medicalization of eating disorders: Melanie A. Katzman and Sing Lee, "Beyond Body Image: The Integration of Feminist and Transcultural

Theories in the Understanding of Self-Starvation," *International Journal of Eating Disorders* 22: 385–394, 1997.

293 Rob Brezsny in his book: Rob Brezsny, *Pronoia Is the Antidote for Paranoia* (Berkeley, CA: Frog, Ltd., distributed by North Atlantic Books, 2005).

297 Sarah Mason: Payson Road viewed online at http://www.paysonroad.com/.

297 Mary Pat: Mary Pat Nally, *Reflecting Grace* (Frederick, MD: PublishAmerica, 2005).

298 Grace Overbake: Sali McSherry, "Play Shows Being Fat Is Something to Laugh At," *The Chagrin Valley Times,* August 17, 2006, viewed online at www.chagrinvalleytimes.com.

298 F.R.E.E.D Foundation: Viewed online at http://www.freedfoundation.org/, Gail Schoenbach, executive director, F.R.E.E.D. Foundation, 18 Chestnut Hill, Warren, NJ 07059.

300 being understood: Katzman and Lee, 1997.

302 mental health parity: Lynn Grefe, CEO of the National Eating Disorders Association, interview with the author, February 15, 2006.

303 Family and Friends Action Council: Viewed online at http://www.eatingdisorderscoalition.org/.

303 appropriated only $21 million: Lynn Grefe, CEO of the National Eating Disorders Association, interview with the author, February 15, 2006.

304 Eating Disorders Coalition: Viewed online at http://www.eatingdisorderscoalition.org/.

304 Lifelines Foundation: Viewed online at http://www.lfed.org/.

304 one woman told her story: Emily Dendinger, "Eating Disorders on Our Campuses: A Student Speaks," *Connections* 10, Issue 2, National Association for Women in Catholic Higher Education, Chestnut Hill, MA, Spring 2002, viewed online at http://www.bc.edu/bc_org/avp/cas/soc/nawche/newsletter/10-2Spring02.pdf.

305 Full of Ourselves: Viewed online at http://www.mclean.harvard.edu/education/youth.

Adult Women with Eating Disorders

Bulik, Cynthia M., and Nadine Taylor. *Runaway Eating: The 8-Point Plan to Conquer Adult Food and Weight Obsessions.* Emmaus, PA: Rodale, 2005.

Fairburn, Christopher. *Overcoming Binge Eating.* New York: Guilford Press, 1995.

Maine, Margo, and Joe Kelly. *The Body Myth: Adult Women and the Pressure to Be Perfect.* Hoboken, NJ: John Wiley & Sons, Inc., 2005.

Relationships and Eating Disorders

Van den Broucke, Stephan, Walter Vandereycken, and Jan Norre. *Eating Disorders and Marital Relationships.* London and New York: Routledge, 1997.

Books on Parenting, Food, and Body Issues

Cederquist, Caroline J. *Helping Your Overweight Child: A Family Guide.* Naples, FL: Advance Medical Press, 2002.

Neumark-Sztainer, Diane. *"I'm, Like, SO Fat!" Helping Your Teen Make Healthy Choices About Eating and Exercising in a Weight-Obsessed World.* New York: Guilford Press, 2005.

Steiner-Adair, Catherine. *Full of Ourselves: A Wellness Program to Advance Girl Power, Health, and Leadership.* New York: Teachers College Press, 2006.

Waterhouse, Debra. *Like Mother, Like Daughter: How Women Are Influenced by Their Mother's Relationship with Food—and How to Break the Pattern*. New York: Hyperion, 1997.

Feminism and Eating Disorders

Chernin, Kim. *The Hungry Self: Women, Eating, and Identity*. New York: Times Books, 1985.

Fallon, Patricia, Melanie A. Katzman, and Susan C. Wooley, eds. *Feminist Perspectives on Eating Disorders*. New York: Guilford Press, 1994.

Pipher, Mary. *Reviving Ophelia: Saving the Selves of Adolescent Girls*. New York: Ballantine Books, 1994.

Memoirs by Adults

Becker, Daniel. *This Mean Disease: Growing Up in the Shadow of My Mother's Anorexia Nervosa*. Carlsbad, CA: Gürze Books, 2005.

Knapp, Caroline. *Appetites: Why Women Want*. New York: Counterpoint, 2003.

Lauren, Jenny. *Homesick: A Memoir of Family, Food and Finding Hope*. New York: Atria Books, 2004.

General Reference

Costin, Carolyn. *The Eating Disorder Sourcebook*. Lincolnwood, IL: Lowell House, 1996.

Erikson, Erik. *Identity and the Life Cycle*. New York: W. W. Norton and Company, 1980.

Thompson, J. Kevin, ed. *Handbook of Eating Disorders and Obesity*. Hoboken, NJ: John Wiley & Sons, Inc., 2005.